Nutrition and Critical Care

This book is dedicated to *Bernard Beaufrère, Chris Pennington, Peter Reeds* and *Arvid Wretlind* who contributed greatly to this field and passed away during 2002.

Nestlé Nutrition Workshop Series
Clinical & Performance Program, Vol. 8

Nutrition and Critical Care

Editors

Luc Cynober, Paris, France

Frederick A. Moore, Houston, Tex., USA

20 figures and 28 tables, 2003

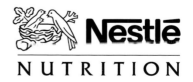

KARGER

Nestec Ltd., 55 Avenue Nestlé, CH–1800 Vevey (Switzerland)
S. Karger AG, P.O. Box, CH–4009 Basel (Switzerland)   www.karger.com

Printed in Switzerland on acid-free paper by Reinhardt Druck, Basel
ISBN 3–8055–7540–8
ISSN 1422–7584

Library of Congress Cataloging-in-Publication Data

Nutrition and critical care / [edited by] Luc Cynober, Frederick A. Moore.
    p. ; cm. – (Nestlé Nutrition workshop series. Clinical & performance program ; v. 8)
    Includes bibliographical references and index.
    ISBN 3–8055–7540–8 (hard cover)
    1. Critically ill–Nutrition–Congresses. I. Cynober, Luc A. II. Moore, Frederick A.,
    1953– III. Nestlé Nutrition workshop series. Clinical & performance programme ; v. 8.
    [DNLM. 1. Critical Illness–Congresses. 2. Nutrition–Congresses. 3. Critical
    Care–Congresses. WB 400 N97425 2003]
    RC86.2.N88 2003
    615.8'54–dc21   2003044604

Contents

Contents

Preface

Over the past 30 years, nutritional support has evolved tremendously. While the beneficial effects of nutritional support have been demonstrated in specific types of patients (e.g. burns, trauma, postoperative cancer resection), it has been difficult to document improved outcomes in less homogenous populations. Intensive care unit (ICU) patients, due to their intense injury stress response, have the potential to benefit most from nutritional support. On the other hand, ICU patients, because of the complexity of their underlying diseases, are especially vulnerable to develop nutritional support-related complications. Despite considerable progress in understanding the optimal route of administration as well as the qualitative and quantitative needs of ICU patients, a lot of controversies and uncertainties exist. In fact, the exact pathophysiologic mechanisms that drive the injury stress response in ICU patients is still a subject of intense research. Over the last decade, a variety of pro- and anti-inflammatory mediators (reactive oxygen metabolites, cytokines, prostaglandins, and nitric oxide) have been identified that modulate hormonal control of nutrient flux. Most recent genomic research has identified a gene polymorphism that results in patients producing different levels of mediators following the same insult. In some, this causes dysregulation of the injury stress response which contributes to adverse outcomes.

This issue is not theoretical, but has important therapeutic implications. A variety of nutritional interventions (e.g. 'immune enhancing diets', β-blockers, antioxidants, and growth hormone) that modulate the immuno-neuro-endocrionologic response to stress are being tested (by necessity in homogenous study populations) and are showing promising results. However, if they are truly modulating the injury stress response, it is quite conceivable that these therapies will be harmful in different subsets of critically ill ICU patients. Obviously, continued epidemiologic study of high risk patients is needed and new risk factors need to better characterized (e.g. the epidemic of obesity).

Since qualitative and quantitative requirements in critically ill ICU patients are different from normal ones, and since nutrition is emerging as an effective intervention in ICU patients, we have to look at nutrients as drugs. This means, for instance, the choice of lipids or specific amino acids (certain being immunostimulating while others might depress immunity), the avoidance of iatrogenic hyperglycemia or the intake of micronutrients must be carefully examined. Also, dose-ranging studies should be considered. Finally, knowledge of the pharmacokinetics of nutrient provided by the enteral or parenteral routes is essential.

The current era of molecular biology offers the potential to truly understand the driving mechanisms of the stress injury response. However, to maximally benefit our patients, translational research cannot be underemphasized. Also, we need to be pragmatic: excellent products disappear from the market if they are not tolerated by our patients. Moreover, we need to take advantage of the expertise of other practitioners who have interests similar to ours. National and international experts have written guidelines and consensus reports in recent years. These documents have been studied in depth resulting in a synthesis presented in the last chapter of this book. In sum, we feel that the chapters of this book and the attached discussions well reflect the outstanding meeting that we had near Paris in September 2002. This book should be of great interest and helpful to everyone working in the field. Good readings!

Luc A. Cynober, Frederick A. Moore

Foreword

Severe metabolic alterations frequently occur in critically ill patients. If nutrition plays an important role in critical care, what are the needs for critically ill patients? Are the requirements organ- and/or age-specific? What is the best route of administration in artificial nutrition? If enteral, what exactly does the gut tolerate? In order to answer these questions and to further understand the pathogenesis of and the therapeutic implications for certain diseases, such as pancreatitis, multiple organ failure and sepsis, the topic 'Nutrition and Critical Care' was chosen for this Workshop, which took place near Paris in September 2002.

I sincerely thank the two chairmen, Prof. Luc Cynober and Prof. Frederick Moore, both outstanding experts in this field, for establishing the program and inviting as speakers the opinion leaders in the experimental and clinical field of nutrition in critically ill patients suffering from various diseases. Scientists from 20 countries contributed to the discussions that are also published in this book.

Furthermore, I would like to express my gratitude to Mrs. Isabelle Babin, Dr. Franck Arnaud-Battandier and their team from Nestlé France who provided the logistical support and their legendary French hospitality. Dr. Philippe Steenhout from the Nutrition Strategic Business Division in Vevey, Switzerland, was responsible for the scientific coordination. His cooperation with the chairpersons was essential for the success of this Workshop.

Prof. Wolf Endres, MD

Vice-President
Nestec Ltd, Vevey, Switzerland

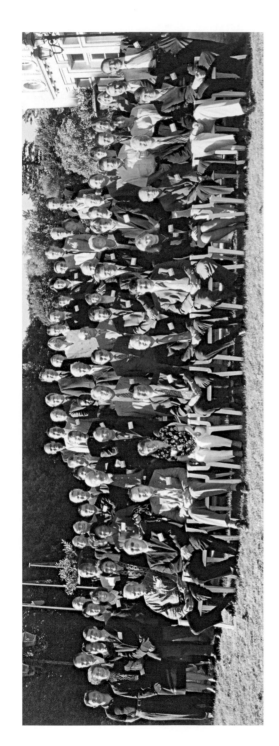

8th Nestlé Nutrition Workshop
Clinical & Performance Program
Paris, France, September 15–19, 2002

Contributors

Chairpersons and Speakers

Prof. Simon P. Allison

Clinical Nutrition Unit
University Hospital
Nottingham NG7 2UH, UK
Tel. +44 115 919 4427
Fax +44 115 919 4427
E-mail: simon.allison@mail.
qmcuh-tr.trent.nhs.uk

Dr. Vickie E. Baracos

Department of Agriculture, Food
and Nutritional Science
University of Alberta
Edmonton, T6G 2P5
Canada
Tel. +1 780 492 7664
Fax +1 780 492 9130
E-mail: vickie.baracos@ualberta.ca

Dr. Mette M. Berger

Surgical Intensive Care Unit
University Hospital (CHUV)
CH–1011 Lausanne
Switzerland
Tel. +41 21 314 2095
Fax +41 21 314 2904
E-mail:
Mette.Berger@chuv.hospvd.ch

Dr. Federico Bozzetti

Instituto Nazionale per lo Studio e
la Cura dei Tumori
Divisione di Chirurgia
dell'Apparato Digerente
Via Venezian 1
I–20133 Milano, Italy
Tel. +39 02 23 903 014
Fax +39 02 23 903 011
E-mail: dottfb@tin.it

Dr. Philip C. Calder

Institute of Human Nutrition
University of Southampton
Bassett Crescent East
Southampton SO16 7PX, UK
Tel. +44 23 8059 4223
Fax +44 23 8059 5489
E-mail: pcc@soton.ac.uk

Prof. René L. Chioléro

Surgical Intensive Care Unit
University Hospital (CHUV)
CH–1011 Lausanne, Switzerland
Tel. +41 21 314 2002
Fax +41 21 314 3045
E-mail:
rene.chiolero@chuv.hospvd.ch

Contributors

Prof. Luc Cynober

Service de Biochimie A
Hôtel Dieu
1, place du Parvis Notre-Dame
F–75181 Paris Cedex 04, France
Tel. +33 1 42 34 82 60
Fax: +33 1 42 34 86 12
E-mail:
luc.cynober@htd.ap-hop-paris.fr

Dr. David N. Herndon

University of Texas Medical
Branch
Shriners Hospital for Children
Department of Surgery
815 Market Street
Galveston, TX 77550, USA
Tel. +1 409 770 6731
Fax: +1 409 770 6919
E-mail: dherndon@utmb.edu

Dr. Kenneth A. Kudsk

University of Wisconsin Hospital
and Clinics
Department of Surgery
H4/736 Clinical Science Center
600 Highland Ave.
Madison, WI 53792-7375, USA
Tel. +1 608 263 1378
Fax +1 608 263 7652
E-mail: kudsk@surgery.wisc.edu

Dr. Robert Martindale

Section of Gastrointestinal Surgery
Department of Surgery
Medical College of Georgia
1120 15th Street
Augusta, GA 30912, USA
Tel. +1 706 721 4686
Fax +1 706 721 6828
E-mail: rmartind@mail.mcg.edu

Prof. Stephen A. McClave

Division of Gastroenterology/
Hepatology
University of Louisville School of
Medicine
550 South Jackson Street
Louisville, KY 40202, USA
Tel. +1 502 852 6991
Fax +1 502 852 0846
E-mail: samcclave@louisville.edu

Prof. Lyle L. Moldawer

Department of Surgery
Room 6116, Shands Hospital
University of Florida College of
Medicine
PO Box 100286
1600 SW Archer Road
Gainesville, FL 32610-0286, USA
Tel. +1 352 265 0494
Fax +1 352 265 0676
E-mail: moldawer@surgery.ufl.edu

Prof. Frederick A. Moore

Department of Surgery
University of Texas
Houston Medical School
6431 Fannin, Suite 4.264
Houston, TX 77030, USA
Tel. +1 713 500 7228
Fax +1 713 500 7232
E-mail:
frederick.a.moore@uth.tmc.edu

Dr. Josef Neu

Department of Pediatrics
University of Florida
Box J-296
1600 S.W. Archer Road
Gainesville, FL 32610, USA
Tel. +1 352 392 3020
Fax +1 352 846 3937
E-mail: neuj@peds.ufl.edu

Dr. Gérard Nitenberg

Institut Gustave Roussy
39, rue Camille Desmoulins
F–94805 Villejuif
France
Tel. +33 1 42 11 45 06
Fax +33 1 42 11 52 12
E-mail: nitenber@igr.fr

Prof. Peter Stehle   Absent

Department of Nutrition Science
University of Bonn
Endenicher Allee 11-13
D–53115 Bonn
Germany
Tel. +49 228 733 680
Fax +49 228 733 217
E-mail: ehw@uni-bonn.de

Moderators

Prof. Paul Bouletreau

Hôpital Edouard-Herriot
Departement Anesthésie-
Réanimation
Pavillon P, Place d'Arsonval
F–69437 Lyon Cedex 03, France
Tel. +33 4 72 11 63 10
Fax +33 4 72 68 46 08
E-mail: paul.bouletreau@chu-lyon.fr

Dr. Jean-Pascal De Bandt

Faculté de Pharmacie
Laboratoire de Biologie de la
Nutrition
4, avenue de l'Observatoire
F–75270 Paris Cedex 06, France
Tel. +33 1 53 73 99 45
Fax +33 1 53 73 99 48
E-mail:
debandt@pharmacie.univ-paris5.fr

Prof. Pierre Déchelotte

Hôpital Charles-Nicolle
Service Polyclinique
1, rue de Germont
F–76031 Rouen Cedex, France
Tel. +33 2 32 88 64 65
Fax +33 2 32 88 83 57
E-mail: pierre.dechelotte@
chu-rouen.fr

Dr. Raymond Peeters

Campus Stuyvenberg
Lange Beeldekenstraat 267
B–2050 Antwerpen, Belgium
Tel. +32 3 217 71 11
Fax +32 3 217 73 60
E-mail:
md.peeters@hetgreetroussaerhuis.be

Dr. Jean Fabien Zazzo

Hôpital Antoine Béclère
Departement Anesthesie-
Réanimation
157, rue Porte de Trivaux
F–92141 Clamart Cedex, France
Tel. +33 1 45 37 49 53
Fax +33 1 45 37 43 42
E-mail: jfzazzo.beclere@invo.edu

Participants

Prof. Kamal Hajiyev / Azerbaijan
Dr. Wim Fassin / Belgium
Dr. Paulo Cesar Ribeiro / Brazil
Dr. Ricardo Rosenfeld / Brazil
Dr. Daren Heyland / Canada
Dr. Khalid Hel Hilal / Dubai
Dr. Alain Bouvet / France
Dr. Cécile Chambrier / France
Dr. Elisabeth Cuchet / France
Dr. Dominique Hanon / France
Dr. Françoise Hanon / France
Dr. Dominique Jusserand / France
Dr. Florence Molenat / France
Dr. Laurent Petit / France
Dr. Jean-Marie Quintard / France
Dr. Pascal Raclot / France
Prof. Christian Löser / Germany
Dr. Ralf-Joachim Schulz / Germany
Prof. Iqbal Moestafa / Indonesia
Dr. Aris Wibudi / Indonesia
Dr. Maria Antonia Fusco / Italy
Dr. Paolo Orlandoni / Italy
Prof. Toshiaki Shimizu / Japan
Dr. Alfonso Fajardo Rodriguez / Mexico
Dr. Fernando Molinar Ramos / Mexico
Dr. Daniel Rodriguez Gonzalez / Mexico
Dr. Robert Tepaske / The Netherlands
Dr. Elizabeth Kanayo Ngwu / Nigeria
Dr. Samuel Yuwa / Nigeria
Prof. Olga Maiorova / Russia
Prof. Demetre Labadarios / South Africa
Prof. Abelardo Garcia de Lorenzo de Mateos / Spain
Dr. Merce Planas Vila / Spain
Dr. Burapat Sangthong / Thailand
Dr. Gordon Carlson / UK
Mrs. Lynne Douglas / UK
Dr. Craig McClain / USA
Dr. Maja Djordevic / Yugoslavia

Nestlé attendees

Dr. Franck Arnaud-Battandier / France
Mr. Laurent Freixe / France
Mr. Hervé Le Henand / France
Mr. Andreas Schläpfer / France
Mrs. Kirsten Christiani / Germany
Mr. Giorgio Giroli / Italy
Mr. Yasuhide Araki / Japan
Mrs. Patricia Anthony / Switzerland
Mr. Denis Breuille / Switzerland
Mr. Claude Cavadini / Switzerland
Prof. Wolf Endres / Switzerland
Dr. Philippe Steenhout / Switzerland
Ms. Theresa Voss / Switzerland
Mrs. Vipapan Panitantum / Thailand
Mrs. Sue Jones / UK
Mrs. Carol Siegel / USA

Cynober L, Moore FA (eds): Nutrition and Critical Care.
Nestlé Nutrition Workshop Series Clinical & Performance Program, Vol. 8, pp. 1–10,
Nestec Ltd.; Vevey/S. Karger AG, Basel, © 2003.

Overview on Metabolic Adaptation to Stress

Vickie E. Baracos

Department of Agriculture, Food and Nutritional Science, University of Alberta,
Edmonton, Alta., Canada

What Do Nutritionists Mean When They Use the Word 'Stress'?

The patients that we wish to feed properly are stressed in different ways
and very often in more than one way. The word 'stress' appears in the
nutrition and clinical nutrition literature attached to a wide variety of
meanings. This usage is a simple reflection of the complexity and diversity of
stressors and stress responses, which are often considered by individual
investigators in a specific, somewhat narrow context. The primary 'stress'
may be a surgical procedure [1–3], an inflammation [4] or injury such as a
burn. The 'stress' is understood to have degrees: surgery is more or less
invasive, and inflammation, infection and burn are more or less extensive.
'Stress' most often connotes a physiological response (neuro – endocrine –
metabolic – immune) to an insult or injury. There are no universally used
indicators or benchmarks of stress (table 1). The 'stress response' evaluated
may be considered to be the activation of the hypothalamic-pituitary-adrenal
(HPA) and sympathetic nervous system (SNS) associated with elevated
secretion of adrenal hormones, particularly epinephrine and glucocorticoids.
The 'stress response' may be considered to consist of inflammation and
activation of the immune system with emphasis on the postoperative or
postinjury 'cytokine storm' [5]. Oxidative 'stress', including reactive oxygen
species and antioxidants, is another manifestation of inflammation and injury
of various types [6]. 'Nutritional stress' refers to a suboptimal preoperative or
predisease nutrient supply, as well as to a depleted state that may evolve
secondarily to another stress type. Stress of all of these types includes
the concomitant psychological response. Nicolaïdis [7] emphasizes the

1

Table 1. Commonly used markers of stress responses

Stress characteristics	Benchmarks
Sympathoadrenal	Epinephrine, norepinephrine
Hypothalamo-pituitary-adrenal	ACTH, cortisol
Inflammatory	Cytokines, cytokine receptor antagonists, soluble cytokine receptors, acute phase proteins, C-reactive protein, immune cell functions, immune cell activation markers, functional tests of immunity
Infectious	Bacterial, viral and fungal organisms, endotoxin, sepsis
Oxidative	Reactive oxygen species, NO, enzymes i.e. superoxide dismutase, antioxidant nutrients
Nutritional	Nutritional markers: anthropometric, biochemical, metabolic, short-lived plasma proteins

importance of the manner in which a stress is perceived by the individual, in the pattern of neuroendocrine activation. 'Stress' includes pain [7, 8].

The broad definition of stress that includes all of these stressors and stress-response elements, is *disruption of homeostasis*. Stress is not a single entity. Stressors can be psychosocial/behavioral, environmental, nutritional, or arise from infectious or neoplastic processes or injury, and are set in a backdrop of genetic makeup and age which may range from varying degrees of prematurity to senescence.

An understanding of the nature of stress is fundamental to the rational design of nutrient mixtures to feed patients whose homeostasis has been altered by one or more stressors. All stresses may be presumed to be associated with characteristic modifications in the metabolism of lipids, carbohydrates, amino acids and micronutrients. A number of alterations may take place. Taking the example of the metabolism of protein and amino acids, multiple modifications of amino acid utilization can occur such that the total and relative amounts of essential amino acids required may change. In some cases, amino acids normally considered nonessential for humans become conditionally essential in the diet. Hepatic or renal insufficiency may limit the tolerance to the total amino acid supply or to imbalanced amino acid mixtures. Similarly, metabolic energy expenditure may increase, but utilization of energy fuels may be substantially limited by factors such as insulin resistance or limited lipoprotein lipase activity. Oxidative stress may place a substantial draw on antioxidant nutrients. A grouping of such changes is associated with stresses, yet we lack a comprehensive formula for the

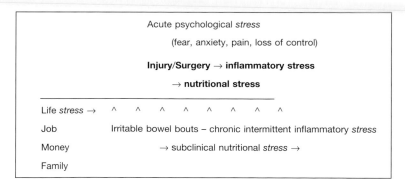

Fig. 1. A constellation of stresses. Primary stress, as viewed by the attending clinical nutritionist, may be surrounded and complicated by a series of concomitant and previously existing stresses of varying degrees. The outcome of a certain dietary intervention contemplated for the primary stress is inevitably colored by these associated stresses.

identification, clinical management and feeding of patients based on their previously existing state of chronic stress, throughout the course of a new stress of an acute or chronic nature.

Many published clinical trials of nutritional support provide evidence for a large degree of heterogeneity in any typical study group of patients. The patients are admitted based on a certain set of inclusion and exclusion criteria, however a constellation of stresses (fig. 1) and related metabolic differences may be hidden below the surface of a group of 'intensive care unit patients with multiple organ failure' or 'patients with advanced cancer defined as locally recurrent or metastatic'. It is thus perhaps not surprising that such studies sometimes lack statistically significant main treatment effects, at the same time that inspection of the results on an individual basis reveals a marked heterogeneity of apparent response. It is the difference between the responders and nonresponders within these cohorts that we need to identify as the basis for prospective study. On some occasions the reason for a positive response in some patients is evident. As often as not, there is no way to determine the difference between responders and nonresponders in a given trial, as the nature of appropriate observations, analysis or samples to take is unknown. Nutritional and metabolic ramifications of each stress variant are indeed what we need to be able to assess.

The Concept of a Stress Classification

A suitable, pathophysiologically based classification of stress responses may aid nutritionists in their efforts to devise diets tailored to deal with specific stress-related problems. A classification of stresses and responses to stressful stimuli will make it possible to test the overall concept by establishing a correspondence between the suggested hormone/mediator profile and the associated clinical picture. A classification of stress will also enable assessment of the benefit of a nutritional strategy designed to fit the particular category of stress response exhibited by the patient.

Building a clinically meaningful categorization of stress requires a broad conceptual base. There is a logarithmic increase in the order of complexity when one moves from the considerations of a single stress response element, such as a glucocorticoid or tumor necrosis factor-α (TNFα), to the multiple elements of the endocrine response to stress. The highly orchestrated interplay amongst the nervous, endocrine and immune systems must be considered for each stress, and the clinical reality of multiple acute or chronic stresses that may be simultaneously present.

A reductionist's approach brings out a comprehensive understanding of an individual stress mediator signal. On the response side there is the regulation of gene expression, synthesis, secretion and eventual degradation of a mediator, and on the reception side, its receptor isoforms, signal transduction and effects upon the metabolism of key nutrients on an organ and whole body basis. By contrast, it is exceedingly difficult to conceptualize the overall sum of a stress response, which can be likened to an orchestra or chorus in terms of the number and types of factors at play. The responses to stress are highly complex and can vary widely. Ideally we would like to know the metabolic alterations in utilization of macro- and micronutrients for each player. In spite of a perhaps daunting conceptual task, the concept of a stress-related classification or taxonomy is emerging, and it is useful to consider current thinking in this regard.

Taxonomy of the Neuroendocrine Aspects of the Response to Stress

It is proposed by Nicolaïdis [7] that classical endocrine criteria could be employed to characterize stress responses in terms of the associated hormonal secretion ratios and their temporal evolution. While this is considered exclusively in the context of the effects of stresses on the activation, the HPA axis and the SNS, it is an interesting perspective. The work of various authors suggests that ratios of the responses to stressors of the sympathoadrenal system and the HPA axis can be either unity (ratio = 1) or dissociated in varying degrees, with dominance of one or the other system and for more or less prolonged periods. 'Balanced' stress types are characterized by a similar level of activation of the HPA and sympathoadrenal systems. Elective surgery is associated with this type of response, and is generally of brief duration. Chronic psychosocial stress, of the type that is associated with renin-dependent hypertension, is another example, and in this case the response may be long-term. Chronic, parallel activation of the HPA and SNS are seen in certain forms of depression.

A second family of stress responses suggested by Nicolaidis [7] are those where the HPA and SNS responses may be dissociated in varying degrees and directions. For example, the fight or flight response is dominated by sympathoadrenal activation. By contrast, the HPA system is activated preferentially in stressful situations where there is a perception of loss of control, and when chronic this state is associated with abnormalities of glucose metabolism and insulin resistance. Some unique patterns emerge, such as in posttraumatic stress syndrome which is usually characterized by increased sympathoadrenal activity together with suppressed activity within the HPA axis with below normal levels of glucocorticoids.

These specific families of stress responses as conceived by Nicolaidis [7] are not yet accompanied in his analysis by a parallel taxonomy of associated changes in the metabolism of key nutrients. He does, however, point out that dysregulation of the HPA axis is known to be associated with the deposition of visceral fat, atherosclerosis, hypertension and insulin-resistant dyslipidemia. It would seem plausible to be able to eventually assemble a map of the corresponding stress types and metabolic changes.

Grading the Severity of Stress

The degree of stress may be exceedingly difficult to grade. For example, with regard to stress within the HPA and sympathoadrenal systems, Nicolaidis [7] has proposed 5 intensities of activation (5 = very high, 4 = high, 3 = moderate, 2 = basal or normal, and 1 = reduced or below normal) but avoids dealing with specific cutoff values due to the highly variable values cited in the literature. To express the magnitude and dimensions of activation of the HPA and SNS, one might elect to use some or all of the factors that are practical and possible to determine in everyday clinical practice using blood and urine samples, such as ACTH, cortisol, epinephrine and norepinephrine. At the same time this sample is under-representative of the vast array of endocrine, neurochemical, electrophysiological and behavioral indices that can only be revealed by analyses specific to a research setting.

A concept of the degree of stress clearly emerges in the clinical nutrition literature with respect to the severity of injury, infection and inflammation. The degree of stress is often ranked using a clinical severity score specific to the insult in question. Direct comparisons of nutritional manipulations have been conducted in populations or severely versus moderately stressed individuals with the same illness or injury, within the same study. For example, Furukawa et al. [1] compared feeding soybean lipid emulsion in

5

'severely stressed' patients undergoing esophagectomy with 'moderately stressed' patients who underwent gastric or colorectal surgery. These authors have studied responses to nutritional intervention after an operative procedure for thoracic esophageal cancer (thoracotomy, laparotomy, and three-field lymph node dissection), a particularly invasive surgery, by itself and in comparison with less invasive surgery [1–3].

The panel of stress-response elements associated with injury, infection and inflammation to be considered could be very large and could contain, for example, acute phase proteins, proinflammatory cytokines, reactive oxygen species, and nitric oxide (NO; table 1). Whatever might be measured, it is an important complication that the magnitude of stress responses may not present on a linear scale. It seems likely that at least some stress responses are intended to have a high amplification factor. The metabolic purpose of such an arrangement would be to have the capacity to develop a large response quickly, and this is typical of many elements of inflammatory and immune responses. This type of regulation can be seen at the cellular level, as well as in the whole organism. For example, skeletal muscle cells respond to proinflammatory cytokines with an increase in basal glucose uptake and oxidation, as well as a large decrease in the insulin-sensitive component of glucose metabolism [9]. The effect on glucose metabolism is mediated by inducible NO synthase (iNOS) and the production of NO. In cultured L6 myoblasts, neither TNFα, interferon-γ or bacterial endotoxin alone induce iNOS, NO production or alterations in basal or insulin-stimulated glucose metabolism. TNFα and interferon-γ together produce a 5-fold increase in NO production and this effect is further enhanced 6-fold by the addition of endotoxin to the mixture. Similarly, the effects of these factors on glucose metabolism emerge only in the presence of multiple effectors and also had a characteristic magnitude that was not directly proportional to NO production. In the presence of TNFα, interferon-γ and bacterial endotoxin, basal glucose metabolism was increased by 125% and the insulin-dependent component of glucose metabolism decreased by 47% [9].

A synergy of stresses and proinflammatory effectors can be seen in vivo, and the magnitude of the reaction to multiple stresses may be difficult to predict. Exposure to stress of one type often alters the subsequent responsiveness of many systems. For example, the presence of a tumor, infection or psychological stress appears to alter the magnitude of the metabolic response to endotoxin. A low dose of 10 μg endotoxin/kg body weight in rats with previous exposure to stress (tail shock) was associated with increased secretion of corticosterone and ACTH, as well as a doubling of serum proinflammatory cytokine levels in response to endotoxin compared to control rats [10]. Servatius et al. [11] provide evidence that some of the changes induced by an initial stress of this type may be relatively long-lived (i.e. days or weeks) when one would have expected acute responses to even intense stressors to end within hours after the end of the stressor.

In tumor-bearing rats challenged with a higher dose (1,000 µg endotoxin/kg), the plasma TNFα 3 h after injection was 45-fold higher than in non-tumor-bearing rats that received the same dose of endotoxin [12]. This would explain why a dose of endotoxin that would only normally be associated with transient anorexia and fever might be fatal if administered to animals bearing a tumor [13], even though the tumor burden was small and otherwise not life-threatening at that point. Arsenijevic et al. [14] show that in mice with chronic toxoplasmosis, a second nonspecific challenge (with endotoxin) exacerbates the hypophagic and hypermetabolic states, the latter being associated with hyperresponsiveness in the production of TNFα and interleukin-10. These data suggest that the superimposition of multiple stresses generates the most difficult situations, both clinically and for the nutritionist.

How Can Advances in Molecular Biology Provide the Tools and New Opportunities for Characterizing the Stress Response and Potential Therapeutic Targets

These are exciting times, as we are able to begin to appreciate responses to stress and to diet in terms of the vast array of gene expression events that follow a disruption of homeostasis. A few examples of this powerful approach are illustrative of the large potential. Studies on tissue stress responses are beginning to emerge. Of these, a particularly interesting example is that of Chinnaiyan et al. [15] who described a gene expression profile of sepsis, in an animal model employing cecal ligation and puncture. These authors identify an organ-specific pattern for sepsis-related gene expression events. Cole et al. [16] examined the gene expression profile of human skin immediately following injury using cDNA microarrays. Specimens of the epidermis and dermis were obtained at 30 min and 1 h after the initial injury. At 30 min, injury resulted in a consistent increase ($>2\times$) in gene expression of 124 of 4,000 genes (3%). These genes were primarily involved in transcription and signaling. One hour after injury only 46 genes were increased in expression (1.15%), but 264 of 4,000 (6.6%) genes were decreased by greater than 2-fold, indicating a silencing of many structural genes. The identification of several previously known as well as novel genes that are highly expressed after injury suggests a key role for certain proteins in regulating the initial inflammatory response.

Gene expression profiling is also being applied to the physiologic responses to stress, such as muscle protein catabolism. Muscle protein serves as a primary reserve of amino acids that can be mobilized during stresses such as fasting and disease to provide a source of carbon for glucose production as well as amino acids for protein synthesis. An important physiological adaptation is thus an increase in the overall rate of breakdown of muscle proteins.

7

This stress response is common to starvation, diabetes, cancer, sepsis, injury, hyperthyroidism, and uremia, and while adaptive in the short-term, depletion of muscle protein is eventually associated with metabolic dysfunction, morbidity and mortality. Although many investigations into this phenomenon have been confined to an individual catabolic state, it emerges that when this response occurs, it is accompanied by a common set of biochemical changes, especially activation of proteolytic processes. Gomes et al. [17] have taken advantage of gene expression microarray technology to more broadly answer the question of which gene transcription events are common to muscle protein catabolism of all types, and which are exclusive to one or a few individual catabolic states. These authors compared gene expression patterns in rodent skeletal muscle after 2 days of starvation versus fed animals, and in tumor-bearing, diabetic and uremic animals versus healthy, fed controls. The initial report by these authors focuses on one highly expressed gene common to all of the studied catabolic states, which they have characterized as a novel muscle-specific ubiquitin ligase with an F-box motif [17]. Ubiquitin ligases are a key element of the major degradative system participating in muscle atrophy, the ATP-ubiquitin-proteasome-dependent pathway. This study design allows identification of gene expression patterns that are common to all of the stress states. In taking this approach, these authors have discovered what may be a critical component in the enhanced proteolysis that leads to muscle atrophy in diverse stress states.

Effects of feeding and diet are also being examined using gene expression microarray approaches. For example, Takahashi et al. [18] examined gene expression profile of liver using high-density oligonucleotide arrays after feeding a high-fat diet (safflower oil or tuna oil) to mice. Similarly, some data for adipose tissue gene expression profile are available for high-fat diet-induced obesity in laboratory animals [19]. During fasting and many systemic diseases, muscle undergoes rapid loss of protein and functional capacity. To define the transcriptional changes triggering muscle atrophy and energy conservation in fasting, Jagoe et al. [20] used cDNA microarrays to compare mRNAs from muscles of control and food-deprived mice. The observed transcriptional changes indicate a complex adaptive program that should favor protein degradation and suppress glucose oxidation in muscle.

A systematic analysis of all of the transcriptional changes in these different conditions is a rather large enterprise, and the results of this analysis will emerge over time. The quantity of information generated by these approaches in the short-term creates a logistical log jam for interpretation. It is a large task to integrate the volume of data generated on expression of known genes, and another huge undertaking to seek the identity and function of novel genes discovered. However, an eventual synthesis of reactions to stress and diet may identify further critical elements that will eventually come into use as key markers related to altered nutrient requirements. This knowledge will guide a multimodal approach to overall patient management, including nutritional support, which may approach the ideals in a manner currently considered to be science fiction.

References

1. Furukawa K, Yamamori H, Takagi K, Hayashi N, Suzuki R, Nakajima N, Tashiro T. Influences of soybean oil emulsion on stress response and cell-mediated immune function in moderately or severely stressed patients. *Nutrition* 2002; 18: 235–40.
2. Takagi K, Yamamori H, Toyoda Y, Nakajima N, Tashiro T. Modulating effects of the feeding route on stress response and endotoxin translocation in severely stressed patients receiving thoracic esophagectomy. *Nutrition* 2000; 16: 355–60.
3. Takagi K, Yamamori H, Morishima Y, Toyoda Y, Nakajima N, Tashiro T. Preoperative immunosuppression: Its relationship with high morbidity and mortality in patients receiving thoracic esophagectomy. *Nutrition* 2001; 17: 13–7.
4. Mercier S, Breuille D, Mosoni L, Obled C, Patureau Mirand P. Chronic inflammation alters protein metabolism in several organs of adult rats. *J Nutr* 2002; 132: 1921–8.
5. Hatada T, Miki C. Nutritional status and postoperative cytokine response in colorectal cancer patients. *Cytokine* 2000; 12: 1331–6.
6. Baines M, Shenkin A. Lack of effectiveness of short-term intravenous micronutrient nutrition in restoring plasma antioxidant status after surgery. *Clin Nutr* 2002; 21: 145–50.
7. Nicolaidis S. A hormone-based characterization and taxonomy of stress: Possible use in management. *Metabolism* 2002; 51 (Suppl): 31–6.
8. Brodner G, Van Aken H, Hertle L, Fobker M, Von Eckardstein A, Goeters C, Buerkle H, Harks A, Kehlet H. Multimodal perioperative management – combining thoracic epidural analgesia, forced mobilization, and oral nutrition – reduces hormonal and metabolic stress and improves convalescence after major urologic surgery. *Anesth Analg* 2001; 92: 1594–600.
9. Bedard S, Marcotte B, Marette A. Cytokines modulate glucose transport in skeletal muscle by inducing the expression of inducible nitric oxide synthase. *Biochem J* 1997; 325: 487–93.
10. Johnson JD, O'Connor KA, Deak T, Spencer RL, Watkins LR, Maier SF. Prior stressor exposure primes the HPA axis. *Psychoneuroendocrinology* 2002; 27: 353–65.
11. Servatius RJ, Natelson BH, Moldow R, Pogach L, Brennan FX, Ottenweller JE. Persistent neuroendocrine changes in multiple hormonal axes after a single or repeated stressor exposures. *Stress* 2000; 3: 263–74.
12. Combaret L, Tilignac T, Claustre A, Voisin L, Taillandier D, Obled C, Tanaka K, Attaix D. Torbafylline [HWA 448] inhibits enhanced skeletal muscle ubiquitin-proteasome-dependent proteolysis in cancer and septic rats. *Biochem J* 2002; 361: 185–92.
13. Grossie VB Jr, Mailman D. Influence of the Ward colon tumor on the host response to endotoxin. *J Cancer Res Clin Oncol* 1997; 123: 189–94.
14. Arsenijevic D, Girardier L, Seydoux J, Pechere JC, Garcia I, Lucas, Chang HR, Dulloo AG. Metabolic-cytokine responses to a second immunological challenge with LPS in mice with *T. gondii* infection. *Am J Physiol* 1998; 274: E439–45.
15. Chinnaiyan AM, Huber-Lang M, Kumar-Sinha C, Barrette TR, Shankar-Sinha S, Sarma VA, Padgaonkar VA, Ward PA. Molecular signatures of sepsis: Multiorgan gene expression profiles of systemic inflammation. *Am J Pathol* 2001; 159: 1199–209.
16. Cole J, Tsou R, Wallace K, Gibran N, Isik F. Early gene expression profile of human skin to injury using high-density cDNA microarrays. *Wound Repair Regen* 2001; 9: 360–70.
17. Gomes MD, Lecker SH, Jagoe TR, Navon M, Goldberg AL. Atrogin-1, a muscle-specific F-box protein highly expressed during muscle atrophy. *Proc Natl Acad Sci USA* 2001; 98: 14440–5.
18. Takahashi M, Tsuboyama-Kasaoka N, Nakatani T, Ishii M, Tsutsumi S, Aburatani H, Ezaki O. Fish oil feeding alters liver gene expressions to defend against PPARalpha activation and ROS production. *Am J Physiol Gastrointest Liver Physiol* 2002; 282: G338–48.
19. Li J, Yu X, Pan W, Unger RH. Gene expression profile of rat adipose tissue at the onset of high-fat-diet obesity. *Am J Physiol Endocrinol Metab* 2002; 282: E1334–41.
20. Jagoe RT, Lecker SH, Gomes M, Goldberg AL. Patterns of gene expression in atrophying skeletal muscles: Response to food deprivation. *FASEB J* 2002; 16: 1697–712.

Discussion

Dr. Moore: I have never come across the term 'nutritional stress', it sounds like a valid concept. In our studies we have attempted to randomize patients but we get mixed signals. How much of this do you believe is due to underlying nutritional stress, or do these patients have a different inflammatory response?

Dr. Baracos: What I mean by the term 'nutritional stress', is that there is some limitation to the availability of essential nutrients, a subclinical deficiency, and I think that can be an underlying factor in a person's response to a major injury. For example we recently completed a study on patients with generalized malignancy: those receiving a fish oil supplementation were compared to controls receiving a placebo containing a different mixture of fatty acids. In this population there was a clear set of responders and a clear set of nonresponders to the fish oil treatment. This study reveals a couple of interesting things. The first one is that there seems to be some abnormality in these patients' ability to assimilate fatty acids, so fatty acids went in the mouth but I don't know where they actually went, maybe they were not absorbed, maybe they were oxidized, but there was a poor correlation between the dietary intake and the appearance of those fatty acids in the plasma phospholipids. If the whole study is restratified according to the actually determined increase in eicosapentaenoic acid or docosahexaenoic acid in plasma or tissue phospholipids, then you have a highly conclusive result which was not seen if you consider the results on an intend-to-treat basis. Some people ate fatty acids but did not show any incorporation and therefore did not manifest a response. This was one instance where it was possible for us to go back and see what happened because we had the means to do so. It was possible to retrospectively analyze the data to determine that there was a problem with nutrient assimilation that explained the failure of the treatment or the appearance of a particular response. I think a deficiency in n-3 fatty acids is a good example of a previously existing nutritional stress, at least in my environment. I live as far away from the ocean as it is possible to be and the diet typically does not contain marine fish. The fatty acid intake is dominated by n-6 fatty acids from vegetable oils and red meats. So I am not certain whether the vast majority of the ill, critically ill or elderly people where I live would suffer from, if not a clinical deficiency, an imbalance in essential fatty acids, that may in part dictate the outcome of a serious illness.

Dr. Cynober: I was very impressed with the data you presented about the protein atrogin-1. I would like to know your feelings about the place of this new mediator in the game. In other words, in your opinion is it just a new transient star in the sky or something very important? For example we remember the cachectic factor discovered by Todorov et al. [1] some years ago and we have absolutely no further news about this cachectic factor which was then presented as something very important.

Dr. Baracos: We now understand that proteasomes are degrading muscle protein in the vast majority of states in which muscle atrophy presents as a problem. Todorov et al. [1] extracted a proteolysis-inducing glycoprotein from tumors, and treated animals and muscle cells with this factor. It causes activation of the protein breakdown process and very strong induction of the proteasome-dependent proteolytic system. Activation of the ubiquitin proteasome system is common to many forms of muscle wasting, regardless of which hormone, cytokine or other factor appears to be the circulating signal for the system's activation.

In the past we had only been aware of the lysosomal and calcium-activated proteolytic systems of muscle, however these systems are of limited importance in the pathogenesis of many forms of muscle atrophy. Now that we have identified the ubiquitin-proteasome system as the major proteolytic system contributing to muscle wasting, we are beginning to learn what is important in that system. Something has to attach ubiquitin to the protein so it can be identified and degraded by the proteasome. Ubiquitin availability is not limiting and the variation in the amount of ubiquitin does not correspond with the rate of the proteolytic process. Several enzymes are possible sites of control, the ubiquitin-activating enzymes, the ubiquitin-conjugating enzymes and then the ubiquitin ligases that participate in eventually making ubiquitinated protein substrate. It cannot yet be stated definitely but I would bet you a bottle of Margaux that because it is the element which confers substrate recognition to the whole pathway, the ubiquitin ligases, including atrogin-1, are likely to emerge as important.

There is another recent ubiquitin ligase discovery [2], very similar in approach to the work of Gomes et al. [3]. Bodine et al. [2] took three kinds of muscle atrophy associated with inactivity (denervation, immobilization, hind-limb suspension), and looked for the most expressed genes. In that approach they independently discovered atrogin-1 and also at the same time discovered a new previously uncharacterized muscle-specific ubiquitin ligase. So a family of ubiquitin ligases is emerging.

Dr. Moldawer: Do you want to comment briefly about the specificity of using the proteasome as a target for therapy of either cachexia? On the market or in clinical testing there are several proteasome inhibitors of primarily NFκB. Some of them are in development for cancer and there is a great deal of toxicity associated with some of the earlier proteasome inhibitors. Do you see attacking the proteasome as a valid therapeutic target for treating protein-wasting syndromes or is it because it is sub-ubiquitous in terms of its function in cells that it will never be a valid target for cachexia-type research?

Dr. Baracos: I think that is an important question. If protein synthesis is completely blocked, death ensues because of the rapid loss of all proteins with short half-lives. When protein catabolism is blocked, something similar occurs. Good inhibitors of the proteasome are lethal because they generate a metabolic catastrophe. If they are given to an animal in a dose efficient to block the activation of that system ubiquitously, the animals will be dead in the morning. Drug development in this area evolved in the direction of modulating these agents so that they are not as toxic or in a way to make them specific to a certain organ or class of protein.

Dr. Moldawer: I guess that is the question. Can you target the specificity of the ligase so that you can distinguish between the degradation of structural protein versus the degradation of the regulatory proteins which seem to be more what confers the toxicity of these inhibitors?

Dr. Baracos: I guess that is what is pleasing about the discovery that there may be muscle-specific ubiquitin ligases, as it may be possible to inhibit proteolysis locally in muscle without affecting other tissues. I think you need to work upstream of the proteasome, you can't just knock that out, it is too dangerous.

One of the things I see as problematic is the heterogeneity of upstream factors that turn on protein breakdown by the proteasome, even with a single disease type. For example, proinflammatory cytokines cause activation of the proteasome through the cytokine receptors on the muscle cell. The proteasome is also activated by an unusual proteolysis-inducing factor that acts on muscle directly [1]. Although both factors activate the proteasome, this is through separate receptor-mediated events. So if you are going to approach this problem right up at the humoral mediation end, you have to be able to identify which specific mediators patients are making – cytokines, the proteolysis-inducing glycoprotein or whatever, and intervene specifically in those cases. If one intervenes downstream, within common (rather than divergent) elements in the pathway leading to proteolysis, a single agent may be effective for multiple forms of muscle atrophy.

11

We are not there yet, but it is encouraging that industry is taking a renewed interest in drug development in the area of muscle protein catabolism, as their investment is very substantial compared to sponsorship from government.

Dr. Chioléro: You have nicely shown that you can have a balanced or an unbalanced response to stress with, for example, a different preponderance, the hypothalamic-pituitary-adrenal (HPA) axis or the sympathoadrenal response, and clearly in our intensive care patients we have different clinical pictures sometimes with a preponderance of one or the other or a very complex tableau. Do you think that we should assess our patients more systematically to know who is a more sympathoadrenal responder or has a more inflammatory response or a more HPA axis response since we have the therapeutic possibilities to influence this response?

Dr. Baracos: I think so. I think it is necessary to pick the panel of stress response elements to measure which, in that case, would be the adrenal-secreted hormones. We need to examine the nutritional changes, and to measure the prognostic significance of the individual elements of the stress response panel, i.e. to link them to the clinical outcome, including survival.

Dr. Déchelotte: To go ahead with this question, what would you suggest for a standard-sized hospital as a reasonable tool for clinical use in direct response of these patients?

Dr. Baracos: I don't think there is a question of looking at this in a standard-sized hospital at this point in time. In Canada with colleagues at the University of Montreal I am presently involved in a study of non-small cell lung cancer patients in advanced stages, so stages IIIB and IV. We are subjecting them to a comprehensive evaluation in a center for nutrition and function. Using a very broad panel of possible stress factors, we are trying to determine those factors which have prognostic significance. But because of the cost, patient burden and the complexity, this can only be accomplished on a limited scale in this patient group, but this should at least give us the opportunity to test these ideas.

Dr. Zazzo: You spoke about the sympathetic profile of one category of patients, and in the intensive care unit (ICU) we have many patients receiving therapy with epinephrine, norepinephrine. Do you think this profile of patients in metabolic response is symmetrical, is the same, if we consider the endogenous sympathetic response and therapeutic sympathetic administration?

Dr. Baracos: That is a very important question to which I don't think we presently have an answer but it would be necessary to figure it in some analysis of those concepts.

Dr. Allison: I greatly enjoyed your combination of analysis and synthesis which you attempted to integrate and as a clinician I could sort of respond to the difficulties you posed to us. A lot of the animal studies are of course necessarily short-term and become the acute event, whereas the ICU experience or the critical care experience is a rather long one and it evolves into different patterns. Whereas I used to look after people in the acute stage I now look after people who have just left the ICU and I can see the continuing stresses to which they are subjected. I was interested in your combination of the psychological and physical because these people have the most colossal psychological stress, of an order which is almost unimaginable, and if you don't inquire of it and measure it you are not aware of it, and this continues. So the challenge therapeutically is how we see what you describe as evolving in a longitudinal way and are we looking at different things? In the acute phase are we looking at actual metabolic support? Let's get away from the term nutrition and nutrition only comes in when you've got over that phase. How do we integrate this longitudinally as well as horizontally in the acute phase?

Dr. Baracos: Your remarks make me think about something that I have encountered in my current work in a palliative care service and has to do with the psychological consequences. The chaplain in our unit is earning her doctorate studying patients who, facing a diagnosis of advanced cancer, face a period of anguish so profound that it obliterates everything else from their conception. You are probably familiar with the term somatization in the psychiatric context, but her area is the understanding of how this horrible anguish can manifest this somatization of pain, and she is interested in identifying clinical markers at the entry into that stage, of the duration of that stage and then the passage through it into a stage of acceptance. The acceptance phase is characterized by a completely different perception of the person's own situation and I cannot believe that it does not have physiologic and metabolic correlates. There are researchers trying to measure this and bring together the understanding of somatization from a spiritual context and a psychological metabolic context.

Dr. Déchelotte: Thank you very much Dr. Allison for addressing this important question that we not only have fat stores and proteins but also the whole body reaction to take into account.

References

1. Todorov P, Cariuk P, McDevitt T, Coles B, Tisdale M. Characterization of a cancer cachectic factor. *Nature* 1996; 379: 739–42.
2. Bodine SC, Latres E, Baumhueter S, et al. Identification of ubiquitin ligases required for skeletal muscle atrophy. *Science* 2001; 294: 1704–8.
3. Gomes MD, Lecker SH, Jagoe TR, et al. Atrogin-1, a muscle-specific F-box protein highly expressed during muscle atrophy. *Proc Natl Acad Sci USA* 2001; 98: 14440–5.

Cynober L, Moore FA (eds): Nutrition and Critical Care.
Nestlé Nutrition Workshop Series Clinical & Performance Program, Vol. 8, pp 15–37,
Nestec Ltd.; Vevey/S. Karger AG, Basel, © 2003.

Genetic Polymorphisms, Functional Genomics and the Host Inflammatory Response to Injury and Inflammation

Robert J. Feezor and Lyle L. Moldawer

Department of Surgery, University of Florida College of Medicine,
Gainesville, Fla., USA

Introduction

The term 'sepsis' refers to the host's systemic inflammatory response to an invasive microbial challenge; when the clinical constellation includes hypotension and/or concurrent end-organ injury, the condition is known as 'severe sepsis' or 'septic shock'. There are more than 750,000 cases and 100,000 deaths each year in the US alone attributable to sepsis and septic shock [1, 2], translating into total costs of USD 16.7 billion annually [3]. Overall, septic patients have a 25–45% mortality [1, 3, 4]. The outcome of patients with sepsis and septic shock has improved minimally in the past 50 years, despite significant overall improvements in intensive care medicine. This systemic inflammatory response, or more explicitly, the interplay between the microbial pathogen and the characteristics of host response, determines the magnitude and diversity of the host response, and ultimately outcome. A growing body of evidence is mounting to suggest that much of the host response is a direct reflection of heritable traits, accounting for interpersonal differences, and allowing for genetic detection.

Supported in part by grants R37-GM-40586–13, and R01-GM-63041–01, awarded by the National Institutes of General Medical Sciences, USPHS. R.J.F. was supported by T32 GM 08721 03, a research training fellowship awarded by the National Institute of General Medical Sciences, USPHS.

15

Systemic Inflammatory Diseases and Immunity

The role of the innate and the acquired immune response in chronic inflammatory diseases is regulated and sustained by the activation of an acquired immune response by antigen-presenting cells, such as macrophages and dendritic cells, with the subsequent release of inflammatory mediators. The inflammatory response is initiated and propagated by an element of immune recognition of self antigens [5], and is sustained by the over-production of inflammatory mediators and T-lymphocyte-derived cytokines. Hence, both the reactive and chronic immune diseases occur as a result (at least at some level) of the dysregulation of the production of these immune mediators.

When these mediators are produced in excess, or when their counteracting receptor antagonists or antagonist-binding proteins are deficient, the protective role of the immune system devolves into a harmful one capable of systemic injury to the host [6].

Recent data have implicated the innate and acquired immune systems as being pivotal for the deleterious effects of acute inflammatory states, such as the systemic inflammatory response syndrome (SIRS). SIRS is defined by the physiological characteristics of the host's response to any of a number of external or internal stimuli, infectious and noninfectious [7], and represents a nonspecific, systemic activation of the innate immune system [8]. SIRS clinically can result from ischemia-reperfusion injury, thermal injury, severe trauma, surgical injury, and microbial infection. Clinically, the SIRS response to an external stimulus is often followed by a compensatory anti-inflammatory response syndrome (CARS), during which there is a state of relative immunocompromise and a concomitant overexpression of genes encoding for anti-inflammatory cytokines (fig. 1) [9]. CARS has been observed for years in clinical practice as patients would develop potentially fatal secondary infections several days after the inciting traumatic injurious event.

The clinical presentation of sepsis and SIRS can be nearly identical, yet sepsis, unlike SIRS, requires the presence of a potentially identifiable microbial stimulus. It is now clear that the common response element for both of these syndromes is activation of the proinflammatory immune system, with a subsequent activation of the anti-inflammatory immune response. The scientific literature has recently become replete with attempts to characterize septic patients in terms of their immune status as a means to complement the clinical parameters (e.g., critical illness scoring systems) which more accurately measure the host's physiological response to the injury and not the cause of the injury per se [10]. In an effort to develop new therapeutic approaches, specific biochemical mediators and cytokines involved in such processes, as well as their genetic control mechanisms have been targeted. Despite a number of successes in animal models, little gains have been

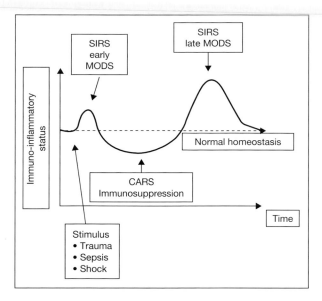

Fig. 1. Clinical course of the systemic inflammatory response syndrome (SIRS). MODS = Multiple organ dysfunction syndrome; CARS = compensatory anti-inflammatory response syndrome. Adapted from Oberholzer et al. [8]. Reprinted with permission.

made with this approach in human studies. There likely are several reasons for the lack of success, including the improper timing of immune-altering measures, the complexity of triggering mechanisms, the redundancy of immune activation pathways, and the heterogeneity of the patient population being studied [11].

Clearly, the current practice of using physiological or immunological scoring systems to risk-stratify septic patients has scientific merit, but such an approach does not account for the underlying health status or predisposition of the individual. The genetic predisposition of patients to develop sepsis following traumatic or surgical injury, as well as their response to sepsis, has only begun to be explored experimentally. Practically speaking, hospital care of the septic patient comprises the bulk of the budget of any intensive care unit: each clinical case of sepsis costs approximately USD 22,100 [3]. Foreknowledge about a particular patient's prognosis could decrease cost and improve the allocation of health care resources, thereby allowing clinicians to 'apply preventative intensive care at lower cost with better outcomes' [12]. If a relationship between the genetic constitution of a patient and the response to a major inflammatory stimulus could be established, better injury-scoring systems could be devised that more accurately predict the clinical trajectory of a patient.

The Triggering Event

The classic stimuli known to cause sepsis and SIRS in humans and animal models are microbial products, predominantly lipopolysaccharide (LPS), which is a component of the cell wall of gram-negative organisms. The innate immune system has been programmed to discriminate self from non-self and has developed elaborate recognition systems to detect the presence of minimal quantities of microbial products [13]. Secretory, acute phase protein products of the liver, including complement, play an integral role in this process. Probably, the best described innate immune system response occurs from the recognition of bacterial LPS. A key acute phase reactant protein involved in the recognition of bacterial LPS is LPS-binding protein (LBP), which is produced by hepatocytes and other cell types, and circulates in the plasma [14]. When bound to LPS, LBP forms a complex with either the soluble or membrane-bound receptor, CD14. This LPS:LPB:CD14 complex, acting via the TLR4 receptor, sets in motion a cascade of reactions which ultimately leads to the recruitment of neutrophils and the release of other inflammatory mediators [15].

This LPS-induced pro-inflammatory cascade is mediated largely by the production of proinflammatory cytokines, including tumor necrosis factor-α (TNFα) and interleukin-1 (IL-1). In animal models, blocking TNFα or IL-1 signaling via its receptors prior to administration of *Escherichia coli* greatly reduces mortality [16, 17]. There is, however, a lack of success at reducing morbidity and mortality in human trials: in over 30 randomized studies with inhibitors of TNFα or IL-1 with more than 12,000 patients enrolled, there has been no proven clinical benefit [18]. 'Merely blocking a single component may be insufficient to arrest the inflammatory process' [18].

The presence of 'non-self' can explain, at least in part, microbe-induced SIRS, but clinical evidence has shown that nonmicrobial stimulation (e.g., mesenteric ischemia-reperfusion, pancreatitis, hemorrhagic shock, thermal injury) will often produce similar clinical outcomes. To reconcile this, Matzinger [19] has proposed that the immune system functions to recognize internal and external 'danger signals' as opposed to the more classical notion that the immune system functions to distinguish 'self' from 'non-self'. In this 'danger signal' theory, the immune system can distinguish not only exogenous microbial products, but also internal endogenous signals such as heat-shock proteins (HSP) or necrotic (but not apoptotic) cells or tissue. In support of this theory, HSP-60 has been shown to be a known ligand for toll-like receptor-4 (TLR4) [20], capable of inducing the same inflammatory cascade as LPS.

The Biological Response

Regardless of the inciting event(s), the key initiators of inflammatory responses are cytokines. As listed by Oberholzer et al. [8], these proximal proinflammatory cytokines function in three primary roles: (1) to induce the production of acute phase proteins by the liver; (2) to cause an elevation in body temperature, and (3) to induce the sequelae of local inflammation, namely an increase in vascular permeability and the chemoattraction of other inflammatory molecules. Most cytokines are not stored within the cell as preformed entities, but rather are synthesized de novo from newly transcribed mRNA. Philosophically, the role of innate immunity and the acute inflammatory response is to prevent the systemic dissemination of the infection while the acquired immune response is being expressed.

The magnitude of the pro- and anti-inflammatory cytokine response is proportional to the severity of tissue trauma [8], and the risk of developing systemic complications. However, it should be noted that the production of these inflammatory mediators may not be uniform throughout the body. In fact, one of the initial responses of the acute inflammation mediated by the innate immune system (and specifically mostly by TNFα is to induce a procoagulant state that serves to thwart the hematogenous spread of the organism or inciting molecule throughout the body, thereby allowing a focused or sequestered inflammatory response to the inciting event. In addition to the circulatory control of the regulation of cytokine distribution, many cytokines are expressed in a 'cell-restricted manner' [21].

There are three principle cytokines that mediate the early acute inflammatory response: IL-1, IL-6, and TNFα. IL-1 primarily serves to mount the febrile response, induces an acute phase reaction, stimulates the proliferation of early hematopoietic progenitor cells, triggers prostanoid release, and regulates 'sickness behavior'; IL-6 stimulates hepatocytes to produce acute phase reactants and causes B-cell proliferation [22]; TNFα is a procoagulant, overlaps with IL-1 in its effects on the hepatic acute phase response, fever and prostaglandin production, and stimulates neutrophil recruitment and activation [22, 23]. TNFα and IL-1 stimulate the production of a variety of secondary proinflammatory and anti-inflammatory cytokines, including IL-6, chemokines (IL-8 superfamily), IL-10, IL-12, and IL-18. Increased levels of TNFα are seen in healthy volunteers after injection of endotoxin [24] as well as in patients with either gram-negative or gram-positive septic shock [25, 26]. The peak TNFα production generally occurs within the first 2 h after endotoxin challenge [24, 27, 28]. In a model of SIRS without microbial infection, elevated levels of TNFα and IL-6 were seen in the serum of patients after thoracoabdominal aneurysm repair, which necessarily includes a period of intraoperative mesenteric ischemia with subsequent reperfusion [29]. Increased frequency and magnitude of multiorgan dysfunction were seen in patients with elevated TNF and IL-6 levels [29].

While most patients survive the initial SIRS response, the proinflammatory mediators that caused the acute physiologic response then contribute to the immune-suppressed state (CARS), which is characterized by T-cell hyporesponsiveness, anergy, a defect in antigen presentation, and increased

T- and B-cell apoptosis [9]. Wood et al. [30] showed that T-cell lymphocytes taken from patients several days after severe injury do not produce IL-2, and furthermore, the degree of suppression of IL-2 production correlated with the likelihood of developing sepsis [30]. Kelly et al. [31] showed that severe thermal injury to mice depressed Th1 cell function, which was manifested by lower levels of IL-2, IFN-γ, and IL-10. Although this relationship was not causative, it gives clear insight into the direct control of the immune system onto clinical outcomes.

Genetic Polymorphisms

The Prophit survey, investigating the concordance of tuberculosis among monozygotic and dizygotic twins, first established the link between genetics and host response to disease states [32]. Links between the presence of genetic markers and the occurrence of common systemic diseases such as coronary artery disease have also been established [33, 34]. Given the converging biological pathways of inflammation, it is unlikely that a single gene will be identified that determines all of the clinical sequelae of sepsis. While a majority of studies have focused on the contribution of single genes or gene products, more recent data have focused on genome wide changes. The Human Genome Project is a large-scale, collaborative effort to sequence the entire human genome. While much of the genome is conserved in all members of the species, approximately 1% is repeatedly and reproducibly variable at a frequency much greater than that which would be expected from random mutations. As opposed to mutations that can occur and likely will be repaired by the cell's defense mechanisms, these areas of variability, called polymorphisms, are stable within the genome. Strictly defined, a polymorphism is the existence of two or more sequence variants occurring at significant frequencies within a population. Common examples of polymorphisms are single nucleotide polymorphisms (SNPs) and variable number of tandem repeats (VNTRs). SNPs are single nucleotides which are substituted for another nucleotide within a sequence of the allele. A VNTR is a duplication of a short run of non-coding DNA arranged in tandem. While research efforts are investigating polymorphisms as genetic markers for disease processes, they are not necessarily causative of that disease, and therefore, afford no immediate therapeutic benefit [4].

Tumor Necrosis Factor

With respect to the host's response to acute inflammation, several of the more well-studied polymorphisms occur within the gene cluster that encodes TNFα and TNFβ on chromosome 6. The TNFα gene is highly conserved

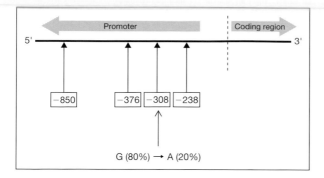

Fig. 2. Locations of the single nucleotide polymorphisms (SNPs) within the tumor necrosis factor-α (TNFα) promoter.

throughout evolution [35] and, therefore, has relatively few known polymorphisms. SNPs are known to occur, however, and some have been identified at positions −850, −376, −308, and −238 (fig. 2) [36]. At position −308 (308 basepairs upstream from the start codon), there is a guanine (G) nucleotide in 80% of the population; this is replaced by an adenosine (A) in the remaining 20% of the population. The sequence with a G is referred to as the TNF1 allele while that with the A is the TNF2 allele. Since each person has two copies of the gene, the relative frequencies of G/G, G/A, and A/A are 65–80%, 15–25%, and 2–5%, respectively [4]. While the TNF2 gene has been associated with the increased production of TNFα, the clinical relevance of this allele has been debated. Mira et al. [37] found that 39% of patients with septic shock had the TNF2 allele as opposed to only 18% of controls, and the frequency of TNF2 was higher among patients who died than those who lived (52 vs. 24%, respectively). Furthermore, stratifying the data according to the severity of clinical illness, there was higher mortality in patients who had at least one copy of the TNF2 allele (71.4 vs. 42.6%) [37]. Overall, there was a 3.7-fold increase in risk of death with at least one copy of TNF2 [37].

The genes for TNFα and TNFβ (LTα and LTβ) are juxtaposed on chromosome 6, within the HLA class-III locus. They are believed to have evolved from a common ancestral gene through duplication [38]. The protein products of these genes have similar functions, although TNFα is produced primarily by macrophages while TNFβ is produced predominantly by lymphocytes. Majetschak et al. [39] examined the frequency of a polymorphism within the first intron of the TNFβ gene in patients who developed post-traumatic sepsis. At position +1069 within the TNFβ gene, 70% of the population have an adenosine (TNFB2 allele) while 30% have a guanine (TNFB1 allele). The odds ratio for developing posttraumatic sepsis in patients with homozygous TNFB2 versus heterozygotes was 5.22 [39]. Reinforcing these results, Fang et al. [40] found that among patients with septic shock, those who were homozygous for the TNFB2 allele had an 81% mortality as opposed to patients who were heterozygous (TNFB2/TNFB1) or homozygous for the TNFB1 allele, who had 42 and 19% mortality, respectively. Stüber et al. [36] reported that patients with severe sepsis who were homozygous for TNFB2 had an increased mortality, a higher circulating concentration of TNFα, and on average, higher multiorgan failure scores than patients who were TNFB2/ TNFB1 heterozygous. These clinical data confirm earlier work that the TNFB2 allele is associated with higher TNFα release from LPS-stimulated monocytes ex vivo [41].

Interleukin-1

The gene for IL-1 is a complex sequence that encodes for 3 distinct protein products, IL-1α, IL-1β, and IL-1ra (a receptor antagonist which acts as a competitive inhibitor of IL-1α and IL-1β) [42]. When activated, the intracellular domain of the IL-1 type-I receptor provides the docking platform for the recruitment of several proteins, including MyD88 and IRAK, whose phosphorylation leads to the activation and translocation of nuclear factor κB (NFκB), which subsequently induces the transcription of IL-1, IL-6, IL-8, as well as other chemokine genes [43].

IL-1ra

IL-1ra is believed to offer some protective role against severe sepsis. In a study comparing 78 patients with severe sepsis, Arnalich et al. [44] found that the plasma concentration of IL-1ra was lower in patients who died compared to those who lived. Although overexpression of IL-1ra has protective effects in murine models of sepsis [45] and administration of IL-1ra protects baboons from bacteremic shock [46], no clinical benefit has been seen with human trials of the administration of recombinant IL-1ra [47].

Within intron 2 of the gene for IL-1ra is an 86 basepair VNTR with 5 known alleles, varying in number of tandem copies from 2 to 6. Seventy percent of the population has 4 copies (the IL-1ra A1 allele), 25% have 2 copies (IL-1ra A2), while the remaining 3 alleles (with 3, 5, and 6 copies of IL-1ra) are seen in less than 5% of the population (fig. 3). The risk of developing immune-mediated diseases, such as ulcerative colitis, alopecia areata, systemic lupus erythematosus, Graves disease, and lichen sclerosis, is higher in patients with the IL-1ra A2 allele [26, 48–52], and this allele has been associated with exaggerated IL-1β secretion [41]. More recently, Fang et al. [40] reported a 2.14-fold greater relative risk of developing severe sepsis for homozygous IL-1ra A2 patients and a 1.73-fold risk for IL-1ra A2 heterozygotes, although the occurrence of the allele did not translate into survival predictability.

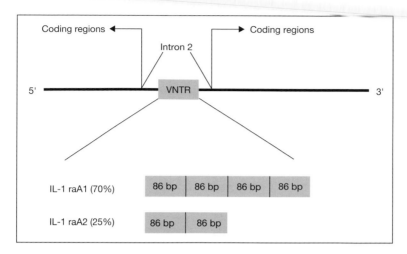

Fig. 3. Scheme showing variable number of tandem repeats (VNTR) polymorphism within intron 2 of the gene encoding IL-1ra.

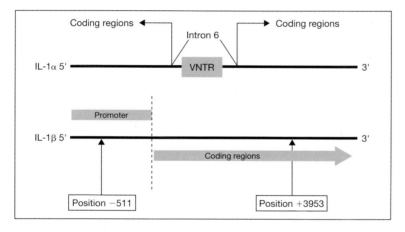

Fig. 4. Diagram of polymorphisms within the genes encoding IL-1α and IL-1β.

This increased incidence of IL-1ra A2 among septic patients was confirmed by Ma et al. [53], further implying a potential susceptibility to sepsis in homozygotes of this allele. Arnalich et al. [54] found that even after adjustment for APACHE II score, homozygosity for the A2 allele was associated with a 6.47-fold increased risk of dying from severe sepsis. Ex vivo studies of peripheral blood monocytes from these same septic patients showed that at least one copy of the IL-1ra A2 allele was associated with elevated production of IL-1ra regardless of the presence or absence of ex vivo stimulation of these cells [54].

IL-1α and IL-1β

Within intron 6 of the gene encoding IL-1α, there is a 46-bp VNTR for which there are 7 known alleles (fig. 4). Ma et al. [53] noted that septic patients homozygous for IL-1α A2 had higher mortality rates than noncarriers or heterozygotes. At position −511 within the gene for IL-1β, there is a polymorphism commonly detected by the restriction enzyme AvaI. Previous work has shown that carriers of IL-1β B2 exhibited exaggerated levels of endotoxin-induced IL-1β [55]. In the same group of septic patients described above by Ma et al. [53], septic patients homozygous for IL-1β B2 had higher mortality than heterozygotes or noncarriers. A second polymorphism of IL-1β exists at position +3953, which likewise has been associated with elevated concentrations of IL-1β (fig. 4) [55].

Interleukin-10

IL-10 has classically been defined as an anti-inflammatory cytokine and serves to downregulate the expression of IL-1, TNFα, and other proinflammatory cytokines. In a murine and primate model, IL-10 has been shown to protect the animals from endotoxin-induced lethality and hypotension [56]. There are three known polymorphisms of the IL-10 gene, all SNPs, which are located within the promoter: at positions −1,082, −819, and −592. Unfortunately, it appears that the three SNPs are in linkage disequilibration, suggesting that their frequency of occurrence is a nonrandom event. Nevertheless, in case-controlled study, Koch et al. [57] found no difference in either the frequency of the alleles or combinations of alleles among patients who had coronary artery disease, a history of a prior myocardial infarction, and normal controls. The allelic frequency of IL-10 polymorphisms in sepsis has not been well described, with the exception of some preliminary reports on meningococcal disease [58].

Interleukin-6

IL-6 has been shown to have both pro- and anti-inflammatory properties; it exerts its biologic effects by binding to its receptor on cell surfaces and then interacting with the gp130 signal-transducing complex. Clinical variation in the level of IL-6 has been noted: high IL-6 production has been shown to adversely affect the survival of human solid organ allografts [59]. Data from the 1997–1998 United Network of Organ Sharing Scientific Registry show that the rate of organ failure for the African-American population is significantly higher than that of the Caucasian population. Ethnicity studies have shown that 98% of African-Americans were 'high IL-6' producers while only 84% of

Caucasians were similarly classified [60]. While this has not been demon-strated to be a causative relationship, it does raise suspicion that genetic variances account for the differences in levels of the production of proin-flammatory cytokines, and may help to identify those patients at increased risk of the untoward clinical sequelae of graft failure.

Systemic levels of IL-6 are believed to be regulated at the level of genetic expression [61]. Several studies have shown a relation between the level of circulating IL-6 and outcome of sepsis [62, 63]. A known polymorphism occurs within the promoter at position -174 at which either a guanine (G) or cytosine (C) nucleotide resides. In a study of 50 septic patients, Schlüter et al. [64] found that among the 25 patients who did not survive, only 2 were homozygous for the G allele (G/G), while 11 of the 25 survivors were G/G. Furthermore, there was good correlation of circulating IL-6 concentration and clinical outcome of these same study patients [64]. The authors concluded that there must be some survival benefit in homozygosity of the G allele. However, the G allele is known to cause spontaneous and inducible genetic expression of the IL-6 gene, and has been associated with elevated levels of circulating IL-6 in healthy adults, as compared to healthy adults without a G allele [65]. Schlüter et al. [64] attempted to explain this apparent incongruity by noting that most of the studies previously performed examining IL-6 production as a function of allelic frequency were done with ex vivo stimulation.

Nuclear Factor κB

NFκB is a DNA-binding protein that incites high-level transcription of several proinflammatory genes including TNFα, IL-1β, IL-2, IL-6, IL-8, IL-12, IFNγ, and others. It is activated by any of a number of inflammatory stimuli or mediators: ischemia-reperfusion, hypoxia, volutrauma, barotrauma, IL-1β, or TNF. The activation of NFκB by TNFα or IL-1β is mediated through a series of kinases, the end result of which is translocation of the heterodimer to the nucleus with subsequent binding to the 6B promoter region. In a study by Bohrer et al. [66], the level of monocyte production of NFκB from patients with sepsis correlated with end organ failure and predicted survival.

CD14

As described above, the CD14 receptor binds to LPS on the surface of monocytes, macrophages, and other peripheral blood mononuclear cells, and thus moderates signals of the innate immune system. The administration of monoclonal antibodies against CD14 has been shown to attenuate organ injury and mortality in rabbits that have been given LPS, even if administered subsequent to the LPS dose [67]. Furthermore, soluble CD14 (sCD14) plays a role in the response of endothelial cells (which lack the CD14 receptor) to microbial stimulation. Within the promoter region for the gene encoding CD14 is a polymorphism at the −159 position. Prior ex vivo studies have shown higher levels of sCD14 (and, incidentally, higher TNFα) from cells of patients who had the T (thymine) nucleotide as opposed to the C (cytosine) allele at this position [68]. Clinically, elevated sCD14 has been associated with higher mortality in patients with septic shock [69, 70]. Gibot et al. [71] examined the frequency of the CD14 polymorphisms in patients with septic shock. They found that the T allele was more common in patients with septic shock as opposed to normal healthy control volunteers (55 vs. 43%). Furthermore, among septic patients, those who were homozygous for the T allele had a higher mortality than those who were either heterozygous or homozygous for the C allele (77% mortality for T/T vs. 26% for C/C). This translated into an odds ratio of 5.3 for death among patients with septic shock in T/T versus C/C [71].

Toll-Like Receptor 4

TLR4 is the major receptor for LPS and gram-negative bacteria, as outlined above. In the mouse strain C3H/HeJ, in which there is an amino acid substitution at position +712 of the TLR4 gene, stimulation with LPS induces an attenuated inflammatory state compared to that which is induced by the stimulation of mice with normal (wild-type) TLR4 [72]. In addition, TLR4$^{-/-}$ mice do not respond to LPS stimulation [73, 74], thereby proving the requirement of this cell surface protein for the induction of the inflammatory state. One known mutation of the TLR4 gene at amino acid position 299 may predispose to septic shock: Lorenz et al. [75] found that 5 of 91 patients with septic shock had this mutation, as opposed to 0 of 73 controls, a difference which reached statistical significance.

Genome-Wide Measurements

If the discovery of markers for systemic disease states represents one level of genetic pathophysiology, the natural sequel is the expression products of the genome. Patients do not die from sepsis because of polymorphisms in their genomic DNA. Presumably, the differential outcome is secondary to altered expression or activity of the protein translated from the expressed gene. The advancement of the Human Genome Project has enabled the development of new wide-scale technologies, not only for screening the human genome, but evaluating the gene expression products. This latter process has been defined as 'functional genomics'. Formerly, it was possible only to measure the level of certain known mediators of systemic inflammation using reductive approaches that focused on single or small numbers of mRNA or proteins, such as Northern or Western analyses, RT-PCR or ELISAs. Now, using oligonucleotide or DNA microarrays, scientists can simultaneously measure the level of expression of thousands of genes from a variety of tissue types in response to various stimuli. This has resulted in the need to challenge how we look at the host response to inflammation. As Lander [76] stated, 'The traditional gene-by-gene approach will not suffice to meet the sheer magnitude of the problem. It will be necessary to take "global views" of biological processes: simultaneous read-outs of all components'. Not only does microarray technology enable simultaneous measurement of thousands of genes, but it also eliminates the need for a priori knowledge of the function of the gene being studied. In this way, the response of a known gene to a given stimulus can be qualified; but furthermore, the function of an unknown gene or expressed sequence tag can be inferred from its expression behavior, relative to thousands of other genes.

The field of oncology is among the first to bring gene expression microarrays into clinical utility. Pathologists are now able to differentiate tumor types based on the RNA expression profile. Golub et al. [77] described the use of gene expression to predict the class of leukemia, even without prior biological knowledge of the cancer. Thus, any class of cell type can be identified not solely by physiologic and phenotypic characteristics, but additionally by its gene expression pattern, the ultimate 'blueprint'.

An overview of the technology and biostatistics associated with this emerging field of functional genomics is complex and beyond the scope of this review. However, Chung et al. [78] provide a succinct summary of the use of microarrays in sepsis and the intensive care setting. They summarize that 'for intensivists, the goal of functional genomics is to better understand [the] integrated molecular response to injury'.

Several groups have begun to investigate the gene expression patterns of antigen-presenting cells of the innate immune system (dendritic cells, DCs) in response to external stimuli [79]. Immature DCs, confined to tissues most suited for immunosurveillance, are capable of detecting pathogens or other immune-activating stressors; once these cells detect such a stimulus, they lose phagocytic capabilities and exhibit enhanced production of cytokines [79]. Granucci et al. [79] compared the gene expression pattern 'transcriptome' of immature and LPS-stimulated and TNFα-stimulated matured DCs from murine bone marrow using a commercial microarray containing oligonucleotide segments representing more than 6,500 murine genes. Previous work has shown that DCs will mature when stimulated with either LPS or TNFα for 18h; their maturity determined by functional traits such as antigen presentation or cytoskeletal characteristics [80, 81]. Despite the phenotypic similarities of DCs matured by either method, microarray analysis revealed

27

diverse genotypes. In fact, only LPS-treated cells, and not TNFα-treated, showed a gene expression pattern consistent with growth arrest and immune activation [79]. This serves to highlight, even at the level of single cell analysis, the increased detection capacity of genome expression analysis over phenotypic analysis.

Similarly, genome-wide analysis on a rat model of sepsis in which the level of expression of over 8,000 genes was quantified in a cecal ligation and puncture model showed that the genetic responses of inflammation are distinct for each organ [82].

Current research efforts are examining the host response to external and internal immunostimulatory triggers at the level of the genome. Such broad-scaled characterization offers a completely novel approach to the problem of systemic inflammation. A recent Large Scale Collaborative Research Program funded by the National Institute of General Medical Sciences seeks to characterize early gene response to major trauma or burns, highlighting the broad interest in this field.

Conclusion

The ability to detect and characterize the immunological status of patients to diseases has illustrated that the host response to the disease affects outcome greatly. In some instances, disease occurs only when there is dysregulation of this response, often at the level of DNA transcription. Several known genetic variants or polymorphisms have been described in an effort to relate genetic constitution and clinical trajectory. Genetic variants may be used to stratify patient response to disease, characterize level of illness, and possibly predict clinical response. Furthermore, continued efforts to characterize genome-wide responses to stimuli will serve to identify heretofore unsuspected genes and potentially novel therapies.

References

1. Sessler CN, Shepherd W. New concepts in sepsis. *Curr Opin Crit Care* 2002; 8: 465–72.
2. Parrillo JE, Parker MM, Natanson C, Suffredini AF, Danner RL, Cunnion RE, Ognibene FP. Septic shock in humans. Advances in the understanding of pathogenesis, cardiovascular dysfunction, and therapy. *Ann Intern Med* 1990; 113: 227–42.
3. Angus DC, Linde-Zwirble WT, Lidicker J, Clermont G, Carcillo J, Pinsky MR. Epidemiology of severe sepsis in the United States: Analysis of incidence, outcome, and associated costs of care. *Crit Care Med* 2001; 29: 1303–10.
4. Tabrizi AR, Zehnbauer BA, Freeman BD, Buchman TG. Genetic markers in sepsis. *J Am Coll Surg* 2001; 192: 106–17; quiz 145–6.
5. Hedley ML. Gene therapy of chronic inflammatory disease. *Adv Drug Deliv Rev* 2000; 44: 195–207.
6. Ksontini R, MacKay SL, Moldawer LL. Revisiting the role of tumor necrosis factor alpha and the response to surgical injury and inflammation. *Arch Surg* 1998; 133: 558–67.

7. American College of Chest Physicians/Society of Critical Care Medicine Consensus Conference. Definitions for sepsis and organ failure and guidelines for the use of innovative therapies in sepsis. *Crit Care Med* 1992; 20: 864–74.
8. Oberholzer A, Oberholzer C, Moldawer LL. Sepsis syndromes: Understanding the role of innate and acquired immunity. *Shock* 2001; 16: 83–96.
9. Bone RC. Toward a theory regarding the pathogenesis of the systemic inflammatory response syndrome: What we do and do not know about cytokine regulation. *Crit Care Med* 1996; 24: 163–72.
10. Oberholzer A, Oberholzer C, Minter RM, Moldawer LL. Considering immunomodulatory therapies in the septic patient: Should apoptosis be a potential therapeutic target? *Immunol Lett* 2001; 75: 221–4.
11. Krishnagopalan S, Dellinger RP. Innovative therapies for sepsis. *Biodrugs* 2001; 15: 645–54.
12. Bion JF. Susceptibility to critical illness: Reserve, response and therapy. *Intens Care Med* 2000; 26: S57–S63.
13. Janeway CA Jr. The immune system evolved to discriminate infectious nonself from noninfectious self. *Immunol Today* 1992; 13: 11–6.
14. Tobias PS, Soldau K, Kline L, Lee JD, Kato K, Martin TP, Ulevitch RJ. Cross-linking of lipopolysaccharide (LPS) to CD14 on THP-1 cells mediated by LPS-binding protein. *J Immunol* 1993; 150: 3011–21.
15. Beutler B. Tlr4: central component of the sole mammalian LPS sensor. *Curr Opin Immunol* 2000; 12: 20–6.
16. Tracey KJ, Fong Y, Hesse DG, Manogue KR, Lee AT, Kuo GC, Lowry SF, Cerami A. Anti-cachectin/TNF monoclonal antibodies prevent septic shock during lethal bacteraemia. *Nature* 1987; 330: 662–4.
17. Fischer E, Van Zee KJ, Marano MA, Rock CS, Kenney JS, Poutsiaka DD, Dinarello CA, Lowry SF, Moldawer LL. Interleukin-1 receptor antagonist circulates in experimental inflammation and in human disease. *Blood* 1992; 79: 2196–200.
18. Glauser MP. Pathophysiologic basis of sepsis: Considerations for future strategies of intervention. *Crit Care Med* 2000; 28: S4–S8.
19. Matzinger P. Tolerance, danger, and the extended family. *Annu Rev Immunol* 1994; 12: 991–1045.
20. Ohashi K, Burkart V, Flohe S, Kolb H. Cutting edge: Heat shock protein 60 is a putative endogenous ligand of the toll-like receptor-4 complex. *J Immunol* 2000; 164: 558–61.
21. Holloway AF, Rao S, Shannon MF. Regulation of cytokine gene transcription in the immune system. *Mol Immunol* 2002; 38: 567–80.
22. Dinarello CA, Moldawer LL. *Proinflammatory and anti-inflammatory cytokines in rheumatoid arthritis: A primer for clinicians.* Thousand Oaks, Amgen, 2002.
23. Fry DE. Sepsis syndrome. *Am Surg* 2000; 66: 126–32.
24. Fong YM, Marano MA, Moldawer LL, Wei H, Calvano SE, Kenney JS, Allison AC, Cerami A, Shires GT, Lowry SF. The acute splanchnic and peripheral tissue metabolic response to endotoxin in humans. *J Clin Invest* 1990; 85: 1896–904.
25. Girardin E, Grau GE, Dayer JM, Roux-Lombard P, Lambert PH. Tumor necrosis factor and interleukin-1 in the serum of children with severe infectious purpura. *N Engl J Med* 1988; 319: 397–400.
26. Cantagrel A, Navaux F, Loubet-Lescoulie P, Nourhashemi F, Enault G, Abbal M, Constantin A, Laroche M, Mazieres B. Interleukin-1beta, interleukin-1 receptor antagonist, interleukin-4, and interleukin-10 gene polymorphisms: Relationship to occurrence and severity of rheumatoid arthritis. *Arthritis Rheum* 1999; 42: 1093–100.
27. Tracey KJ, Beutler B, Lowry SF, Merryweather J, Wolpe S, Milsark IW, Hariri RJ, Fahey TJ 3rd, Zentella A, Albert JD, et al. Shock and tissue injury induced by recombinant human cachectin. *Science* 1986; 234: 470–4.
28. Dinarello CA. Proinflammatory and anti-inflammatory cytokines as mediators in the pathogenesis of septic shock. *Chest* 1997; 112: S321–S9.
29. Welborn MB, Oldenburg HS, Hess PJ, Huber TS, Martin TD, Rauwerda JA, Wesdorp RI, Espat NJ, Copeland EM 3rd, Moldawer LL, Sooger IM The relationship between visceral ischemia, proinflammatory cytokines, and organ injury in patients undergoing thoracoabdominal aortic aneurysm repair. *Crit Care Med* 2000; 28: 3191–7.

30. Wood JJ, Rodrick ML, O'Mahony JB, Palder SB, Saporoschetz I, D'Eon P, Mannick JA. Inadequate interleukin 2 production. A fundamental immunological deficiency in patients with major burns. *Ann Surg* 1984; 200: 311–20.
31. Kelly JL, O'Suilleabhain CB, Soberg CC, Mannick JA, Lederer JA. Severe injury triggers antigen-specific T-helper cell dysfunction. *Shock* 1999; 12: 39–45.
32. Comstock GW. Tuberculosis in twins: A re-analysis of the Prophit survey. *Am Rev Respir Dis* 1978; 117: 621–4.
33. Wilson PW, Schaefer EJ, Larson MG, Ordovas JM. Apolipoprotein E alleles and risk of coronary disease. A meta-analysis. *Arterioscler Thromb Vasc Biol* 1996; 16: 1250–5.
34. Gerdes LU, Gerdes C, Kervinen K, Savolainen M, Klausen IC, Hansen PS, Kesaniemi YA, Faergeman O. The apolipoprotein epsilon4 allele determines prognosis and the effect on prognosis of simvastatin in survivors of myocardial infarction: A substudy of the Scandinavian simvastatin survival study. *Circulation* 2000; 101: 1366–71.
35. Gray PW, Aggarwal BB, Benton CV, Bringman TS, Henzel WJ, Jarrett JA, Leung DW, Moffat B, Ng P, Svedersky LP, et al. Cloning and expression of cDNA for human lymphotoxin, a lymphokine with tumour necrosis activity. *Nature* 1984; 312: 721–4.
36. Stuber F. Effects of genomic polymorphisms on the course of sepsis: Is there a concept for gene therapy? *J Am Soc Nephrol* 2001; 12(suppl 17): S60–S4.
37. Mira JP, Cariou A, Grall F, Delclaux C, Losser MR, Heshmati F, Cheval C, Monchi M, Teboul JL, Riche F, Leleu G, Arbibe L, Mignon A, Delpech M, Dhainaut JF. Association of TNF2, a TNF-alpha promoter polymorphism, with septic shock susceptibility and mortality: A multicenter study. *JAMA* 1999; 282: 561–8.
38. Nedwin GE, Naylor SL, Sakaguchi AY, Smith D, Jarrett-Nedwin J, Pennica D, Goeddel DV, Gray PW. Human lymphotoxin and tumor necrosis factor genes: Structure, homology and chromosomal localization. *Nucleic Acids Res* 1985; 13: 6361–73.
39. Majetschak M, Flohe S, Obertacke U, Schroder J, Staubach K, Nast-Kolb D, Schade FU, Stuber F. Relation of a TNF gene polymorphism to severe sepsis in trauma patients. *Ann Surg* 1999; 230: 207–14.
40. Fang XM, Schroder S, Hoeft A, Stuber F. Comparison of two polymorphisms of the interleukin-1 gene family: Interleukin-1 receptor antagonist polymorphism contributes to susceptibility to severe sepsis. *Crit Care Med* 1999; 27: 1330–4.
41. Pociot F, Wilson AG, Nerup J, Duff GW. No independent association between a tumor necrosis factor-alpha promotor region polymorphism and insulin-dependent diabetes mellitus. *Eur J Immunol* 1993; 23: 3050–3.
42. Dinarello CA. Is there an interleukin-1 genetic predisposition to developing severe sepsis? *Crit Care Med* 1999; 27: 1397–8.
43. Christman JW, Lancaster LH, Blackwell TS. Nuclear factor kappa B: A pivotal role in the systemic inflammatory response syndrome and new target for therapy. *Intens Care Med* 1998; 24: 1131–8.
44. Arnalich F, Garcia-Palomero E, Lopez J, Jimenez M, Madero R, Renart J, Vazquez JJ, Montiel C. Predictive value of nuclear factor kappaB activity and plasma cytokine levels in patients with sepsis. *Infect Immun* 2000; 68: 1942–5.
45. Hirsch E, Irikura VM, Paul SM, Hirsh D. Functions of interleukin 1 receptor antagonist in gene knockout and overproducing mice. *Proc Natl Acad Sci USA* 1996; 93: 11008–13.
46. Fischer E, Marano MA, Van Zee KJ, Rock CS, Hawes AS, Thompson WA, DeForge L, Kenney JS, Remick DG, Bloedow DC, et al. Interleukin-1 receptor blockade improves survival and hemodynamic performance in *Escherichia coli* septic shock, but fails to alter host responses to sublethal endotoxemia. *J Clin Invest* 1992; 89: 1551–7.
47. Opal SM, Fisher CJ Jr, Dhainaut JF, Vincent JL, Brase R, Lowry SF, Sadoff JC, Slotman GJ, Levy H, Balk RA, Shelly MP, Pribble JP, LaBrecque JF, Lookabaugh J, Donovan H, Dubin H, Baughman R, Norman J, DeMaria E, Matzel K, Abraham E, Seneff M. Confirmatory interleukin-1 receptor antagonist trial in severe sepsis: A phase III, randomized, double-blind, placebo-controlled, multicenter trial. The Interleukin-1 Receptor Antagonist Sepsis Investigator Group. *Crit Care Med* 1997; 25: 1115–24.
48. Blakemore AI, Tarlow JK, Cork MJ, Gordon C, Emery P, Duff GW. Interleukin-1 receptor antagonist gene polymorphism as a disease severity factor in systemic lupus erythematosus. *Arthritis Rheum* 1994; 37: 1380–5.
49. Hurme M, Lahdenpohja N, Santtila S. Gene polymorphisms of interleukins 1 and 10 in infectious and autoimmune diseases. *Ann Med* 1998; 30: 469–73.

50. Mansfield JC, Holden H, Tarlow JK, Di Giovine FS, McDowell TL, Wilson AG, Holdsworth CD, Duff GW. Novel genetic association between ulcerative colitis and the anti-inflammatory cytokine interleukin-1 receptor antagonist. *Gastroenterology* 1994; 106: 637–42.

51. Tarlow JK, Clay FE, Cork MJ, Blakemore AI, McDonagh AJ, Messenger AG, Duff GW. Severity of alopecia areata is associated with a polymorphism in the interleukin-1 receptor antagonist gene. *J Invest Dermatol* 1994; 103: 387–90.

52. Tarlow JK, Cork MJ, Clay FE, Schmitt-Egenolf M, Crane AM, Stierle C, Boehncke WH, Eiermann TH, Blakemore AI, Bleehen SS, Sterry W, Duff GV. Association between interleukin-1 receptor antagonist (IL-1ra) gene polymorphism and early and late-onset psoriasis. *Br J Dermatol* 1997; 136: 147–8.

53. Ma P, Chen D, Pan J, Du B. Genomic polymorphism within interleukin-1 family cytokines influences the outcome of septic patients. *Crit Care Med* 2002; 30: 1046–50.

54. Arnalich F, Lopez-Maderuelo D, Codoceo R, Lopez J, Solis-Garrido LM, Capiscol C, Fernandez-Capitan C, Madero R, Montiel C. Interleukin-1 receptor antagonist gene polymorphism and mortality in patients with severe sepsis. *Clin Exp Immunol* 2002; 127: 331–6.

55. Pociot F, Molvig J, Wogensen L, Worsaae H, Nerup J. A TaqI polymorphism in the human interleukin-1 beta (IL-1 beta) gene correlates with IL-1 beta secretion in vitro. *Eur J Clin Invest* 1992; 22: 396–402.

56. Yamano S, Scott DE, Huang LY, Mikolajczyk M, Pillemer SR, Chiorini JA, Golding B, Baum BJ. Protection from experimental endotoxemia by a recombinant adeno-associated virus encoding interleukin 10. *J Gene Med* 2001; 3: 450–7.

57. Koch W, Kastrati A, Bottiger C, Mehilli J, von Beckerath N, Schomig A. Interleukin-10 and tumor necrosis factor gene polymorphisms and risk of coronary artery disease and myocardial infarction. *Atherosclerosis* 2001; 159: 137–44.

58. van der Pol WL, Huizinga TW, Vidarsson G, van der Linden MW, Jansen MD, Keijsers V, de Straat FG, Westerdaal NA, de Winkel JG, Westendorp RG. Relevance of Fcgamma receptor and interleukin-10 polymorphisms for meningococcal disease. *J Infect Dis* 2001; 184: 1548–55.

59. Marshall SE, McLaren AJ, Haldar NA, Bunce M, Morris PJ, Welsh KI. The impact of recipient cytokine genotype on acute rejection after renal transplantation. *Transplantation* 2000; 70: 1485–91.

60. Hoffmann SC, Stanley EM, Cox ED, DiMercurio BS, Koziol DE, Harlan DM, Kirk AD, Blair PJ. Ethnicity greatly influences cytokine gene polymorphism distribution. *Am J Transplant* 2002; 2: 560–7.

61. Castell JV, Geiger T, Gross V, Andus T, Walter E, Hirano T, Kishimoto T, Heinrich PC. Plasma clearance, organ distribution and target cells of interleukin-6/hepatocyte-stimulating factor in the rat. *Eur J Biochem* 1988; 177: 357–61.

62. Hack CE, De Groot ER, Felt-Bersma RJ, Nuijens JH, Strack Van Schijndel RJ, Eerenberg-Belmer AJ, Thijs LG, Aarden LA. Increased plasma levels of interleukin-6 in sepsis. *Blood* 1989; 74: 1704–10.

63. Schluter B, Konig B, Bergmann U, Muller FE, Konig W. Interleukin 6 – A potential mediator of lethal sepsis after major thermal trauma: Evidence for increased IL-6 production by peripheral blood mononuclear cells. *J Trauma* 1991; 31: 1663–70.

64. Schluter B, Raufhake C, Erren M, Schotte H, Kipp F, Rust S, Van AH, Assmann G, Berendes E. Effect of the interleukin-6 promoter polymorphism (−174 G/C) on the incidence and outcome of sepsis. *Crit Care Med* 2002; 30: 32–7.

65. Fishman D, Faulds G, Jeffery R, Mohamed-Ali V, Yudkin JS, Humphries S, Woo P. The effect of novel polymorphisms in the interleukin-6 (IL-6) gene on IL-6 transcription and plasma IL-6 levels, and an association with systemic-onset juvenile chronic arthritis. *J Clin Invest* 1998; 102: 1369–76.

66. Bohrer H, Qiu F, Zimmermann T, Zhang Y, Jllmer T, Mannel D, Bottiger BW, Stern DM, Waldherr R, Saeger HD, Ziegler R, Bierhaus A, Martin E, Nawroth PP. Role of NFkappaB in the mortality of sepsis. *J Clin Invest* 1997; 100: 972–85.

67. Schimke J, Mathison J, Morgiewicz J, Ulevitch RJ. Anti-CD14 mAb treatment provides therapeutic benefit after in vivo exposure to endotoxin. *Proc Natl Acad Sci USA* 1998; 95: 13875–80.

68. Baldini M, Lohman IC, Halonen M, Erickson RP, Holt PG, Martinez FD. A polymorphism* in the 5' flanking region of the CD14 gene is associated with circulating soluble CD14 levels and with total serum immunoglobulin E. *Am J Respir Cell Mol Biol* 1999; 20: 976–83.

69. Landmann R, Zimmerli W, Sansano S, Link S, Hahn A, Glauser MP, Calandra T. Increased circulating soluble CD14 is associated with high mortality in gram-negative septic shock. *J Infect Dis* 1995; 171: 639–44.
70. Burgmann H, Winkler S, Locker GJ, Presterl E, Laczika K, Staudinger T, Knapp S, Thalhammer F, Wenisch C, Zedwitz-Liebenstein K, Frass M, Graninger W. Increased serum concentration of soluble CD14 is a prognostic marker in gram-positive sepsis. *Clin Immunol Immunopathol* 1996; 80: 307–10.
71. Gibot S, Cariou A, Drouet L, Rossignol M, Ripoll L. Association between a genomic polymorphism within the CD14 locus and septic shock susceptibility and mortality rate. *Crit Care Med* 2002; 30: 969–73.
72. Poltorak A, He X, Smirnova I, Liu MY, Huffel CV, Du X, Birdwell D, Alejos E, Silva M, Galanos C, Freudenberg M, Ricciardi-Castagnoli P, Layton B, Beutler B. Defective LPS signaling in C3H/HeJ and C57BL/10ScCr mice: mutations in Tlr4 gene. *Science* 1998; 282: 2085–8.
73. Takeuchi O, Hoshino K, Kawai T, Sanjo H, Takada H, Ogawa T, Takeda K, Akira S. Differential roles of TLR2 and TLR4 in recognition of gram-negative and gram-positive bacterial cell wall components. *Immunity* 1999; 11: 443–51.
74. Hoshino K, Takeuchi O, Kawai T, Sanjo H, Ogawa T, Takeda Y, Takeda K, Akira S. Cutting edge: Toll-like receptor 4 (TLR4)-deficient mice are hyporesponsive to lipopolysaccharide: evidence for TLR4 as the Lps gene product. *J Immunol* 1999; 162: 3749–52.
75. Lorenz E, Mira JP, Frees KL, Schwartz DA. Relevance of mutations in the TLR4 receptor in patients with gram-negative septic shock. *Arch Intern Med* 2002; 162: 1028–32.
76. Lander ES. Array of hope. *Nat Genet* 1999; 21: 3–4.
77. Golub TR, Slonim DK, Tamayo P, Huard C, Gaasenbeek M, Mesirov JP, Coller H, Loh ML, Downing JR, Caligiuri MA, Bloomfield CD, Lander ES. Molecular classification of cancer: Class discovery and class prediction by gene expression monitoring. *Science* 1999; 286: 531–7.
78. Chung TP, Laramie JM, Province M, Cobb JP. Functional genomics of critical illness and injury. *Crit Care Med* 2002; 30: S51–S7.
79. Granucci F, Vizzardelli C, Virzi E, Rescigno M, Ricciardi-Castagnoli P. Transcriptional reprogramming of dendritic cells by differentiation stimuli. *Eur J Immunol* 2001; 31: 2539–46.
80. Winzler C, Rovere P, Rescigno M, Granucci F, Penna G, Adorini L, Zimmermann VS, Davoust J, Ricciardi-Castagnoli P. Maturation stages of mouse dendritic cells in growth factor-dependent long-term cultures. *J Exp Med* 1997; 185: 317–28.
81. Rescigno M, Citterio S, Thery C, Rittig M, Medaglini D, Pozzi G, Amigorena S, Ricciardi-Castagnoli P. Bacteria-induced neo-biosynthesis, stabilization, and surface expression of functional class I molecules in mouse dendritic cells. *Proc Natl Acad Sci USA* 1998; 95: 5229–34.
82. Chinnaiyan AM, Huber-Lang M, Kumar-Sinha C, Barrette TR, Shankar-Sinha S, Sarma VJ, Padgaonkar VA, Ward PA. Molecular signatures of sepsis: multiorgan gene expression profiles of systemic inflammation. *Am J Pathol* 2001; 159: 1199–209.

Discussion

Dr. Baracos: One of the things that really blows my mind in trying to appreciate all this comes from a couple of presentations where the investigators presented changes in gene expression using microarray approaches after an acute stimulus over time. The first question that I saw related to that has to do with a simple experimental model in which muscles were stimulated to contract and the pattern of gene expression at 1, 2 and 6 h following stimulation has genes that go up and up and up, and and then go back down again and stay down or go down and come back up again on a time frame which leads you to believe that a snap shot might even be taken of these arbitrarily chosen gene expression changes. This would lead you to have a huge amount of traffic that escapes your perception. How do you work around that?

Dr. Moldawer: Your point is exactly correct. These sophisticated procedures to assess mRNA levels have really become very simple analytical tools, and we routinely have surgical residents and graduate students perform the analyses. There is a required learning curve, and the techniques require someone with analytical sophistication, but the techniques are relatively straight-forward. The problem is that the cost to perform these studies is enormous. The Affymetrix instrument costs about USD 250,000 to purchase and USD 30,000 a year to maintain. Each chip, even with a University discount like ours, is approximately USD 400 per sample. The costs associated with sample preparation are about USD 350. So we estimate an analytical cost of approximately USD 750 for each data point. In a 13-patient study in which we have performed approximately 40 chips, the estimated cost for materials alone is about USD 35,000. So when designing these studies, we are limited by the overall number of time points and replicates available to examine changes in the pattern of expression over time. Single interval snapshots tend to be misleading, but the reality is that it is difficult to design the optimal study with all of the required time intervals. So as investigators, we are faced with a conundrum which is that you generate a great deal of incomplete data which really can either lead you astray or towards enlightenment. The challenge is how do you handle the data and how do you use the data to generate a hypothesis, and that is not an easy challenge.

Dr. Baracos: I guess I should additionally ask if that is an argument for having a presentation venue for that information, or can someone sit down and look over it on a Sunday afternoon. I mean what if you get a phone call from somebody who is reading the results of microarray analysis and asks you what you think about x protein? This gene expression has increased, and I don't see how we can have a venue for discussion even for the volume of results which might be generated by such an approach. What is not obvious to you on inspection of that list of expressed genes might be plain and evident to someone else who has a larger understanding of what those different proteins might be doing.

Dr. Moldawer: You are exactly correct. For example, we generated a list of 37 genes which seem to predict the outcome in this patient population. Several of these genes were for cytokines or inflammatory proteins that I am unfamiliar with, so I am looking at the expression profile of genes which I essentially have no knowledge of their function. I have to go to GenMapp and GenBank even to figure out their identity and function. Even with these limitations, however, there is immense power with these techniques. The power first of all is I can now take that list of genes and I can ask a specific question and test it prospectively. This is a supervised statistical method to extract data retrospectively. We do not need to know the function of these genes to use their expression for class prediction. Now the first question we need to ask is whether the genes whose expression predicted outcome, can be confirmed prospectively. So we are now going back and prospectively testing whether those 37 genes are actually predictive in the next 30 patients that we are studying. We are validating the expression by other techniques as well, because microarrays are not as good qualitatively as RT- or real-time PCR, so you need to go back and validate the expression levels with the polymerase chain reaction. Once you have validated the results, then the power of bioinformatics can be directed to start querying those pathways and networks that are invoked. In this manner, we can start to query which pathways or networks are involved in the sepsis response. Can I learn something about pathways? Is there a preferential hypothetical pathway which seems to be involved? Based on these results, you can formulate the questions to ask. And these studies can be performed quickly. The challenge is in the bioinformatics and dissecting the information from literally 800,000 data points.

Dr. Déchelotte: You said that there is a lot of convincing evidence that gene expression may be altered in various ways in these patients, but with the final products, the protein itself, do you think we can draw anything from this gene approach without having the proteomics approach together?

Dr. Moldawer: There are groups who have looked at high throughput proteomics and tried to correlate them with changes in functional genomics, and have generally shown a rather poor correlation between proteomics and genomic analyses. Now that does not negate the value of the genomics as a diagnostic tool, because it still reveals that changes in expression may not be cause and effect, but they may be prognostic. But you are indeed correct, and the problem from an analytical point of view is that the proteomics field is probably about 5 years behind the genomics field. We do have high throughput mass spectrometry techniques that can separate between 50 and 100 thousand peptide fragments from human blood, but the ability to annotate the human data base for the protein fragments is much more limited and much cruder than we have for the genornics.

Dr. Martindale: Do you feel that some day we will be doing a preoperative genetic analysis prior to a patient undergoing major surgery to predict and tell them that the risk of developing sepsis from the same insult is much higher than others?

Dr. Moldawer: Yes, I think this is inevitable. We will be doing two things. We will be doing genetic profiling in terms of single nucleotide polymorphisms (SNPs). The cost of a single SNP measurement can be reduced down to about 10 cents. Now if you have 100,000 SNPs, that is still approximately USD 10,000 per patient to profile, but these costs will undoubtedly decline, and genetic analyses will become routine. It is my belief that in the future we will not only examining SNPs in our patients and generating databases for our patients, but we will also be routinely doing transcriptome profiling, gene expression profiling, in the same patients. The technology is improving, and the costs are coming down; my belief is that it will be some time in the forseeable future.

Dr. Martindale: Then if we think about the cost of giving Xigris™, the drug you mentioned, the activated protein C is USD 7,000 per patient and we have to give it to 13 patients to see 1 responder. If we are looking at USD 7,000 dollars for the delivery of a drug, it is not really that unreasonable to think that perhaps we should look preoperatively or in the immediate to postoperative phase, saying that this person is perhaps a responder versus a nonresponder, and then treat the responders.

Dr. McClain: You are assuming that polymorphisms are playing a major role in outcome. Could it also be that the body responds in only a limited number of ways to a variety of different insults? In my particular area of expertise, the liver for example, if you have a hepatic infection, the hepatocytes undergo apoptosis with subsequent release of cytokines such as IL-8 and IL-18. These cytokines then play a role in killing the invading bacteria in a beneficial response. However, if you have hepatocyte apoptosis due to toxins such as alcohol, then the cytokine release does not kill invading bacteria but instead just amplifies a toxin-induced liver injury in a maladaptive response. Thus my question is whether polymorphisms are the major factor determining outcome. Could it also not be the particular insult, and possibly a maladaptive response to that insult, which plays a role in outcome?

Dr. Moldawer: My statement was an oversimplification. I think what we do know is that the polymorphisms will alter the level of *expression* of certain genes and that will contribute to outcome. How that contributes to outcome will be determined not only by the polymorphism of that gene, but polymorphism in other genes as well as the nature of the inflammatory stimulus. The host has what we call a common *response* element, in the liver. The acute phase response is a classic example of a common response element to a variety of different inducing stimuli. But what I think the microarray data have told us and what we are beginning to learn when we look at genome-wide and proteosome-wide scans, is that this common response element is probably greater in diversity than we had anticipated. If we look genome-wide, the diversity of the response is either determined by the genetic predisposition of the patient or the inflammatory stimulus is much broader than we had anticipated.

Dr. Cynober: I understand that there is a poor correlation between research coming from genomics and proteomics with regard to this factor. I would like to know if, in that case, it may be correct to feel that a key control point could be transcription factors, such as IP1 or NFκB, which could explain this?

Dr. Moldawer: I think there are several places where expression is regulated post-transcriptionally, and can not be detected with these microarrays. Expression can be regulated at the level of message stability but it is more likely to be at the level of protein processing. Functional genomics has no way of dealing with that issue. The activation state of kinases for I-κB as you mentioned, has nothing to do with the message expression level, it has to do with post-transcriptional processes. So the supposition that genomics will give us the entire answer is really naïve and over simplistic. What genomics gives us is another set of questions.

Dr. Cynober: You did not comment on gene polymorphism as a gene encoding for nitric oxide synthesis. Can it be of importance?

Dr. Moldawer: I did not comment a lot about gene polymorphism because it is not my strength relative to the other aspects of the presentation. My expertise on this subject is probably no better than many people present in this room. What I have seen is that there has been compelling evidence suggesting a role for these polymorphisms on outcome. The problem has been that the background frequency for the polymorphism is always unique to the population studied and the ability to translate these results to other populations is frequently difficult. For example, I know the tumor necrosis factor (TNF) gene better than nitric oxide gene, and the ability to translate the -308 polymorphism from the Finnish population to the American population has been difficult. Stuber's staff with the TNF-β locus is another example where there seem to be correlations between outcome from sepsis in some subpopulations, but not with others. Clearly, we have evaluated just the tip of the iceberg, from which we have picked out just enough information to feel comfortable that there is some importance in understanding the polymorphisms, but we haven't been able to dissect those factors which lead to the importance in outcome.

Dr. Kudsk: In the 1970s prostaglandins were the main topic and in the 1990s cytokines were the main topic and created a certain amount of enthusiasm. For example, you used samples of serum or blood cells. How do you know that this is the correct window as opposed to liver or muscle?

Dr. Moldawer: Excellent question. Dr. Baracos mentioned the studies in which they studied 12 tissues and did not identify the correct one. So we don't know the appropriate tissue compartment to sample. First of all, in hospitalized patients, we assume that it is easy to obtain peripheral blood leukocytes. It is really the only one immune cell population that you can sample reproducibly and easily. Dr. David Herndon in Texas has the ability to sample a number of other tissues from burn patients, but we don't have that capability. We sample leukocytes as a marker of the reiculoendothelial and lymphoid systems, and we admit that in fact it may not be optimal because we know that the gut and the liver are the primary organs which are involved in the immune response to endotoxemia. The issue of compartmentalization of response is a fundamental question we have not fully addressed.

Dr. Berger: We are clearly not equal when facing sepsis. In the intensive care unit we have much fewer females coming in with sepsis and they generally do better. Many reasons have been given for that. Have genomics brought any new insights to this aspect?

Dr. Moldawer: It is such a new field. I think there have probably been only 25–30 reports in the field that have applied microarrays to sepsis in critical illness. So I think it is too early to answer your question. You know the seven stages of an experiment where the first one is euphoria and the last one is recrimination, we are still in the euphoria stage with microarrays. Anti-cytokine therapies for sepsis are definitively in the recrimination stage. With microarrays, we see only the potential, we don't see the limitations yet.

Dr. Moore: From our standard epidemiology assessment, we have developed prediction modals using host factors, injury severity and indices of shock that fairly accurately predict the clinical trajectory of trauma patients within 6 to 12 hours of injury. I am struggling with how you would put genomics in such a data base and I am not quite sure how a patient who has sepsis goes on to get multiple organ failure. Exactly what causes patients to go into multiple organ failure? What do you think all those proteins are doing?

Dr. Moldawer: That is a good question without a ready answer. In fact the reason we did the study is because we don't know why so many of these patients go on to develop single-organ or multiple organ failure. You look at the comorbidities preoperatively, you look at the surgical events, and there are some patients who have a rough surgical course, they lose blood and you know they are going to have a rough post-operative course. But in the majority of patients who undergo this surgical procedure, you don't know what the outcome is going to be. In fact the general phenomenon is that on the first post-operative day these patients do pretty well, and then around days 2–4 you start seeing problems. We don't know why, we only know that if we have long ischemia times they have a worse prognosis. So the idea was to go in early, look at the leukocytes and see if the gene expression pattern would give us something that might tell us which patients are going to crash and burn, and for what reason. You have to do a lot of statistics to get 37 genes and it is a supervised statistical approach. In this regard, you have to tell the analysis who got sick and who didn't to draw out those genes. So I don't want to say that is going to be the answer, it has to be tested prospectively. But I guess the reason we took this direction, very much like some of the things we are doing with sepsis and trauma, is to try to find techniques which tell us, a little better than now, what track the patients are going to take.

Dr. Nitenberg: Your presentation is very fascinating. I don't know if you remember the Monty Python movie, The Life of Brian. When the people were coming in, those on the right were told that they were to be crucified, and those on the left that they were to be saved. It is almost the same and I don't like this idea. I prefer to keep our work in searching for what we can do in terms of therapeutic goals. Do you think that by identifying patients at risk we can modify the treatment according to genetics?

Dr. Moldawer: I am not a clinician so I can stand up here and pontificate, and not have any clinical consequences to what I say. Whereas, there are those of you who deal with these patients daily and have to live with the consequences. The only point I can make is that there was never an attempt to say we are going to withhold therapy on individual patients because their genetic background is such that their likely outcome is worse or better. What these tools really gives us is an opportunity to relatively comfortably say, look, here is a *group of patients* who, as a group, are likely to have a better or worse clinical trajectory. The way I envision their use, is we have patients whose genetic polymorphism or the microarrays, for whatever reason, suggest that they are at high risk. As a physician, you will have that additional information, and say perhaps we need to watch this patient a little more aggressively.

Dr. Déchelotte: We discussed that between genes and proteins there is a great gap and perhaps we should come back to nutrients in that field because we all know that there is a lot of evidence now that nutrients, even in the weeks before injury, may condition the expression of several genes and final products. So in your study, where we have seen these profiles predicting bad or good issues in these patients, were you able to correlate these genotypes also with some basic nutritional parameters such as body mass index or fat stores or antioxidant vitamin stores?

Dr. Moldawer: I started my talk with the apology that I haven't done nutrition research for about 10 or 15 years: I was headed out the door when one of my post-doctorates gave me an article showing the importance of TNF polymorphism in response to fish oil diets. Unfortunately I didn't have the opportunity to review the results for this group, but here is an example of where are we going. It was a study showing that the ability of fish oil to suppress ex vivo TNF production was dependent upon the polymorphism for the −308 TNF locus. I purpose we let our fish oil lover, Dr. Calder, make the final comments.

Dr. Calder: Yes, what we found was that the −308 polymorphism made people more sensitive to fish oil but so does the polymorphism in the TNF-β gene, −252 I think it is, but we don't really understand the interplay between the TNF-β gene and TNF-α production.

Dr. Moldawer: The TNF gene is located right in the middle of the major histocompatibility (MHC) class 3 complex and the linkage equilibrium between the TNF gene and MHC is not fully resolved. So the ability to dissect the contribution of the TNF polymorphism is very difficult. I apologize if I did not include your paper in the presentation.

Dr. Allison: Ljungqvist gives a simple carbohydrate drink 2 h before surgery, and this profoundly affects the metabolic and clinical changes after surgery. Is this linked through this kind of system, and if we are going to drive our car should we be sure to have a good breakfast?

Dr. Moldawer: I think technology will demand we move in this direction.

Cynober L, Moore FA (eds): Nutrition and Critical Care.
Nestlé Nutrition Workshop Series Clinical & Performance Program, Vol. 8, pp. 39–56,
Nestec Ltd.; Vevey/S. Karger AG, Basel, © 2003.

Modulation of the Post-Burn Hypermetabolic State

Jong O. Lee and David N. Herndon

University of Texas Medical Branch, Shriners Hospital for Children,
Galveston, Tex., USA

Physiologic Basis of the Hypermetabolic Response in Burn Patients

Burn patients have the highest metabolic rate of all critically ill or injured patients. The metabolic response to a severe burn injury is characterized by a hyperdynamic cardiovascular response, increased energy expenditure, accelerated glycogen and protein breakdown, lipolysis, loss of lean body mass and body weight, delayed wound healing, and immune depression [1, 2]. This response is mediated by increases in circulating levels of the catabolic hormones, catecholamines, cortisol, and glucagon [3]. Catecholamines increase up to 10 times normal. Catabolism after major burn injury begins on the 5th day after injury and continues up to 9 months later [4]. Increasing age, weight, and delay in definitive surgical treatment predict increased catabolism in children. In adults, the response increases up to age 50 where it plateaus [5]. The body surface area burned increases catabolism until a 40% body burn is reached. The magnitude of metabolic expenditure is 1.5 to twice normal in burns of greater than 40% total body surface area (TBSA). Catabolism is further increased by 50% with environmental cooling or the development of sepsis.

Hypermetabolism and muscle protein catabolism continue long after completion of wound closure [4]. Protein breakdown continues 6 and 9 months after severe burn. There is almost complete lack of bone growth for 2 years after injury resulting in long-term osteopenia which may adversely affect peak bone mass accumulation [6, 7]. Severely burned children with a burn size of >80% have a linear growth delay for years after injury [8].

Therapeutic attempts to manipulate the hypermetabolic response to severe burn injury should be sustained for at least 9 months after burn.

Nutritional and Environmental Support of Burn Patients

There is a change in the hypothalamic temperature set point after major burns such that patients are striving for a core temperature 2 °C above normal [9]. Warming rooms from 20 °C to 33 °C decreases the metabolic rate from 100% above normal to 40% above normal in burns over 40% of the body.

Despite nutritional manipulation, weight loss of up to 30% of body mass was common in burn patients prior to the use of continuous feeding [10]. Nutritional support of the hypermetabolic response in severely burned patients is best accomplished by early enteral feeding. Burn-induced intestinal ileus is not nearly as pervasive a problem as once commonly believed. Early enteral feeding with whole milk or complete elemental formulas (100% free amino acids) preserves gut mucosal integrity and improves intestinal blood flow and motility.

Caloric needs are estimated using formula created by the retrospective analysis of the calories required to maintain body weight in large patient series or by direct measurement of metabolic rate using indirect calorimetry. Overfeeding causes increases in carbon dioxide production, fatty infiltration of liver, and blood urea nitrogen. Underfeeding results in increased loss of lean body mass, muscle wasting, poor wound healing, and increased susceptibility to infection. Indirect calorimetry is performed using a mobile metabolic cart measuring the concentration of oxygen and carbon dioxide in the inspired and expired gas to determine oxygen consumption and carbon dioxide production. This can be performed at the bedside.

Total energy expenditure measured over the hospital course by stable isotope techniques is 1.2 times the resting energy expenditure (REE) measured by a metabolic chart [11]. Caloric delivery beyond $1.2 \times$ REE results in increased fat mass without attenuation of loss of lean body mass [12]. REE/predicted basal metabolic rate correlates directly with burn size, time of surgical grafting, sepsis, ventilator dependence, and muscle protein catabolism [12].

One of the most commonly used formulas for calculating caloric needs in burn patients estimates caloric needs to be 25 kcal/kg/day plus 40 kcal/% TBSA burn/day in adults; there are separate formulas for children of different ages (table 1) [13–16].

Enteral nutrition, supplied predominantly as carbohydrate and protein rather than as fat-based formula such as milk and the majority of available hospital diets, improves the net balance of skeletal muscle protein in severely burned children [17]. Muscle protein degradation is decreased with a high-carbohydrate protein diet due to increased endogenous insulin production.

Table 1. Commonly used formulas for estimating caloric requirements in pediatric burn patients at Shriners Burns Hospital in Galveston, Texas

Formula name	Age years	Formula kcal/m^2/day + kcal/m^2 burn
Galveston Infant	0–1	2,100 + 1,000
Galveston Revised	1–11	1,800 + 1,300
Galveston Adolescent	12	1,500 + 1,500

Burn patients may require exogenous insulin to control hyperglycemia. Tight euglycemic control with insulin improves wound healing and decreases infection and mortality [18, 19].

Protein breakdown is elevated in the acute, flow, and convalescent phases of burn injury [20]. Increasing protein delivery from 1.5 to 3 g nitrogen/kg/day, however, shows little benefit on whole-body protein breakdown and muscle protein synthesis rates [21].

Arginine and glutamine are not considered essential amino acids, but under severe stress they become essential dietary nutrients. Arginine is known to stimulate T lymphocytes and enhance natural killer cell function, and to stimulate synthesis of nitric oxide, which is important in communication and host resistance to infection. Arginine appears to improve immune responsiveness and promote wound healing when given as a supplement. Glutamine is a primary fuel for enterocytes. It appears to play an integral role in wound healing as well. Muscle glutamine formation is suppressed in severely hypercatabolic burned patients. There is increasing evidence that supplementation of arginine and glutamine is of benefit in critically ill patients [22].

A small quantity of fat is an essential component of nutritional support. A substantial proportion of calories delivered as fat improves glucose tolerance and decreases CO_2 production, but the hormonal environment of the burn patient causes such a great degree of endogenous lipolysis that the extent to which lipid can be utilized in the burned patient is limited.

Increased peripheral lipolysis, a principal component of the metabolic response to injury, results in fatty infiltration of the liver. This can be exacerbated by overfeeding and the use of total parenteral nutrition. Released free fatty acids are oxidized for energy and re-esterified to triglyceride in the liver. They are either deposited in the liver or further packaged for transport to other tissues. The liver weight of burn children is increased up to 2 times the liver weight of age- and sex-matched controls [23]. Mochizuki et al. [24] demonstrated an adverse effect on immune function in burned guinea pigs when diets contained more than 15% lipids. n-6 fatty acids, from vegetable and animal oils, are metabolized to yield PGE_1 and PGE_2 which have immunosuppressive properties. n-3 fatty acids from fish oil are metabolized to yield PGE$_3$, which is immunologically inert. Post-burn immunosuppression might be improved by replacing n-6 fatty acids with n-3 fatty acids. Alexander et al. [25] showed that burned guinea pigs fed a diet high in fish oil compared to safflower oil had better cell-mediated immune responses.

Electrolyte disturbances are common in burn patients and must be corrected frequently, particularly calcium and potassium. Albumin supplementation may also be necessary during the acute phase since protein loss is extensive and hepatic synthesis of constitutive proteins is decreased as the liver accelerates its production of acute-phase proteins.

Prevention of Infection, Excision and Closure of the Burn Wound

Prevention of infection and sepsis are critical therapeutic maneuvers to decrease the hypermetabolic response. The patients who develop sepsis, as defined either by a burn-specific score or one modified from the American Academy of Chest Physicians and the Society of Critical Care Medicine, have an increased metabolic rate determined by metabolic chart and an increase in protein catabolism determined by stable isotope techniques of 40% greater than that of like-sized burns throughout the hospital course and well into the time of rehabilitation [5]. The other major therapeutic modulation that has been shown to have a marked effect on metabolic rate is early excision and closure of the burn wound. Early burn wound excision with coverage using a widely meshed autograft covered with cadaver skin, and cadaver skin being used to cover all other remaining areas, results in decreased operative blood loss, decreased length of stay, fewer septic complications and decreased mortality in children and young burned adults relative to patients treated by serial debridement [5, 26–28]. Comparing patients who had total burn wound excision and coverage within 72 h of injury (early group) to a group in whom excision and coverage of wound was performed within 3–10 days after injury (middle group) and to a group whose excision was performed 10–21 days after the time of injury (late group), the net protein loss across the patients' legs increased from 0.03 (early) to 0.05 (middle) to 0.07 (late) µmol phenylalanine/min/100 cm^3 of leg blood volume, a doubling of catabolism results from delay in wound excision. It was also demonstrated that bacterial log counts in quantitative tissue cultures increased from 3 in the early treatment group to 3.5 in the middle treatment group to 4.2 in the late treatment group. The incidence of burn wound sepsis also increased during the hospital course from 20% in those excised early to 35% in those excised in a middle period and to 50% in those excised late [29].

The metabolic rate markedly increases with activity, pain and anxiety. Burn care (debridement, range of motion exercises, dressing changes and application of topical antimicrobials) increases already nearly unbearable pain levels. Maximum utilization of narcotics, sedatives, and supportive psychology help reduce these effects.

Pharmacologic Modulation of the Hypermetabolic Response in Burn Patients

Pharmacological agents have been used to attenuate catabolism and to stimulate growth in burn injury. Growth hormone, insulin, insulin-like growth hormone (IGF)/IGF-binding protein-3 (IGFBP-3), testosterone, and oxandrolone improve nitrogen balance and promote wound healing [30–34]. Tachycardia is sustained for many weeks in massively burned patients even after they are covered with autografts. The use of propranolol decreases cardiac work, myocardial oxygen consumption, resting energy consumption, lipolysis and also contributes to the maintenance of lean body mass [35].

Recombinant Human Growth Hormone

Recombinant human growth hormone (rhGH) has shown efficacy in improving muscle protein kinetics and wound healing [3, 30]. In adults, plasma growth hormone levels have been shown to decrease after severe burn [30]. rhGH administration leads to an increase in catecholamines, glucagon, and free fatty acids [3]. Administration of 0.2 mg/kg/day of rhGH accelerates donor site healing by up to 30% by increasing epithelial mitosis and synthesis of structural proteins such as collagen [36]. Accelerated healing leads to earlier burn wound coverage, decreased length of hospital stay, and decreased septic morbidity and death. Growth hormone has also been shown to increase type-1 T-helper cytokine production and decrease type-2 T-helper cytokine production [37].

Questions have been raised about the safety of administration of rhGH to adults in intensive care units by European trials that reported a significant increase in mortality among catabolic patients (exclusive of burns) treated with rhGH compared to a control group [38]. However, Ramirez et al. [39] demonstrated that rhGH treatment of severely burned children is safe and efficacious. A 2% mortality was observed in both rhGH and placebo groups, with no differences in complications or mortality. The requirements for albumin supplementation to maintain serum albumin levels above 25 g/l was reduced by more than 50% in the group receiving rhGH. Growth hormone given during acute hospitalization maintains growth in severely burned children who would otherwise experience a significant growth delay [40]. There is a significant improvement in height velocity during the first 2 years after burn in growth hormone-treated groups compared to controls [40], rhGH stimulates bone formation and muscle protein synthesis via insulin-like growth factor-I [7] successfully abating muscle catabolism and osteopenia [7, 40].

Insulin

Submaximal insulin administration produces muscle anabolism by stimulating net muscle protein synthesis in severely burned patients [18]. Insulin also improves skin graft donor site healing and improves wound matrix formation [31]. Clinical studies are underway using exogenous insulin infusions to produce euglycemic hyperinsulinemia for the duration of hospital stay in an attempt to reduce muscle breakdown and improve outcomes.

IGF-1/IGFBP-3

Administration of IGF-1/IGFBP-3 attenuates catabolism [28] and results in a decrease in interleukin-1β, tumor necrosis factor-α, and type-I acute phase protein (C-reactive protein, α$_1$-acid glycoprotein, and complement C-3) production in burned patients [32, 41].

Other anabolic agents are being investigated, such as testosterone and oxandrolone, in a search for safe and less expensive alternatives to recombinant growth hormone, IGF-I/IGFBP-3, or insulin for the treatment of burn patients.

Testosterone

Testosterone production is greatly decreased after severe burn injury, which can last for several months afterwards. Testosterone administration has been shown to ameliorate the catabolism of fasting by increasing net protein synthesis in normal men. Increased protein synthesis with testosterone is accompanied by a more efficient utilization of intracellular amino acids derived from protein breakdown and an increase in inward transport of amino acids [33]. An increase in net protein synthesis is attainable in adult men with large burns by restoring testosterone concentrations to the physiologic range [33]. Total testosterone increases significantly from baseline to the low normal range after 1 week of testosterone administration, protein synthetic efficiency increases 2-fold and protein breakdown decreases almost 2-fold resulting in an improvement in net amino acid balance [33].

Oxandrolone

Oxandrolone, an analogue of testosterone (with less androgenic effect), has been used therapeutically in Turner's syndrome and other constitutional delays of growth, in cachectic alcoholic hepatitis patients, and AIDS patients [42]. It also has been used in acute and rehabilitating adult burn patients with promising results in terms of weight gain [42]. Oxandrolone improves muscle protein metabolism in severely burned children through enhanced protein synthetic efficiency [34].

Adrenergic blockade has been used with success in pathologic hypercatecholamine states and thyrotoxicosis by decreasing myocardial workload, whole-body irritability, and tremulousness. Herndon [1] showed in 1980 that total catecholamine absence in 60% burned rats, induced by either adrenalectomy or chronic reserpine administration decreased hyper-metabolism. Wilmore et al. [43] were able to show significant decreases in metabolic rate with combined α- and β-blockade and with β-blockade alone in burned patients. This decrease in metabolic rate is associated with a decrease in pulse rate, blood pressure, minute ventilation, and free fatty acids. Several studies have demonstrated that limited β-blockade can be safely used in severely burned patients throughout the hospital course [35, 44]. No significant side effects or complications were noted in these studies. Maggi et al. [45] showed that selective β_1-blockade decreased cardiac work without adverse side effects using intravenous metoprolol administration. Five days of metoprolol administration (2.0 ± 1.1 mg/kg/day) significantly reduced heart rate and the rate-pressure product in large burns without affecting protein metabolism or lipolysis.

Nonselective β_1 and β_2 Antagonist

The most frequently used antiadrenergic agent is propranolol. Studies have shown that propranolol administered in doses of 1–2 mg/kg/day can produce a reduction in heart rate and left ventricular work of approximately 20%. In addition to decreasing heart rate and left ventricular work, propranolol administration causes decreased peripheral lipolysis, decreased tremulousness, and irritability. Propranolol treatment is a safe and effective means for mitigating the hyperdynamic cardiovascular and catabolic response to thermal injury [44].

In children with severe burns, treatment with propranolol during hospitalization attenuates hypermetabolism and reverses muscle-protein catabolism [35]. β-Blockade decreases heart rates and REE. In propranolol-treated patients muscle protein net balance improved by 82% compared to pretreatment baseline values, where it decreased by 27% in untreated controls [35]. Lean body mass was maintained by propranolol treatment compared to a 9% loss in controls [35].

Increases in metabolic rate and core temperature are characteristic responses to severe injury. Increased substrate cycling contributes to the increased thermogenesis and energy expenditure following severe burns. Increased triglyceride-fatty acid cycling is due to β adrenergic stimulation [46]. Administration of propranolol decreases peripheral lipolysis and decreases fat deposition in the liver of burn patients [8, 47].

Table 2. Cost of a daily dose of anabolic agents for a 70-kg patient

	USD[a]
rhGH, 0.2 mg/kg/day	490
Oxandrolone, 15 mg/day	21.42
Insulin, 240 units/day i.v.	83.28
Propranolol, 200 mg/day	2.56

[a] Rate in June 2002.

Table 3. Potential complications and identified incidence of anabolic agents

Drug	Complication	Incidence %
rhGH	Hyperglycemia	50[a]
	Growth arrest	0
Insulin	Hypoglycemia	50[a]
IGF-1	Hypoglycemia	25[a]
	Neuropathy	23
Oxandrolone	Hirsuitism	0
	Hepatic dysfunction	0
Propranolol	Bronchospasm	0[a]
	CV collapse	0[a]

[a] Dose-dependent.

Insulin, β-blockade with propranolol and use of the synthetic testosterone analog oxandrolone are the most cost-effective and least toxic pharmacotherapies for the treatment of the hypercatabolic responses to trauma (table 2, 3) [48].

Conclusion

Hypermetabolism is a characteristic response to severe burn which lasts up to 1-year after injury. Persistent catabolism slows rehabilitative efforts, which in turn slows meaningful return of individuals to society. Hypermetabolism can be attenuated by nutritional treatments that include enteral feeding with high-carbohydrate, high-protein feeding, possibly supplemented with n-3 fatty acids, arginine and glutamine, calcium and specific vitamins [49]. Early excision and grafting, prevention of sepsis, maintenance of a warm environment, and pain and anxiety reduction also attenuate hypermetabolism [26–29]. Growth hormone is an anabolic treatment which has been used for the last 15 years in burns and has been shown to improve wound and donor site healing, to increase growth in growth-stunted pediatric burn survivors and to increase accretion of lean body mass and bone mineral content. It can cause hyperglycemia due to peripheral insulin resistance. But these problems have been shown to be easily manageable by most groups reporting their experience with growth hormone. Recently questions have been raised about the safety of growth hormone in adult patients in the intensive care unit. A significant increase in the mortality rate of critically ill patients who were given growth hormone has been reported from two large prospective randomized trials from Europe. These results were in direct contrast to the results of many studies carried out in burn populations. While the cause of increased mortality in these European studies has not been identified, clinicians have sought other possibly safer adjunctive anabolic therapies such as insulin, IGF-1, alone or in combination with IGFBP-3, testosterone, oxandrolone and propranolol. The simplest effective anabolic strategies for severe burn injuries are early excision and grafting of the burn wound, maintenance of environmental temperature at 30–32 °C and continuous enteral feeding of a high carbohydrate, high protein diet. To further minimize erosion of lean body mass, administration of rhGH, insulin, oxandrolone or propranolol is a reasonable approach. Exogenous continuous insulin infusion, β-blockade with propranolol, and administration of the synthetic testosterone analog, oxandrolone, are the most cost-effective and least toxic pharmacotherapies to date [48].

References

1. Herndon DN. Mediators of metabolism. *J Trauma* 1981; 21: 701–5.
2. Takagi K, Suzuki F, Barrow RE, Wolf SE. Recombinant human growth hormone modulates Th1 and Th2 cytokine response in burned mice. *Ann Surg* 1998; 228: 106–11.
3. Fleming RYD, Rutan RL, Jahoor F, Barrow RE, Wolfe RR, Herndon DN. Effects of recombinant human growth hormone on catabolic hormones and free fatty acids following thermal injury. *J Trauma* 1992; 32: 698–702.
4. Hart DW, Wolf SE, Mlcak R, Chinkes Dl, Ramzy PI, Obeng MK, Wolfe RR. Persistence of muscle catabolism after severe burn. *Surgery* 2000; 128: 312–9.
5. Hart DW, Wolf SE, Chinkes DL, Gore DC, Mlcak RP, Beauford RB, Obeng MK, Lal S, Gold WF, Wolfe RR, Herndon DN. Determinants of skeletal muscle catabolism after severe burn. *Ann Surg* 2000; 232: 455–65.
6. Klein GL, Herndon DN, Langman CB, Rutan TC, Young WE, Pembleton G, Nusynowitz M, Barnett JL, Broemeling LD, Sailer DE, McCauley RL. Long-term reduction in bone mass after severe burn injury in children. *J Pediatr* 1995; 126: 252–6.
7. Klein GL, Wolf SE, Goodman WG, Phillips WA, Herndon DN. The management of acute bone loss in severe catabolism due to burn injury. *Horm Res* 1997; 48: 83–7.
8. Rutan RL, Herndon DN. Growth delay in postburn pediatric patients. *Arch Surg* 1990; 125: 392–5.
9. Herndon DN, Captain MD, Wilmore DW, Mason AD. Development and analysis of a small animal model simulating the human postburn hypermetabolic response. *J Surg Res* 1978; 25: 394–403.
10. Newsome TW, Mason AD, Pruitt BA. Weight loss following thermal injury. *Ann Surg* 1973; 178: 215–7
11. Goran MI, Peters EJ, Herndon DN, Wolfe RR. Total energy expenditure in burned children using the doubly labeled water technique. *Am J Physiol* 1990; 259; E576–E85.
12. Hart DW, Wolf SE, Herndon DN, Chinkes DL, Lal SO, Obeng MK, Beauford RB, Mlcak RP. Energy expenditure and caloric balance after burn: Increased feeding leads to fat rather than lean mass accretion. *Ann Surg* 2002; 235: 152–61.

13. Curreri PW. Assessing nutritional needs for the burned patient. *J Trauma* 1990; 30: S20–S3.
14. Hildreth M, Herndon DN, Desai MH, Broemeling LD. Caloric requirement of patients with burns under one year of age. *J Burn Care Rehabil* 1993; 14: 108–12.
15. Hildreth M, Herndon DN, Desai MH, Broemeling LD. Current treatment reduces calories required to maintain weight in pediatric patients with burns. *J Burn Care Rehabil* 1990; 11: 405–9.
16. Hildreth M, Herndon DN, Desai MH, Duke M. Caloric needs of adolescent patients with burns. *J Burn Care Rehabil* 1989; 10: 523–6.
17. Hart DW, Wolf SE, Zhang XJ, Chinkes DL, Buffalo MC, Matin SI, DebRoy MA, Wolfe RR, Herndon DN. Efficacy of a high-carbohydrate diet in catabolic illness. *Crit Care Med* 2001; 29: 1318–24.
18. Ferrando AA, Chinkes DL, Wolf SE, Matin S, Herndon DN, Wolfe RR. A submaximal dose of insulin promotes net skeletal muscle protein synthesis in patients with severe burns. *Ann Surg* 1999; 229: 11–8.
19. Van Der Berghe G, Wouters P, Weekers F, VerAqest C, Bruyninckx F, Schetz M, Vlasselaers D, Ferdniande P, Lauwers P, Bouillon R. Intensive insulin therapy in critically ill patients. *N Engl J Med* 2001; 345: 1359–67.
20. Jahoor F, Desai M, Herndon DN, Wolfe RR. Dynamics of the protein metabolic response to burn injury. *Metabolism* 1988; 37: 330–7.
21. Patterson BW, Nguyen T, Pierre EJ, Herndon DN, Wolfe RR. Urea and protein metabolism in burned children: Effect of dietary protein intake. *Metab Clin Exp* 1997; 46: 573–8.
22. Biolo G, Fleming RYD, Maggi SP, Nguyen TT, Herndon DN, Wolfe RR. Inhibition of muscle glutamine formation in hypercatabolic patients. *Clin Sci* 2000; 99: 189–94.
23. Barret JP, Jeschke MG, Herndon DN. Fatty infiltration of the liver in severely burned pediatric patients: autopsy findings and clinical implications. *J Trauma* 2001; 51: 736–9.
24. Mochizuki H, Trocki O, Dominioni L, Ray MB, Alexander JW. Optimal lipid content for enteral diets following thermal injury. *JPEN J Parenter Enteral Nutr* 1984; 638–46.
25. Alexander JW, Saito H, Trocki O, Ogle CK. The importance of lipid type in the diet after burn injury. *Ann Surg* 1986; 204: 1–8.
26. Herndon DN, Barrow RE, Rutan RL, Rutan TC, Desai MH, Abston S. A comparison of conservative versus early excision therapies in severely burned patients. *Ann Surg* 1989; 209: 547–53.
27. Gray DT, Pine RW, Horner TJ, Marvin J, Engrav L. Early surgical excision versus conventional therapy in patients with 20 to 40% burns – A comparative study. *Am J Surg* 1982; 144: 76–80.
28. Moral SW, Saffle SR, Sullivan JJ, Larsen CM, Warden GD. Increased survival after major thermal injury. A nine-year review. *Am J Surg* 1987; 154: 623–7.
29. Hart DW, Wolf SE, Chinkes DL, Beauford RB, Mlcak RP, Heggers JP, Wolfe RR, Herndon DN. Effects of early excision and aggressive enteral feeding on hypermetabolism, catabolism and sepsis after severe burn. *J Trauma*, in press.
30. Wolf SE, Barrow RE, Herndon DN. Growth hormone and IGF-I therapy in the hypercatabolic patient. *Baillieres Clin Endocrinol Metabol* 1996; 10: 447–63.
31. Pierre E, Barrow R, Hawkins H, Nguyen TT, Sakurai Y, Desai M, Wolfe RR, Herndon DN. Effects of insulin on wound healing. *J Trauma* 1998; 44: 342–5.
32. Herndon DN, Ramzy PI, DebRoy MA, Zheng M, Ferrando AA, Chinkes DL, Barret JP, Wolfe RR, Wolf SE. Muscle protein catabolism after severe burn: Effect of IGF-1/IGFBP-3 treatment. *Ann Surg* 1999; 229: 713–20.
33. Ferrando AA, Sheffield-Moore M, Wolf SE, Herndon DN, Wolfe RR. Testosterone administration in severe burns ameliorates muscle catabolism. *Crit Care Med* 2001; 29: 1936–42.
34. Hart DW, Wolf SE, Ramzy PI, Beauford RB, Ferrando AA, Wolfe RR, Herndon DN. Anabolic effects of oxandrolone after severe burn. *Ann Surg* 2001; 233: 556–64.
35. Herndon DN, Hart DW, Wolf SE, Chinkes DL, Wolfe RR. Reversal of catabolism by beta-blockade after severe burns. *N Engl J Med* 2001; 345: 1223–9.
36. Herndon DN, Barrow RE, Kunkel KR, Broemeling LD, Rutan RL. Effects of recombinant human growth hormone on donor-site healing in severely burned children. *Ann Surg* 1990; 212: 424–31.
37. Takagi K, Suzuki F, Barrow RE, Wolf SE, Herndon DN. Recombinant human growth hormone modulates Th1 and Th2 cytokine response in burned mice. *Ann Surg* 1998; 228: 106–11.

38. Takala J, Ruokonen E, Webster NR, Nielsen MS, Zandstra DF, Vundelinckx G, Hinds CJ. Increased mortality with growth hormone treatment in critically ill adults. *N Engl J Med* 1999; 341: 785–92.
39. Ramirez RJ, Wolf SE, Barrow RE, Herndon DN. Growth hormone treatment in pediatric burns: A safe therapeutic approach. *Ann Surg* 1998; 228: 439–48.
40. Low JFA, Barrow RE, Mittendorfer B, Jeschke MG, Chinkes DL, Herndon DN. The effect of short-term growth hormone treatment on growth and energy expenditure in burned children. *Burns* 2001; 27: 447–52.
41. Jeschke MG, Barrow RE, Herndon DN. Insulin-like growth factor I plus insulin-like growth factor binding protein 3 attenuates the proinflammatory acute phase response in severely burned children. *Ann Surg* 2000; 231: 246–52.
42. Sheffield-Moore M, Urban RJ, Wolf SE, Jiang J, Catlin DH, Herndon DN, Wolfe RR, Ferrando AA. Short-term oxandrolone administration stimulates net muscle protein synthesis in young men. *J Clin Endocrinol Metab* 1999; 84: 2705–11.
43. Wilmore DW, Long JA, Mason AD, Skreen RW, Pruitt BA. Catecholamines: Mediator of the hypermetabolic response to thermal injury. *Ann Surg* 1974; 180: 653–69.
44. Minifee PK, Barrow RE, Abston S, Desai MH, Herndon DN. Improved myocardial oxygen utilization following propranolol infusion in adolescents with postburn hypermetabolism. *J Pediatr Surg* 1989; 24: 806–11.
45. Maggi SP, Biolo G, Muller MJ, Barrow RE, Wolfe RR, Herndon DN. B1 blockade decreases cardiac work without affecting protein breakdown or lipolysis in severely burned patients. *Surg Forum* 1993; 44: 25–7.
46. Wolfe RR, Herndon DN, Jahoor F, Miyoshi H, Wolfe M. Effect of severe burn injury on substrate cycling by glucose and fatty acids. *N Engl J Med* 1987; 317: 403–8.
47. Aarsland A, Chinkes D, Wolfe RR, Barrow RE, Nelson SO, Pierre E, Herndon DN. Beta-blockade lowers peripheral lipolysis in burn patients receiving growth hormone. *Ann Surg* 1996; 223: 777–89.
48. Hart DW, Wolf SE, Chinkes DL, Wolfe RR. Anabolic strategies after severe burn. *J Am Coll Surg,* in press.
49. Jeschke MJ, Hendon DN, Ebener C, Barrow RE, Jauch KW. Nutritional intervention high in vitamins: Protein, amino acid and omega-3 fatty acids improves protein metabolism during the hypermetabolic state after thermal injury. *Arch Surg* 2001; 136: 1301–6.

Discussion

Dr. Moldawer: You made the statement earlier on that a 40% full-thickness burn was your threshold for intervention. Is that all right, is that across all comers depending upon age, prior initial nutritional status, co-existing morbidity, does that 40% hold up?

Dr. Herndon: Certainly not, the answer to your question is that co-morbidity, pre-existing starvation, pre-existing sepsis or other traumas will increase or change that threshold. I meant to say that only in pure burn is the threshold around 40%. With other pre-existing diseases or co-morbidities or co-traumas that threshold changes greatly. What I would suggest practically is to determine the resting energy expenditure after the first 5 days after injury to determine whether a patient is hypermetabolic, then you should introduce therapy or you should get genetic profiles and see what the single nucleotide variation is.

Dr. Moldawer: What is it about 40%? Is it the resting energy expenditure, is that the inflexion point, is that the criteria then that you use?

Dr. Herndon: Over the many burns that we have studied, it takes this size of injury alone to cause the increase in resting energy expenditure and the protein catabolism which have been our phenotypic markers in the past, and we can't correct upon the endogenous responses in smaller burns. However, a 30% burn with a fracture we can; a 30% burn with a small keenolation injury we can, and a 30% burn with delay in

49

resuscitation which causes a perfusion-reperfusion injury, like aortic aneurysm for example, we can.

Dr. Moore: I spoke to you a bit earlier about the study by van den Berghe et al. [1] in the *New England Journal of Medicine* on the use of intensive insulin therapy in critically ill patients. They randomized about 1,500 patients and showed reductions in sepsis, mortality, and poly-neuropathy of critical illness. They propose that by keeping the glucose low that they are somehow modulating the immune response. I don't know if this is true, what are your thoughts? And the second question, is just how aggressive do you need to be? We are placing people on continuous insulin drips of roughly 7 to 10 units of insulin an hour, and there have been some problems with hypoglycemia.

Dr. Herndon: Yes, I think the continuous use of insulin throughout the hospital course in appropriately monitored ICUs is a very potentially useful therapy. Its primary effect, as I have measured it, has been general improvement in protein synthesis and an improvement in protein synthesis in healing wounds. The needed dose for these effects is much lower than we originally had found. We studied hyper-insulinemic euglycemic clamps in which we were initially giving 10–20 units/h throughout the hospital course and this was efficacious. But if, for instance, the nurse turned off the enteral feeding for some reason, if you use total parenteral nutrition (TPN) and somebody shut that off, then you get a hyperglycemic person developing sepsis and ileus and becoming hyperglycemic unless continuously monitored. We have recently found that in burn patients just to maintain type euglycemia, their plasma glucose should be 8.4–9.0 mmol/l throughout the hospital course, presumably because of the increase in glucose flow and not necessarily insulin resistance. But if you give them 2–4 units of insulin/h throughout the hospital course they don't become hyperglycemic, their plasma glucose is around 5.6 mmol/l type euglycemic control considering that they are continuously getting 1,500 kcal/m^2 plus 1,500 kcal/m^2 burn they get a high carbohydrate protein diet. The difficulties come with ileus or therapeutic mistakes or turning the feeding off during operation, then you can have disastrous hyperglycemic episodes. So it is only under purely control conditions that I think this is a psiatory effect and I do think that looking at immune responsiveness in this setting is also required. I think there are psiatory effects.

Dr. Martindale: I am interested in your comments about hypercaloric feeding when you are monitoring the patient so they have more adipose tissue. What about hypocaloric feeding in the burn population in the critical care setting? We feed our obese population hypocalorically, and we are now leading towards feeding normal-sized patients hypocalorically. What about in the burn population?

Dr. Herndon: How do you define hypocaloric? I think you need to feed sufficiently to maintain lean body mass, to have sufficient protein delivery and glucose delivery to maximize the host-defense mechanism. What that threshold is, in any particular disease state, remains to be seen. Hypocaloric relative to what we use to think was appropriate certainly, absolutely hypocaloric definitively not.

Dr. Cynober: You got very impressive results with different anabolic agents. From a practical point of view I would like to know which ones you are using routinely in your clinical practice.

Dr. Herndon: I don't really have a routine clinical practice in that everybody who comes to our institute is involved in some sort of clinical trial. But if I would recommend what I would routinely use today on other people, it would be oxandrolone and propranolol in combination during the acute hospital stay, except in ICUs where insulin can be given safely in low monitored doses, then perhaps that would be a more psiatory agent than oxandrolone. Insulin also causes epithelial mitosis and production of proteins that are psiatory by the epithelium and are important to me. It may well be that both oxandrolone and propranolol will have immunological effects, but if you believe that we do worse with oxandrolone and go the wrong way, insulin would be the better and preferred agent in combination with propranolol in units that can handle it.

Dr. Cynober: I think this is an important issue because this type of research is in principle to improve the care of the patient and if, for example, you have a 40% improvement in protein synthesis with IGF-1, logically we should try to further improve and provide IGF-1 to all the patients and to look at what happens even, for example, in addition to propranolol.

Dr. Herndon: I think that those are psiatory benefits in the data I did not have time to show today. I believe that we have to treat our patients not just during the acute hospital course but we must look hard at their convalescence, 6, 9 and 12 months after injury, the use of exercise and anabolic agents can markedly improve protein mass, lean body mass and growth in children if we refocus our efforts away from just the ICU towards convalescence.

Dr. Cynober: Of course to make anabolism you need anabolic agents but you also need amino acids to make proteins. Have you some special view and recommendation about amino acids in burn patients and the potential synergistic effect between amino acids and anabolic agents?

Dr. Herndon: I don't have a lot to say about that scientifically. The studies that we have performed show that 1 g/kg/day of protein is as efficacious as 3 g/kg/day of amino acids, that you can only handle so much amino acid before it just flows over, similar to glucose. As far as which amino acid is best, I do have some papers on that but it goes a little bit out of the scope. But glutamine and arginine do have a place as supplements but I don't want to plug that too much right now.

Dr. Berger: Two questions, one about the timing of oxandrolone. Clearly our patients change with time and there is worry about hepatic function with early oxandrolone. While insulin is currently used early on, would you use an early time point for initiating oxandrolone? What would your criteria be?

Dr. Herndon: We have not been instituting any of these anabolic agents until the 5th day after the first operation which would be about day 5 after ICU admission, and day 7 after admission, bearing in mind that my patients are in hospital for a month or so. Oxandrolone is an agent that we are using for long-term treatment to try to improve muscle mass over time, insulin is a better ICU agent theoretically.

Dr. Berger: So you would agree with starting with insulin and, when the acute phase response fails, to introduce oxandrolone or something like that.

Dr. Herndon: That is probably a reasonable strategy.

Dr. Berger: The second question is about growth hormone in children and the difference with adults. It is known that in children there is a depression in growth hormone and so on. Would you think this could be an explanation for the better response to growth hormone in children than in the adults who are not obviously deficient?

Dr. Herndon: There are probably many reasons for differences with age and response to this. Quite clearly children who are growth hormone-deficient an bringing their levels back up improve their growth, improve their albumin synthesis, decrease the acute phase response, improve the wound healing.

Those results, not being been translatable to adults, may have any number of reasons. Clearly adults get more hyperglycemic, they get more hyperlipidemic, their cardiac output effects of growth hormone may actually be deleterious to an older population whereas children love it. They already have a fixed tachycardia and growth hormone helps the cardiac output and improves oxygen and substrate delivery. Those things can't happen in adults.

Dr. Berger: When would you start them on it, just timing?

Dr. Herndon: In children again I don't start any anabolic agent until Dr. Cuthbertson has said the ebb phase is over. So about 5 days; his findings have guided me for a long time.

Dr. Kudsk: I should comment on studies that we did when I was in Tennessee. I think that the findings you have are relevant. They have to be tested in individual populations. We tried growth hormone and IGF-1 and oxandrolone in our trauma population. Growth hormone had a real effect upon constitutive proteins but did not have much of an effect on nitrogen balance. Hyperglycemia was only a problem when the patients developed an infection. IGF-1 also had an effect on constitutive proteins. We did a study with the University of Kentucky. The patients had positive nitrogen balance at least until the binding proteins were inhibited. Oxandronole had no effect. These findings were recently published [2]. This has to be tested in individual patient populations.

Dr. Chioléro: I have an additional question concerning anabolic therapy since you have nicely shown that there are a lot of possibilities. But when you combine drugs there is the possibility of interaction, for example insulin and β-blockade. Have you done any studies on combined therapy?

Dr. Herndon: I have many currently running studies on combined therapy. In the last one that was published in the *Annals of Surgery*, I gave growth hormone and propranolol and found that when I gave propranolol the growth hormone effects were inhibited, but conversely the growth hormone effects did not inhibit the propranolol effects. So your comment is well taken that combination therapies need to be studied for interactions and this alphametric technique also helps you a lot in seeing what genes are regulated and not regulated by each individual therapy, and how the combination therapies can affect it. You can then go on and look at the proteins that were varied in those experiments and that might help us come to grips more quickly with the drug interactions.

Dr. McClain: Many of your patients had fatty liver. Do you think this is analogous to the fatty liver that you see with obesity where an over-production of cytokines is seen and the patients are insulin-resistant?

Dr. Herndon: I think that there may be major corollaries between those. The fatty infiltration in liver seen after major injuries has been seen as a non-phenomenon or something that really does not cause morbidity. I think it is a very significant and a huge phenomenon. Most people have said it is due to TPN or overfeeding, but I am not sure that this bears out either. I think it is more a catecholamine effect which causes profound peripheral lipolysis and the liver cannot export fat in the form of very low density lipoproteins. We recently published a paper in the *Annals of Surgery* showing that there is too much fat coming into the liver and you can't get rid of it under these circumstances. Whether you hypocalorically feed or not, this phenomenon occurs: just feeding pure protein and sugar and no fat it still occurs, and it is something that needs to be addressed by specific purpose. I don't think it is a non-phenomenon, I think it leads to liver failure and to multiple organ failure in the debts of disease.

Dr. McClain: It is a critical phenomenon because when you try to transplant those livers, the patients die because those are dysfunctional or 'bad' livers.

Dr. Herndon: Our thoughts for the last 40 years that the livers were alright are wrong, I think there are bad livers.

Dr. McClave: The comment you made about the effects of these hormonal therapies on protein metabolism and propranolol reducing the phenotypic expression of the response: the question is are these really surrogated end points, how many of these hormonal therapies actually affected outcome parameters? Oxandrolone for alcoholic hepatitis did all of the things on proteins that you mentioned but really had almost no effect on outcome.

Dr. Herndon: I think that is an absolutely key sort of question. Of course my outcome parameters are very long-term. Short-term enhanced acute outcome parameters, there is virtually no effect in these small studies that I am describing. There have been huge effects on growth and huge effects on strength when you look at people at 6, 9, 12 and 24 months. So my outcome parameters, unlike many in the literature on trauma, go beyond this charge and well into the convalescence. I think we need to do that when we are looking at an inflammatory hypermetabolic response that sets up when an acute insult establishes itself, and maintains itself for very prolonged periods of time. So all of these have had profound effects on long-term outcome indicators, they have had very little effect on short-term mortality infectious disease-type indicators, though there are many biochemical indicators that show that it is doing something in the acute phase.

Dr. Nitenberg: Just to make a point, you are specially dealing with burn patients?

Dr. Herndon: Children with burns.

Dr. Nitenberg: We are talking about critical care in this meeting, so I want to be sure that there is no confusion because I have some experience with β-blockade in ICU patients and I can say that I have killed patients with this practice. We tried that with Bekins 20 years ago and that was the result. We have had the same experience with growth hormone and, as Dr. Kudsk said, I think we have to modulate our experience with this type of hormone and hormone manipulation in acutely ill patients depending on the level of trace. Do you agree with that?

Dr. Herndon: I certainly agree that you need to be very careful translating results in children to adults. I do think the burn patients are definitely critically ill individuals and are a superb example of critically ill individuals. I am very sorry that you killed people with propranolol, I would point out that this is due to a little lack of attention to details, and I would also say that killing people with growth hormone is due to a lack of attention to detail. So I would advise in any study to be very conscious about utilizing these profound modulators of the response.

Dr. Cynober: To react to Dr. Nitenberg's statement. You were abrupt in saying that human growth hormone killed adult patients in the ICU because, among various reasons I have read, the Takala et al. [3] study showed that the nitrogen support of the patients was very low, 0.15 mg/kg/day, and there are some speculations open for discussion. Of course the speculation about the fact that by blocking muscle the amino acid was an insult for the patient because there was no sufficient amount of amino acids to synthesize in the liver some of the proteins which are required in response to injury. Those results were published 2 years.

Dr. Nitenberg: I agree with you. I don't say that growth hormone is especially lethal in every patient. I said that in this type of patients in this type of experiment it killed patients. My point was we must be careful in using this type of hormone in patients. That is the only thing I want to say because, for example, to use β-blockade in septic patients is clearly dangerous. Dr. Herndon is dealing with children who are in a stable situation over a long time. In this type of patient you can probably manipulate the hormones very easily. In acutely ill patients with one hint, a second hint, a third hint, you can't do that very easily and you are probably being harmful. That is the point.

Dr. Herndon: I would like to respond just briefly to the comment. Many evidence-based articles, including a very large one in the *New England Journal of Medicine* showing the decreased mortality with β-blockade, not only during acute hospitalization but with a long-term outcome, have shown that the use of β-blocking agents in individuals undergoing major operative trauma, pre- and peri-operatively, causes the overall decrease in myocardial advance with the utilization of that agent over time. So I am not arguing with you that a drug was certainly misused causing difficulties with it, but I think that careful utilization can be safe and done for great benefit to patients.

Dr. Zazzo: A few years ago, in major surgery Kelhet and Kolics demonstrated a positive metabolic effect of epidural analgesia and early nutrition. Have you any data on the strict use of analgesia without other drugs and do you think that good analgesia could be added to your list?

Dr. Herndon: Absolutely, I think that the apherin stimulators that cause the central hyperdynamic response, the stress response, are greatly augmented and modulated by pain and any technique that can ameliorate the pain response will down-regulate the apherin stimulator, and it should be studied and tried and encouraged.

Dr. Moore: Your data on TPN being harmful supports my bias. You are dealing with very hypermetabolic patients and, if you are not using TPN, how do you meet their caloric goals and is that important early in their hospital course or do you just feed them high protein enteral diets and as time goes on you are able to get up to a reasonable rate?

Dr. Herndon: Actually in burn patients if you start feeding them immediately after the burn injury you can get to full caloric maintenance within 24 or 36 h at the time of injury. The ileus that has been described in the past immediately after injury is, I believe, generally an edema problem that can be greatly reduced by using the gut, stimulating it with food earlier on and increasing blood flow, and perhaps by not giving as much lactate as you are known to do in the other parts of Texas.

Dr. Moore: Do you feed into the stomach or post-pyloric?

Dr. Herndon: I feed into the stomach initially because it takes a while to get post-pyloric. I used to feed entirely just the stomach and not post-pylorically, and it has become a fad to feed post-pylorically and I do it sort of 50/50.

Dr. Moore: So you try to get people on positive caloric balance as soon as possible.

Dr. Herndon: That is correct.

Dr. Allison: It is sort of reassuring that if you stick around long enough you come back into fashion again. We started using insulin in the 1960s and 1970s and published data [4], and I want to echo Dr. Cynober's point that one of the effects of insulin is that you are limiting the endogenous amino acid supply, so you should not only give enough glucose to prevent hyperglycemia, and as a diabetologist I would suggest that if you are getting hyperglycemia you may not be managing the situation very well, you should also give adequate protein or amino acid with your insulin. The other thing we showed was that one of the major responses to injury which has not been mentioned is that you get salt and water retention, and you just mentioned the edema problem. One of the things we showed with insulin was that not only maintaining an adequate intravascular volume was important in enabling patients to excrete an excess salt and water load but, in contrast to the effect of insulin in obesity which causes the salt and water retention, these people had massive diuresis of salt and water following the insulin, and so that is another way in which insulin might be effective in this situation. I don't know whether with modern management you get much problem in that direction but I would be interested to know if you have any observations on this.

Dr. Herndon: Our earlier studies are still right on and we appreciate them.

Dr. Ngwu: From a dietetic point of view we know that patients have some factors affecting their nutrient intake, something like appetite, something like stress. Should we target giving them diets that are recommended dietary allowances, especially in areas where TPN is not very active, or do you have other standards to measure their nutrient intake?

Dr. Herndon: This is a very important comment. I think that you can give continuous enteral feeding to populations with great efficacy but you need to be very careful about measuring how much that is because it is often exaggerated, from self reporting and reporting of others. I think we are going to have a debate about TPN versus other feedings later. Maybe we can expand on them.

Dr. Baracos: I would like to ask you, with so much success with therapies that are both anti-catabolic and hyper-anabolic, where do you have any catabolic patients left? I don't mean to be cynical, what I want to ask really is do you have any patients that you believe are intractable to those things that you do? Are you presently aware of and what do you think might be going on in those instances? What fraction of your patients do you believe have an anabolic or catabolic problem that you don't presently have the means to manage?

Dr. Herndon: Quite clearly those individuals who become septic are more catabolic than patients just catabolic from the injury itself, and we and others in this room have read extensively about such patients making it hard to handle glucose and protein and other regular nutrients. So a septic patient is very difficult to handle with anabolic agents and is more intransigent to anabolic agents though insulin seems to be the one to use particularly in septic individuals, you get another inter-current stress and it remains problematic. I did not mean to say we have conquered the mountain here. We cannot maintain lean body mass except by assiduous utilization of anabolic agents in those patients who cannot tolerate enteral feeding and require TPN. We still develop exacerbation of immune suppression and do not reach anabolic goals.

Dr. Baracos: In addition to that you have your benchmark at a reasonable expectation of promoting the lean body mass, i.e. skeletal muscles in instances where the patients are completely bedridden.

Dr. Herndon: I have put up this slide just to point out that exercise and physical therapy are absolutely required to maintain lean body mass, early institution of physical therapy and exercise are critical in that effort. You can maintain nitrogen balance with anabolic agents but I would say not without some form of physical therapy.

Dr. Allison: Boulder in Buffalo was eccentric, he used to exercise his patients in the ICU, bag them as they walked up and down.

Dr. Herndon: He was eccentric but smart.

Dr. Rosenfeld: Welhara and Hill almost 2 years ago demonstrated that septic and trauma patients increased their metabolic rate about 2-fold after the first week. Have you observed this in burn patients and have you observed a necessity to change the anti-catabolic strategy you planned?

Dr. Herndon: Yes, our time course for seeing the increase in metabolic rates in the data of Dr. Cuthbertson shows an ebb phase for about a week or so after injury then it reaches a maximum at 7–15 days after injury and remains elevated, at least I hope I have shown here not just throughout the hospital course but well into the 1st year or 2 after injury. I generally do not begin anti-catabolic or anabolic agents until the ebb phase or the relatively hypermetabolic phase has been completed. Some of the studies by Dr. Moldawer and others show that the genetic evidence, the genetic effects that may set up this inflammatory response, may occur in the first minutes or hours after injury and the typical endocrinologic phenotypic response is maximized in your studies at 1–2 weeks after injury.

Dr. Chioléro: An additional comment on the route of feeding since we all agree that enteral feeding should be implemented in burn patients, there is no question about that. However, concerning the statement that TPN is a poison in such patients, I am not sure it is supported by the literature, since most of the papers that were published on the bad effect of TPN are old papers, the patients received hyper-alimentation, and they had too much fat with all solutions. So, at least in adults, when enteral nutritional support is difficult in our units, we sometimes add TPN to patients and they do well.

Dr. Herndon: I certainly don't want to be dogmatic about the paper, when I tried TPN augmentation and maximal enteral feeding that was 10–15 years ago, and clearly more reason than superior techniques may modify those results and don't have to be repeated. We fortunately have been able to get away with just enteral feeding in the last 20 years in the treatment of burns without TPN, but there is no question and no disrespect intended to current practices elsewhere.

Dr. Allison: Could you speculate on something that has always been a mystery to me. As you just said, how this inflammatory store perpetuates this metabolic response for such a period of time long beyond the point where the neuroendocrine and the inflammatory storm is over is unknown. Maybe there is some persistent neuroendocrine effect. Why do you, particularly in burns, get this very prolonged effect?

Dr. Herndon: I am currently stupefied by that question and terribly interested in trying to gain some insight into it. It might be the persistent development of hypertrophic care in this patient population providing persistent inflammatory foci, sufficient to cause an already revved up engine to rise, but that is hypothesis and certainly not a fact, which continues to intrigue me and I will continue to look.

References

1. Van den Berghe G, Wouters P, Weekers F, et al. Intensive insulin therapy in critically ill patients. *N Engl J Med* 2001; 345: 1359–67.
2. Gervasio JM, Dickerson RN, Swearingen J, et al. Oxandrolone in trauma patients. *Pharmacotherapy* 2000; 20: 1328–34.
3. Takala J, Ruokonen E, Webster NR, et al. Increased mortality associated with growth hormone in critically ill adults. *N Engl J Med* 1999; 341: 785–92.
4. Hinton P, Allison SP, Littlejohn S, Lloyd J. Insulin and glucose to reduce catabolic response to injury in burned patients. *Lancet* 1971; i: 767–9.

Cynober L, Moore FA (eds): Nutrition and Critical Care.
Nestlé Nutrition Workshop Series Clinical & Performance Program, Vol. 8, pp. 57–73,
Nestec Ltd.; Vevey/S. Karger AG, Basel, © 2003.

Nutrition Support in Critical Illness: Amino Acids

Peter Stehle

Department of Nutrition Science, University Bonn,
Bonn, Germany

Introduction

The general approach to the nutritional care of the catabolic, malnourished or critically ill patient involves delivery of a balanced diet including energy (in the form of carbohydrates and lipids), an adequate amount of nitrogen, all essential nutrients (amino acids, fatty acids, vitamins, electrolytes) and fluid [1]. Traditionally, the qualitative and quantitative composition of dietetic measures in patients was derived from recommended daily allowances for healthy adults with addition of a so-called 'safety margin'. In the past 2 decades, this view has been fundamentally modified. Firstly, overwhelming evidence has been brought forward that critical illness is associated with profound alterations in carbohydrate, lipid, and protein metabolism [2, 3]. Consequently, nutrient demands of patients can considerably differ in comparison with healthy adults. Presently, great efforts are being undertaken to define 'disease-related' recommendations and, in line with this novel concept, to provide 'tailor-made' formulas for specific patient groups like children, renal and liver diseases, and critical illness. Secondly, evidence was found that various nutrients including amino acids and fatty acids possess more than the well-known 'nutritive' effects on body function and metabolism [4]. In vitro and in vivo studies showed that nutrients can modify the immune response as well as the integrity of organs and tissues in health and disease in a dose-dependent manner. Moreover, the extent and target of this 'pharmacological' effect can be controlled by the timing and the way (oral/enteral, intravenous) of substrate administration. Indeed, this approach opens the possibility to modulate the metabolic response to stress.

This chapter briefly reviews the role of selected amino acids as conditionally indispensable substrates (*nutritive approach*) and as modifying agents (*pharmacological approach*) in the therapy of critically ill patients.

The Nutritive Approach: Conditionally Indispensable Amino Acids

On the basis of long-term clinical studies and with the availability of improved analytical technologies, it became evident that some clinical conditions are associated with particular amino acid deficiencies, antagonisms or imbalances which then cause specific changes in amino acid metabolism and requirements. Accordingly, amino acids are nowadays classified as *indispensable, conditionally indispensable* and *dispensable* substrates [5, 6] (table 1). This new approach of categorizing amino acids recognizes the functional and physiological properties of a given substrate under various pathological states as well as the ratio of supply to demand. Accordingly, certain amino acids known as nonessential substrates for healthy adults have to be reconsidered as 'conditionally indispensable' substrates in stressed patients and, thus, must be part of nutritional support.

In this respect, *glutamine* seems to be of utmost importance for the critically ill. There are numerous data available showing that hypercatabolic and hypermetabolic situations are accompanied by glutamine deprivation. During prolonged starvation [7], after elective operations, major injury, burns, infections [8] and pancreatitis [9], intramuscular glutamine concentrations declined considerably regardless of nutritional efforts. This reduction in the muscle-free glutamine pool (about 50% of normal) can be seen as a typical feature of injury and malnutrition; the extent and duration of the depletion being proportional to the severity of the illness [10]. Recent studies underlined that glutamine deprivation is mainly caused by trauma-induced alterations in the interorgan glutamine flow [10]. Muscle and, as postulated,

Table 1. New classification of nutritive amino acids

Indispensable amino acids
  Amino acids which cannot be synthesized endogenously

Conditionally indispensable amino acids
  Amino acids which exhibit a considerably increased need in certain diseased situations
  Amino acids which cannot be synthesized in adequate amounts due to disease-dependent limited/impaired synthesis

Dispensable amino acids
  Amino acids which can be sufficiently synthesized by transamination

---

Table 2. Consumers and producers of endogenous glutamine during metabolic stress

Consumers	
Gastrointestinal tract, g/day	11–15
Kidneys, g/day	4
Immunecompetent cells, g/day	2–4
Producers	
Muscle, g/day	8–10
Lung (?), g/day	1–2
Balance, g/day	minus 12

lung glutamine efflux are accelerated to provide substrate for the gut, immune cells, and the kidneys [11, 12] explaining the profound decline in muscle-free glutamine concentration. Even under maximum glutamine efflux from the muscle, endogenous provision cannot meet the increased demands of glutamine consumers. Based on recent calculations, glutamine balance is negative with approximately 12 g/day (table 2).

Numerous studies in different patient groups have convincingly shown that inadequate glutamine supply contributes to impaired cell metabolism [for references see 8]. Exogenous provision of glutamine is, thus, a necessary replacement of a deficiency rather than a supplementation.

While the role of glutamine as an indispensable substrate in the critically ill is widely accepted, the way and the timing of glutamine administration is still under discussion. Two unfavorable chemical properties hamper the use of free glutamine itself as nutrition substrate in routine clinical setting [13]: (1) instability especially during heat sterilization and prolonged storage, and (2) limited solubility (~3 g/100 ml at 20 °C). The rate of breakdown of free glutamine depends on temperature, pH, and anion concentration. Indeed, this decomposition of free glutamine is quantitative and yields the cyclic product pyroglutamic acid and ammonia.

Among the approaches discussed [14], the implication of stable and highly soluble synthetic dipeptides shows great promise as an effective route for the provision of amino acids otherwise difficult to deliver [15]. Dipeptides with a glutamine residue at the C terminal position reveal high solubility in water (glycyl-*L*-glutamine, Gly-Gln, 154 g/l; *L*-alanyl-*L*-glutamine, Ala-Gln, 568 g/l) and sufficient stability during heat sterilization and prolonged storage. These properties qualify the dipeptides to be approved by the authorities as suitable constituents of liquid nutritional preparations.

In various clinical studies, the beneficial effects of parenteral glutamine dipeptide administration on the metabolic response to stress and patient outcome and recovery have been shown [for references see 8]. A recent multicenter study performed between 1997 and 1998 in 11 centers in Europe with a total of 126 patients showed better daily and cumulative nitrogen balances with glutamine dipeptide than in the control group [16, 17]. Despite the heterogenous material, the length of hospital stay was 2.0 days shorter in the test group (21%) as compared with the controls. Plasma-free glutamine was in the low normal range before operation and showed a significantly higher concentration with supplemental Ala-Gln, while in the controls plasma glutamine levels remained unchanged. The length of hospital stay could be calculated in one of the centers with similar degrees of illness showing significantly reduced hospitalization with glutamine peptide [17]. The time of hospitalization for both test and control groups is also depicted by the Kaplan-Meier probability diagram, clearly demonstrating a reduction in hospital stay with Ala-Gln. Group stratification, length of operation, intraoperative blood loss and type of operation were considered independent variables for entry into the model of the Cox regression. This analysis revealed clearly that hospital stay was significantly dependent on the total parenteral nutrition (TPN) regimen and was not influenced by the type of surgery, length of operation or intraoperative blood loss.

In a current study, 95 patients were randomized and treated for more than 5 days and 68 patients for 9 days or more to receive either standard parenteral nutrition or supplemented TPN with Ala-Gln (0.3 g/kg body weight). Fourty-six patients received the dipeptide supplement and 49 served as controls. Six-month survival was improved for patients treated for 9 days or longer with glutamine supplementation (66.7%) vs. patients receiving standard TPN (40%; fig. 1). In the dipeptide-treated group plasma-free glutamine concentrations increased after 6–9 days. These results support the notion that replacement of glutamine deficiency may correct excess mortality in intensive care unit (ICU) patients due to inadequate parenteral nutrition [18].

A novel finding is the striking influence of supplemental glutamine dipeptide on cysteinyl-leukotriene (Cys-LT) metabolism. Cys-LTs are potent lipid mediators. It has been emphasized that diminished release of these mediators is accompanied by an attenuated endogenous host defense [19]. After surgery, the low Cys-LT concentration in isolated polymorphonuclear leukocytes was completely restored with supplemental dipeptide while remaining low with conventional TPN [20]. It is well known that the highly charged glutamic acid molecule, one of the direct precursors of glutathione, is poorly transported across the cell membrane whereas glutamine is readily taken up by the cell. Glutamine is then deaminated and can, thus, be used as a glutamic acid precursor. Accordingly, it is proposed that the capacity of cysteinyl-leukotriene generation might be normalized with supplemental glutamine [21].

In contrast to the beneficial results seen with parenterally supplemented glutamine, there was no improvement in nitrogen balance, protein synthesis and other variables relating to nitrogen economy when glutamine-enriched tube feeds were administered in short-term trials in ICU patients [22, 23]. Enteral tube feeds supplemented with L-glutamine failed to increase or even

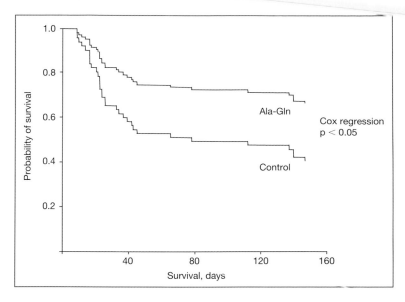

Fig. 1. Survival plot of a subgroup of parenterally fed patients treated for 9 days and longer under standardized conditions. Ala-Gln = 1.2 g/g body weight standard amino acid solution plus 0.3 g/g body weight/day alanyl-glutamine; control = 1.5 g/g body weight standard amino acid solution. Reproduced with permission from Goeters et al. [18].

to normalize plasma glutamine levels in adult or pediatric ICU patients [24]. Oral glutamine supplementation in cancer patients did not prevent the occurrence of doxifluridine-induced diarrhea and had no impact on tumor response to chemotherapy [25]. The results are somewhat at variance with the findings of Conversano et al. [26], who reported a decrease in both the duration and severity of gastrointestinal symptoms with oral glutamine supplementation.

In adult patients glutamine has been shown to have a beneficial effect on intestinal barrier function when given orally (30 g/day) for several weeks following high-dose chemotherapy or radiotherapy for esophageal cancer [27]. In a pilot study, 'swish and swallow' therapy with 4 × 2 g glutamine/day for 28 days reduced the symptoms of severe stomatitis following extensive chemotherapy [28]. Following this pilot study, a large randomized clinical trial was done on the effects of oral glutamine on stomatitits in 195 bone marrow transplant patients [29]. Less mouth pain, less difficulties in eating, and a reduction in the use of opioids were found with a low dose of glutamine, and the 28-day survival rate was improved in the glutamine group. In contrast, a randomized, placebo-controlled, double-blind study in 24 mucositis patients showed no benefit of oral glutamine (16 g/day) over placebo [30].

The possible reasons for the less favorable results with enteral glutamine supplementation are multifactorial. The presence of bacterial overgrowth in stressed patients might in part explain the observed low circulating glutamine concentrations, as it is well known that bacteria readily consume glutamine as a preferred substrate. It is also possible that prompt splanchnic glutamine utilization may contribute to the inability of glutamine-enriched enteral feeds to increase the plasma glutamine levels. Glutamine is absorbed in the upper part of the small intestine and subsequently metabolized in the liver, and thus it may not be available in sufficient quantity for the target mucosal tissue at the lower sites of the intestine.

In a current study of a more heterogenous group of ICU patients capable of tolerating enteral feeding [31], many of whom were already infected on admission, there was no suggestion of reduced mortality, but overall postintervention hospital costs were significantly reduced in both enteral and parenteral glutamine recipients. In a randomized, double-blind study oral and parenteral glutamine supplementation was evaluated in 66 bone marrow transplant patients. Unfortunately, the investigators did not distinguish between enteral (oral) and parenteral treatment. Nevertheless, there was a suggestion of a possibly improved long-term survival [32].

In conclusion, it is to mention that lack of glutamine supply in glutamine-deprived critically ill patients will be associated with symptoms such as impaired gut barrier function, immune response and protein economy which then unfavorably influence outcome. An adequate provision of this indispensable amino acid (about 15 g glutamine corresponding to about 25 g glutamine dipeptide) is, thus, mandatory.

The Pharmacological Approach: Amino Acids with Additional Functions

As already outlined in the Introduction, several amino acids possess additional 'pharmacological' functions on the molecular/cellular level. Provision of these amino acids outside a potential metabolic need can beneficially modify the metabolic response to a given trauma. Within the ICU, the use of arginine and cysteine as modulating agents are extensively discussed.

Arginine may be of significance in the critically ill because of its potential role in immunomodulation [33, 34]. It is hypothesized that (high-dose) arginine enhances the depressed immune response of individuals suffering from injury, surgical trauma, malnutrition or sepsis. In experimental animals as well as in human studies, supplementation with arginine resulted in an improved cellular response, a decrease in trauma-induced reduction in the T-cell function and a higher phagocytosis rate [33]. Innate host cellular cytotoxicity, mediated in part by natural killer (NK) and lymphokine-activated killer (LAK) cells, is thought to play an important role in the inhibition of tumor growth and the reduction in metabolic spread. Arginine supplementation has been shown to enhance NK and LAK cytotoxicity [for references see 34]. Interestingly, a daily supply of 30–35 g of arginine is claimed to retard tumor growth and to diminish tumor metastasis [35, 36]. On the other hand, it has been reported that substituting ornithine for arginine in parenteral regimens will ameliorate an arginine-related increase in growth of a Ward colon tumor [37].

Clinical studies administering arginine enterally have demonstrated moderately improved net nitrogen retention and protein synthesis compared to isonitrogenous low arginine diets in critically ill and injured patients. Following surgery for certain malignancies in elderly postoperative patients, supplemental arginine (25 g/day) enhanced T-lymphocyte responses to phytohemagglutinin and concanavalin A and increased the CD4 phenotype number. Interestingly, IGF-1 levels were about 50% higher reflecting the growth hormone secretion induced by arginine supplementation. A high load of oral arginine (30 g/day) improved wound healing [35] and enhanced the blastogenic response to several mitogens [38]. On the other hand, some of these studies were also associated with in vitro evidence of enhanced immunoactivity [33, 39, 40]. However, these results did not demonstrate improvements in overall patient outcome or length of hospital stay [41].

Recently, arginine was shown to be the unique substrate for the production of the biological effector molecule nitric oxide (NO). NO is formed by oxidation of one of the two identical terminal guanidino groups of L-arginine by the enzyme NO synthase (NOS). Of the three NOS isoenzymes characterized, two are constitutive, Ca^{2+}-dependent (endothelial, eNOS, and neuronal, nNOS), and generate lesser levels of NO than their inducible counterpart (iNOS) [42]. iNOS is prominent in inflammatory conditions and it is also most often implicated as the producer of NO during the immune response. According to recent reports, NO plays an essential role in the regulation of inflammation and immunity. Interestingly, parenteral arginine may improve myocardial ischemia in patients with obstructive coronary artery disease by producing nonstereospecific peripheral vasodilation thereby improving endothelium-dependent vasodilation. This effect is certainly due to stimulation of insulin-dependent NO release or nonenzymatic NO generation [43].

There are some highly interesting studies elucidating the potential role of the sulfur-containing amino acid *cysteine* as a modulating substrate [44]. Macrophages act as cysteine transporters under the action of inflammatory stimuli such as endotoxin and TNF. The uptake of cysteine in macrophages is competitively inhibited by glutamate [45]. During episodes of immunosuppression or in diseases with compromised immunocompetence such as AIDS and malignancy, increased extra- and intracellular glutamate concentrations are observed [46].

Cysteine also enhances a number of lymphocyte functions, such as cytotoxic T-cell activity. A high glutamate/cysteine ratio is associated with a low share of T-helper cells [47]. N-Acetyl-cysteine, reduced glutathione and

Table 3. Provision of amino acids in critical illness – a personal suggestion

Basic nutritive support (about 1.2–1.5 g amino acids/kg body weight)	
Indispensable amino acids, %	45–50
Dispensable amino acids, %	30–35
Conditionally indispensable amino acids	
Glutamine, %	10–15
Modulation of stress response (depending on individual situation)	
Arginine, g/day	8–12
Cysteine, g/day	about 2

cysteine inhibit the expression of the nuclear transcription factor in stimulated T-cell lines [48]. This observation might provide an interesting approach in the treatment of viral diseases like AIDS, since the transcription factor is necessary to express the human immunodeficiency virus (HIV) mRNA. In fact, in vitro studies demonstrate that the stimulatory effects on tumor necrosis factor, induced by free radicals, on HIV replication in monocytes can be inhibited by sulfhydryl compounds [47]. These basic studies indicate that treatment of inflammatory diseases and AIDS with sulfhydryl compounds may be beneficial, and powerful arguments have been advanced in favor of such treatment [47]. Clinical studies using this strategy are not yet available. One reason might be the lack of suitable preparations.

Conclusion

According to our present knowledge, an adequate provision of amino acids in the ICU is based on two approaches (table 3). (1) It is now widely accepted that a balanced nutritional support (oral/enteral and/or parenteral) considering all indispensable and conditionally indispensable amino acids is a prerequisite to improve/maintain the metabolic stauts of the ICU patient thereby beneficially influencing patient outcome. (2) The (high-dose) supplementation of specific 'modulating' amino acids can help to optimize healing processes. Since these effects are influenced by timing and way of administration as well as the situation of the patient, these measures must be planned and performed individually.

References

1. Wilmore DW. The practice of clinical nutrition: How to prepare for the future. *JPEN J Parenter Enteral Nutr* 1989; 13: 337–43.
2. Fürst P. Intracellular muscle free amino acids – Their measurements and function. *Proc Nutr Soc* 1983; 42: 451–62.

3. Fürst P. Carbohydrate, lipid, and protein metabolism in the critically ill patient. In: Ronco C, Bellomo R, eds. *Critical care nephrology*. Amsterdam: Kluwer Academic, 1998; 355–73.
4. Stehle P, Grimble RF. Neutraceutics: A novel approach in nutrition prevention and therapy. *Curr Opin Clin Nutr Metab Care* 1998; 1: 525–6.
5. Laidlaw SA, Kopple JD. Newer concepts of the indispensable amino acids. *Am J Clin Nutr* 1987; 46: 593–605.
6. Stehle P, Kuhn KS, Fürst P. From structure to function: What should be known about building blocks of protein. In: Pichard C, Kudsk KA, eds. *From nutrition support to pharmacologic nutrition in the ICU. Update in intensive care and emergency medicine*. Berlin: Springer, 2000; 34: 26–37.
7. Elwyn DH. Nutritional requirements of stressed patients. In: The Society of Critical Care Medicine, ed. *Textbook of critical care*. Philadelphia: Saunders, 1988; 223–7.
8. Fürst P, Stehle P. Glutamine and glutamine-containing dipeptides. In: Cynober L, ed. *Amino acid metabolism and therapy in health and nutritional disease*. Boca Raton: CRC Press, in press.
9. Karner J, Roth E. Alanylglutamine infusions to patients with acute pancreatitis. *Clin Nutr* 1990; 9: 43–5.
10. Fürst P. Regulation of intracellular metabolism of amino acids. In: Bozzetti F, Dionigi R, eds. *Nutrition in trauma and cancer sepsis*. Basel: Karger, 1985; 21–53.
11. Souba WW. Glutamine – A key substrate for the splanchnic bed. *Annu Rev Nutr* 1991; 11: 285–308.
12. Windmueller HG, Spaeth AE. Respiratory fuels and nitrogen metabolism in vivo in small intestine of fed rats. Quantitative importance of glutamine, glutamate and aspartate. *J Biol Chem* 1980; 255: 107–12.
13. Meister A. Metabolism of glutamine. *Physiol Rev* 1956; 36: 103–27.
14. Fürst P. New developments in glutamine delivery. *J Nutr* 2001; 131: S2562–S8.
15. Fürst P, Pogan K, Stehle P. Glutamine dipeptides in clinical nutrition. *Nutrition* 1997; 13: 731–7.
16. Fürst P. Effects of supplemental parenteral L-alanyl-L-glutamine (Ala-Gln) following elective operation. A European multicenter study. *Clin Nutr* 1999; 18: 16.
17. Mertes N, Schulzki C, Goeters C, Winde G, Benzing S, Kuhn KS, Van Aken H, Stehle P, Fürst P. Cost containment through L-alanyl-L-glutamine supplemented total parenteral nutrition after major abdominal surgery: A prospective randomized double-blind controlled study. *Clin Nutr* 2000; 19: 395–401.
18. Goeters C, Wenn A, Mertes N, Wempe C, Van Aken H, Stehle P, Bone HG. Parenteral L-alanyl-L-glutamine improves 6-month outcome in critically ill patients. *Crit Care Med* 2002; 30: 2032–37.
19. Köller M, König W, Brom J, Raulff M, Gross-Weege W, Erbs G, Müller FE. Generation of leukotrienes from human polymorphonuclear granulocytes of severely burned patients *J Trauma* 1988; 28: 733–40.
20. Morlion BJ, Stehle P, Wachtler P, Siedhoff HP, Köller M, König W, Fürst P, Puchstein C. Total parenteral nutrition with glutamine dipeptide after major abdominal surgery. *Ann Surg* 1998; 227: 302–8.
21. Morlion BJ, Torwesten E, Kuhn KS, Puchstein C, Fürst P. Cysteinylleukotriene generation as a biomarker for survival in the critically ill. *Crit Care Med* 2000; 28: 3655–8.
22. Long CL, Nelson KM, DiRienzo DB, Weiss JK, Stahl RD, Broussard TD, Theus WL, Clark JA, Pinson TW, Geiger JW, et al. Glutamine supplemented enteral nutrition: Impact on whole body protein kinetics and glucose metabolism in critically ill patients. *JPEN J Parenter Enteral Nutr* 1995; 19: 470–6.
23. Jensen GL, Miller RH, Talabiska DG, Fish J, Gianferante L. A double-blind, prospective, randomized study of glutamine-enriched compared with standard peptide-based feeding in critically ill patients. *Am J Clin Nutr* 1996; 64: 615–21.
24. Houdijk AP, Rijnsburger ER, Jansen J, Wesdorp RI, Weiss JK, McCamish MA, Teerlink T, Meuwissen SG, Haarman HJ, Thijs LG, van Leeuwen PA. Randomised trial of glutamine-enriched enteral nutrition on infectious morbidity in patients with multiple trauma. *Lancet* 1998; 352: 772–6.
25. Bozzetti F, Biganzoli L, Gavazzi C, Cappuzzo F, Carnaghi C, Buzzoni R, Dibartolomeo M, Baietta E. Glutamine supplementation in cancer patients receiving chemotherapy. A double-blind randomized study. *Nutrition* 1997; 13: 748–51.

26. Conversano L, Muscaritoli M, Petti MC. Effects of oral glutamine on high-dose chemotherapy (HDCT)-induced gastrointestinal toxicity in acute leukaemia patients: A pilot study. *Clin Nutr* 1995; 14: 6.
27. Yoshida S, Matsui M, Shirouzu Y, Fujita H, Yamana H, Shirouzu K. Effects of glutamine supplements and radiochemotherapy on systemic immune and gut barrier function in patients with advanced esophageal cancer. *Ann Surg* 1998; 227: 485–91.
28. Skubitz KM, Anderson PM. Oral glutamine to prevent chemotherapy induced stomatitis: A pilot study. *J Lab Clin Med* 1996; 127: 223–8.
29. Anderson PM, Ramsay NK, Shu XO, Rydholm N, Rogosheske J, Nicklow R, Weisdorf DJ, Skubitz KM. Effect of low-dose oral glutamine on painful stomatitis during bone marrow transplantation. *Bone Marrow Transplant* 1998; 22: 339–44.
30. Houdijk APJ. Glutamine-enriched enteral nutrition in patients with multiple trauma. *Lancet* 1998; 352: 1553.
31. Powell-Tuck J, Jamieson CP, Bettany GE, Obeid O, Fawcett HV, Archer C, Murphy DL. A double-blind, randomized, controlled trial of glutamine supplementation in parenteral nutrition. *Gut* 1999; 45: 82–8.
32. Schloerb PR, Skikne BS. Oral and parenteral glutamine in bone marrow transplantation: A randomized double-blind study. *JPEN J Parenter Enteral Nutr* 1999; 23: 117–22.
33. Kirk SJ, Barbul A. Role of arginine in trauma, sepsis, and immunity. *JPEN J Parenter Enteral Nutr* 1990; 14: S226–S9.
34. Evoy D, Lieberman MD, Fahey TJ III, Daly JM. Immunonutrition: The role of arginine. *Nutrition* 1998; 14: 611–7.
35. Barbul A. Arginine and immune function. *Nutrition* 1990; 6: 53–8.
36. Daly JM, Reynolds J, Sigal RK, Shou J, Liberman MD. Effect of dietary protein and amino acids on immune function. *Crit Care Med* 1990; 18: S86–S93.
37. Grossie VBJ. Citrulline and arginine increase the growth of the Ward colon tumor in parenterally fed rats. *Nutr Cancer* 1996; 26: 91–7.
38. Sodeyama M, Gardiner KR, Regan MC, Kirk SJ, Efron G, Barbul A. Sepsis impairs gut amino acid absorption. *Am J Surg* 1993; 165: 150–4.
39. Brittenden J, Park KG, Heys SD, Ross C, Ashby J, Ah-See A, Eremin O. L-Arginine stimulates host defenses in patients with breast cancer. *Surgery* 1994; 115: 205–12.
40. Beaumier L, Castillo L, Ajami AM, Young VR. Urea cycle intermediate kinetics and nitrate excretion at normal and 'therapeutic' intakes of arginine in humans. *Am J Physiol* 1995; 269: E884–E96.
41. Lin E, Goncalves JA, Lowry SF. Efficacy of nutritional pharmacology in surgical patients. *Curr Opin Clin Nutr Metab Care* 1998; 1: 41–50.
42. Nathan C, Xie Q. Nitric oxide synthases: Rolls, tolls and controls. *Cell* 1994; 78: 915–8.
43. Quyyumi AA. Does acute improvement of endothelial dysfunction in coronary artery disease improve myocardial ischemia? A double-blind comparison of parenteral D- and L-arginine. *J Am Coll Cardiol* 1998; 32: 904–11.
44. Grimble RF, Grimble GK. Immunonutrition: Role of sulfur amino acids, related amino acids, and polyamines. *Nutrition* 1998; 14: 605–10.
45. Grimble RF. Nutritional antioxidants and the modulation of inflammation: Theory and practice. *New Horiz* 1994; 2: 175–85.
46. Ollenschläger G, Jansen S, Schindler J, Rasokat H, Schrappe-Bächer M, Roth E. Plasma amino acid pattern of patients with HIV infection. *Clin Chem* 1988; 34: 1787–9.
47. Dröge W. Cysteine and glutathione deficiency in AIDS patients: A rationale for the treatment with N-acetyl-cysteine. *Pharmacology* 1993; 46: 61–5.
48. Mihm S, Ennen J, Pessagra U. Inhibition of HIV-1 replication and NFkB activity by cysteine and cysteine derivatives. *AIDS* 1991; 5: 497–503.

Discussion

Dr. De Bandt: I don't know if we have to thank you or Dr. Stehle. Perhaps some of his opinions are not exactly yours, when you state in your first slide that we must see glutamine in the context of balanced nutrition and arginine as an immunonutrient, because you said that you have to test an isonitrogenous diet to assess the effect of this nutrient and, if we take your word, we have to supply a very large amount of nitrogen in order to obtain an isonitrogenous diet compared with a glutamine-supplemented diet. So do you really consider it as a balanced diet?

Dr. Cynober: It is a balanced diet if you are providing extra nitrogen in both groups. This is a matter of controversy and it is an important point which can explain discrepancies in the literature. There are two ways to achieve an isonitrogenous diet. The first one is to provide an amount of nitrogen which will cover the basal requirements and then in 1 group you add the amount of glutamine required, for example 20 g/day, and in the other group you add a mixture of nonessential amino acids to avoid pharmacological or toxic effects. The second way to achieve an isonitrogenous intake is to include glutamine in the basal regimen as well as for the mixture of nonessential amino acids, but by making that you are in fact decreasing the amount of all essential amino acids and also nonessential amino acids, making the glutamine group clearly disadvantaged. This may explain why, for example if we consider that glutamine is efficient in modulating the response to stress and even if there is some pharmacokinetic difference between glycyl-glutamine and alanyl-glutamine, in fact most of the studies indicate positive results with alanyl-glutamine and not with glycyl-glutamine. The difference between the two peptides from a practical point of view is that alanyl-glutamine is a powder you have to add to a standard solution. It is the first way to proceed as I described. On the contrary glycyl-glutamine is included in parenteral nutritional solutions and included in the total nitrogen intake.

Dr. Allison: Let me provoke you on a tendentious part. Overcoming that nitrogen problem you could perhaps give α-ketogluterate. Can I provoke you on that one?

Dr. Cynober: About what results?

Dr. Allison: As an alternative to glutamine.

Dr. Cynober: It is certainly an interesting molecule for several reasons. One is the fact that it is not only a precursor of glutamine but also a precursor of arginine, polyamines, and also it elicits very strong growth hormone secretion when provided by the parenteral route, and insulin secretion when given by the oral and enteral route. Clearly this molecule appears to be very efficient, for example in burn injury, because 3 different reports indicated that α-ketoglutarate administration in the range of 20 g/day dramatically improved wound healing [1–3]. Note that there is no report on glutamine in burn patients. I don't know why but it is the fact. Of course it is my point of view and not Dr. Stehle's.

Dr. Rosenfeld: You talked about balanced nutritional support and I feel like an imbalanced solution with this recommendation. I would like your comment about the promotion of ureagenesis or increasing urea production and the necessity of dialysis in these patients with these recommendations, principally in older patients.

Dr. Cynober: You mean about patients suffering organ failure such as kidney failure?

Dr. Rosenfeld: Some patients are not really in renal failure but they have a decrease in renal function.

Dr. Cynober: I am not really competent on the problem of nutrition in kidney insufficiency, but what I heard recently at a congress was that the decreased intake of amino acids in such a situation was a dogma, and the fact that, except in certain cases, these patients can very well support a balanced mixture of amino acids and there is no reason to restrict these patients. I don't know if more competent people agree with that or not.

Dr. Déchelotte: I would like to add some recent experience in this field because at ASPEN we recently presented a prospective study of 114 patients treated with glutamine dipeptide as glutamine or standard isonitrogenous control. Of course at the beginning we selected patients without renal insufficiency, above 250 µmol/l creatinine for any contraindication of parenteral nutrition, but afterwards during the treatment period, about 5–10 days, we were not able to detect any impairment in renal function even with these patients receiving 1.5 g/kg/day amino acids plus 0.5 g dipeptide/kg/day. So as far as renal function is concerned I think this safety margin with dipeptide was rather high, probably higher than we thought because of the nitrogen intake. And there are some experimental data that could at least lead one to think that glutamine may have beneficial effects on renal function because it increases acid output for instance.

Dr. Planas Vila: Due to the interference between glutamine and growth hormone treatment in the anabolic response, do you know if there are some clinical studies in ill patients on the association of growth hormone and glutamine?

Dr. Cynober: There are some studies dealing with gastrointestinal patients, studies by Scolapio et al. [4, 5] and by Byrne et al. [6]. A total of 4 or 5 studies, and I saw the first study performed by Byrne et al. [6] which provided positive results combining glutamine and growth hormone, and the last one is a French study by Messin et al. (unpublished). I think, all the subsequent studies failed to show any advantage of providing glutamine and growth hormone together.

Dr. Baracos: I need you to help me out with an explanation of something. In one of Dr. Stehle's slides you have two categories, balanced nutritional support I understand that for amino acids, that is only amino acids in the rate balance according to some requirements. And then you have something that you call pharmaconutrition, or immunological nutrition, and since it is not in the category of balanced I think that means imbalanced, and that is the interpretation people take away from that categorization. And I, quite frankly, don't understand this definition. I think some amino acid feeding is balanced nutritional support and someone is always telling me, oh no, that is pharmaconutrition, and in fact there are other people who are telling me that a certain supplementation of fatty acids is not actually nutritional support, it is pharmaconutrition, and I still don't understand the distinction.

Dr. Cynober: I will try to answer. I did not have the opportunity to read Dr. Stehle's manuscript and I did not discuss it with him but I feel that I understand what he means by this distinction. Clearly glutamine supplementation is helpful and useful when there is glutamine deficiency. If you are providing a glutamine-enriched diet to healthy subjects nothing happens. For example, there was a study some years ago by Fox et al. [7] in healthy subjects or in healthy rats and they provided glutamine-enriched nutrition to rats treated by methotrexate or to control rats. In the control rat group glutamine had absolutely no effect on any parameter but, providing a glutamine-enriched diet in methotrexate-treated animals dramatically improved nitrogen balance and a certain number of other parameters. Clearly glutamine displays anabolic properties, regulatory properties, but when the glutamine levels are normal there is absolutely no reason for these properties to work. There is another example with the administration of a glutamine-enriched diet in heavy sport training, and in that situation the decrease in the glutamine pool is very moderate, and almost all authors failed to identify any improvement in immunological function and so on by providing a glutamine-enriched diet, except perhaps the preliminary study by Parry-Billings et al. [8] some years ago. Now with arginine it is very different because the studies by

Yu et al. [9] with stable isotopes indicate that there is clearly an increase in arginine turnover in stress situations, for example after burn injury, but the requirements of arginine are not fulfilled by de novo synthesis at 80 or 85%, and the arginine pool is very dependent on regular protein intake. And what we are researching by providing a high amount of arginine is to have a true pharmacological effect because by providing a high amount of arginine we are upregulating plasma levels, and therefore the intracellular production of nitric oxide is parallel with arginine availability in plasma in such a situation. This explains this pharmacological effect. This is also the case with the production of growth hormone following an intravenous arginine secretion because this effect on growth hormone secretion is only dependent on the arginine plasma levels. Therefore I feel that we are following two different logics with these two amino acids. And finally I mentioned that to my knowledge there is no positive effect in providing glutamine to healthy subjects. On the contrary, there are several reports, especially from Barbul [10], indicating the benefit of high arginine intake in healthy subjects.

Dr. De Bandt: I will make myself the devil's advocate in saying that there are some situations, perhaps not in critically ill patients, where small amounts of arginine have beneficial effects, for example in diabetes and atherosclerosis. There can be decreased availability of arginine in this situation, though I don't think we can make a clear black and white distinction between the two categories.

Dr. Bouletreau: Could you comment a little more on whether something is known about the optimal dosage of arginine in our intensive care unit (ICU) patients and the optimal moment to give it, regarding its role in nitric oxide production?

Dr. Cynober: To date to the best of my knowledge there is no study ranging those effects and there are discussions about the fact. Dr. Stehle presented only the wide side, the study by Gianotti et al. [11], but there are several experimental studies in the same model which clearly indicate that huge amounts of arginine actually decrease survival, and there is a metaanalysis by Heyland et al. [12]. There are a lot of papers, but I am not willing to start such a debate because I know that Dr. Martindale will give a lecture on this topic and it will be unfair to discuss this now, but I will be happy to discuss this fascinating point after Dr. Martindale's lecture.

Dr. Heyland: I look forward to that further discussion on arginine but I did want to ask you some questions related to glutamine. One point is that none of our critically ill patients are the same and if we say that glutamine deficiency is a result of catabolic stress and, we talked about this this morning, that there are various forms of stress and variations in individual patients' responses to those stressors, I am just wondering if there is a better way of identifying or characterizing those patients who are truly glutamine-deficient and therefore would benefit from glutamine supplementation, than thinking that all critically ill patients may benefit from glutamine supplementation? Do we need to measure plasma glutamine levels or are there some other biochemical or clinical parameters that would help us discriminate what populations with critical illness would benefit the most?

Dr. Cynober: We can look at proteomics and so on, but the measurements of plasma concentrations of amino acids are very debatable because as you know it is just a reflection between the rate of appearance and the rate of disappearance. In my lecture, I will present some results which indicate that when we are making true kinetics we can have much more interpretable and interesting results. However, I think we can look to plasma glutamine levels to identify patients who are depleted. This is a personal point of view. I want to be clear because probably Dr. Stehle would give another answer. But I am basing this feeling on an article by Parry-Billings et al. [13] published some years ago showing that there was a relationship between plasma glutamine in burn patients and the intensity of stress, and also there was an increased morbidity in patients with lower glutamine levels, and therefore we can probably look at plasma glutamine levels. Also just to tell a story, and this has not really any scientific value but it is absolutely clear. When I was a young intern in St. Antoine Hospital I was working with the burn center head of department, and in my laboratory we performed amino acid chromatography on a routine basis and patients with a glutamine level of <200 μmol/l systematically displayed complications. Therefore I think that it is a simple reliable way to assess the disequilibrium between the rate of appearance from muscle and perhaps the rate of consumption by central organs. Otherwise we can look at some immunological markers but you know very well that it is not specific.

Dr. Neu: I just want to express a little heresy here. It is a dogma in these kinds of studies to have isonitrogenous controls and I think that that can actually lead to a lot of trouble because the isonitrogenous controls can actually have effects of their own. If we are going to do this correctly we should have a real world control group compared to the experimental treatment group. So if one has to do this totally correctly you will have 3 groups, one is the supplemented group, one is the isonitrogenous control, and the other is the real world group.

Dr. Cynober: I agree totally, I published that in the *Journal of Nutrition* 3 years ago and I will be pleased to send you a reprint with exactly 3 such groups [14]. But more seriously I think that it is a key issue and we have to be very careful. For this reason a certain number of research groups, including Déchelotte's and mine, are actually using as an isonitrogenous control a mixture of 6 or 8 amino acids because, by providing huge amounts of glycine, you cannot exclude a positive or negative effect which could mask or reinforce the effect of the so-called immunonutrient. But fundamentally, although it probably doesn't matter in the final results, I believe that we need an isonitrogenous group in order not to have this point obscure the results.

Dr. Neu: In certain situations the isonitrogenous control can actually cause problems. When we were doing some studies in baby rats a few years ago we tried to use glycine as the isonitrogenous control, and we killed more rats using glycine.

Dr. Cynober: I agree.

Dr. Moore: I am surprised by the comment that enterally delivered glutamine does not get absorbed since we did a randomized study using a product that was supplemented with glutamine and glutamine levels went up. So maybe you could educate me on that. My second comment is that glutamine as an enteral nutrient in the critical ill may be beneficial because it increases the perfusion to the mucosa and it is an amino acid that, once it is absorbed, the enterocyte can use it to produce ATP. In a recent study, we showed that glutamine actually protected against ischemia reperfusion by maintaining these ATP levels.

Dr. Cynober: There are several aspects in your question. The first one, it is absolutely true that most of studies providing glutamine by the enteral route to adult patients provide negative results. This is a matter of fact. Secondly, this is very different to what has been repeatedly observed in very low weight infants with at least two reports providing efficiency. From studies performed on piglets we think that there is some evolution in the enzymatic equipment of the intestine, and this was the last hypothesis by Dr. Stehle, and I think that it must be considered. You know, in a given cell, trafficking has a lot of possibilities and you cannot imagine that the substrate in the cell is looking like that to search an enzyme, and this leads to the concept of compartmentalization. This means that once an amino acid and probably other substances are taken up by a specific transporter, it is immediately metabolized by a given associated enzyme. This allows a reduction in the loss of intermediary nutrient, to drive the substrates in a given pathway, and by the way this explains why, for example, an amino acid such as arginine may be taken up by 4 different transporters. Therefore you can imagine that in adults, but perhaps not in very low birth weight infants, glutamine taken up at the luminal side is transformed into glutamate which could be associated immediately to a transaminase of dehydrogenase and used for energy purposes, and nothing happens. You can imagine that on the vascular side the transporter is associated with the enzymes which channel glutamine from glutamate to arginine and further to polyamines because if you carefully read the article by Rhoads et al. [15], it indicates that glutamine has a trophic effect in the intestine, stimulating the MAP kinase system. In fact this is a cAMP-dependent inhibitable system, and what makes glutamine is to release the inhibition exerted by cAMP. But what is interesting in the discussion section of this article is that when glutamine metabolism is blocked using amino-oxoacetate, this leads to the disappearance of the glutamine effect. Rhoads speculated that in fact the effect of glutamine at the intestinal level was due to the generation of aliphatic polyamines, which can make sense because this molecule is known to have a very important effect in this tissue. Therefore in my opinion, to explain why in humans and in animals enteral glutamine is not as efficient on the intestinal mucosa as parenteral glutamine, it is the different behavior in the cell. But now we cannot exclude that by providing a very high amount of glutamine a part of the glutamine escapes intestinal metabolism and then returns to the cells via the general circulation and has such an effect. I will present these data later in my lecture, a single article showing a very positive effect with only a supplementation of glutamine, not a mixture. It is the article by Houdijk et al. [16] published in the *Lancet*. I made the calculation, the patients actually received 33 g glutamine/day, whereas in most of the studies, such as those of Long et al. [17] and Jensen et al. [18], the dose given to the patients was around 15–28 g/day.

Dr. Déchelotte: To go with this point I agree with Dr. Moore that glutamine is very well absorbed. Some years ago with Dr. Baugerie, we made a study in both volunteers and in very short bowel patients; it was published in the *American Journal of Clinical Nutrition.* Even patients with only 30–40 cm of small bowel left were able to absorb a very high amount of glutamine. That is the first point. The second point, I agree with Dr. Cynober, is that probably most of the studies published previously with enteral glutamine were performed at rather low dosages, about 20 g/day which is quite near to that used by the parenteral route in previous postoperative studies, and we know now that with 30 g enteral glutamine/day we are able to inhibit the de novo synthesis of glutamine both in healthy humans with hypercatabolism and postoperative patients. So it is efficient to influence the endogenous metabolism of glutamine, and if we go ahead with further dosages of enteral glutamine then we are able to detect a quite clear enhancement of the glutamine concentration which means that it is bioavailable. The problem with the previous studies is that perhaps we did not exactly measure the right things with enteral glutamine. We now have effects on several mechanisms of heat shock protein production in the gut or protein synthesis and other mechanisms which are difficult to measure in patients. So I am pretty sure we can go ahead with this enteral supply of glutamine, maybe with higher dosages and maybe other issues too.

Dr. Bozzetti: Are you aware of any study in surgical patients where glutamine was administered prior to the surgical operation? I am asking this because if you look at the experience in preoperative nutrition both total parenteral or enteral nutrition were more successful when support was started preoperatively.

Dr. Cynober: The answer is yes but at this moment I am not able to remember in which recent article I have read such a manipulation with positive results. But I think that there are some recent data providing glutamine preoperatively, yes.

Dr. Labadarios: Thank you for a very nice presentation. In one slide you made a recommendation which I find a little bit too general, in relation to glutamine, arginine and cysteine. What type of evidence do we have at present in relation to the safety of this proposal that you are making, in relation to the type of patients who would benefit, and also in relation to the course of the illness? At what point of a given course of illness do you think that this recommendation would be appropriate?

Dr. Cynober: It is Dr. Stehle who should answer the question. With regard to safety, studies published in 1990 by Ziegler et al. [19] indicate that even by providing a very high amount of glutamine there is absolutely no toxicity with this amino acid. Perhaps, but this is only a hypothesis because to the best of my knowledge nobody has checked. It may be toxic in liver failure, but for reasons we can imagine nobody has tried to give high amounts of glutamine to patients suffering from liver failure. Now I should say that unfortunately we have absolutely no dose ranging studies available in patients, so that the suggested dose is a sort of compromise of what is available in the literature. And with regard to the subtype of patients, probably glutamine is very efficient in groups of postoperative patients, but I am not certain that these patients require a glutamine-enriched diet to get better. It probably has marginal effects, but we have to consider that in some groups of sick patients there is an advantage of providing glutamine. Then there is an important question arising from Griffiths et al. [20] with no improvement during the ICU stay, but it was a very short period of administration, 3–5 days, with low glutamine intake, 15 g/day. However, these authors observed a clearly decreasing mortality at 6 months and an associated reduced cost in surviving people. Now this is magical but can perhaps be explained. Just to recall, a former Swedish study by Petersson et al. [21] indicated that in cholecystectomized patients a short period of postoperative administration of glutamine decreased fatigue 1 month after the surgery. I don't know what the mechanism of this action is, perhaps it is related to glutathione and oxidative stress. And then to finish answering your question we have to remember that some studies in very sick patients, patients with major sepsis, with very high levels of stress, did not respond at all to glutamine therapy, and I especially refer to the study of Roth et al. [22] providing a high amount of glutamine by the parenteral route, and they were even not able to restore the muscle glutamine concentrations. To summarize my answer there is clearly a need for further work to designate subgroups of patients who can benefit most from such therapy, and in any case we cannot give an absolute recommendation of dosage.

Dr. Déchelotte: Just to add to the body of knowledge, a French multicenter trial with dipeptide, reported in ASPEN, showed that we are able to reduce the incidence of infectious complications by about 40% and to half the number of cases of pneumonia in very severe ICU patients. So I think it is also another step in the story, which is not quite finished.

Dr. Cynober: Sorry, I should have remembered these very impressive results.

References

1. Coudray-Lucas C, Le Bever H, Cynober L, et al. Ornithine alpha-ketoglutarate improves wound healing in severe burn patients: A prospective randomized double-blind trial versus isonitrogenous controls. *Crit Care Med* 2000; 28: 1772–76.
2. Donati L, Ziegler F, Pongelli G, Signorini MS. Nutritional and clinical efficacy of ornithine alpha-ketoglutarate in severe burn patients. *Clin Nutr* 1999; 18: 307–11.
3. De Brandt JP, Coudray-Lucas C, Lioret N, et al. A randomized controlled trial of the influence of the mode of enteral ornithine alpha-ketoglutarate administration in burn patients. *J Nutr* 1998; 128: 563–9.
4. Scolapio JS, Camilleri M, Fleming CR, et al. Effect of growth hormone, glutamine, and diet on adaptation in short-bowel syndrome: A randomized, controlled study. *Gastroenterology* 1997; 113: 1074–81.

5. Scolapio JS. Effect of growth hormone, glutamine, and diet on body composition in short bowel sydrome: A randomized, controlled study. *JPEN J Parenter Enteral Nutr* 1999; 23: 309–13.
6. Byrne TA, Morrissey TB, Nattakom TV, et al. Growth Hormone, glutamine and a modified diet enhance nutrient absorption in patients with severe short bowel syndrome. *JPEN J Parenter Enteral Nutr* 1995; 19: 296–302.
7. Fox AD, Kripke SA, De Paula J, et al. Effect of a glutamine-supplemented enteral diet on methotrexate induced enterocolitis. *JPEN J Parenter Enteral Nutr* 1988; 12: 325–31.
8. Parry-Billings M, Budgett R, Koutedakis Y, et al. Plasma amino acids concentrations in the overtraining syndrome: Possible effects on the immune system. *Med Sci Sports Exerc* 1992; 24: 1353–8.
9. Yu YM, Ryan CR, Burke JF, et al. Relations among arginine, citrulline, ornithine, and leucine kinetics in adult burn patients. *Am J Clin Nutr* 1995; 62: 960–8.
10. Barbul A. Arginine and immune function. *Nutrition* 1990; 6: 53–8.
11. Gianotti L, Braga M, Fortis C, et al. A prospective, randomized clinical trial on perioperative feeding with an arginine-, omega-3 fatty acid-, and RNA-enriched diet: Effect on host response and nutritional status. *JPEN J Parenter Enteral Nutr* 1999; 23: 314–20.
12. Heyland DK, Novak F, Drover JW, et al. Should immunonutrition become routine in critically ill patients? *JAMA* 2001; 286: 22–9.
13. Parry-Billings M, Evans J, Calder PC, Newsholme EA. Does glutamine contribute to immunosuppression after major burns? *Lancet* 1990; 336: 523–5.
14. Chambon-Savanovitch E, Felgines C, Farges MC, et al. Comparative study of glycine, alanine or casein as inert nitrogen source in endotoxemic rats. *J Nutr* 1999; 129: 1866–70.
15. Rhoads JM, Argenzio RA, Chen W, et al. Glutamine metabolism stimulated intestinal cell MAPKs by a cAMP-inhibitable. Raf-independent mechanism. *Gastroenterology* 2000; 188: 90–100.
16. Houdijk AP, Rijnsburger ER, Jansen J, et al. Randomised trial of glutamine-enriched enteral nutrition on infectious morbidity in patients with multiple trauma. *Lancet* 1998; 352: 772–6.
17. Long CL, Borghesi L, Stahl R, et al. Impact of enteral feeding of a glutamine-supplemented formula on the hypoaminoacidemic response in trauma patients. *J Trauma* 1996; 40: 97–102.
18. Jensen GL, Miller RH, Talabiska DG, et al. A double-blind, prospective, randomized study of glutamine-enriched compared with standard peptide-based feeding in critically ill patients. *Am J Clin Nutr* 1996; 64: 615–21.
19. Ziegler TR, Benfell K, Smith RJ, et al. Safety and metabolic effects of *L*-glutamine administration in humans. *JPEN J Parenter Enteral Nutr* 1990; 14: 137S–46S.
20. Griffiths RD, Jones C, Palmer TE. Six-month outcome of critically ill patients given glutamine-supplemented parenteral nutrition. *Nutrition* 1997; 13: 295–302.
21. Peterson B, Waller SO, Vinnars E, Wernerman J, Long-term effect of glycyl-glutamine after elective surgery on free amino acids in muscle. *JPEN J Parenter Enteral Nutr* 1994; 18: 320–5.
22. Roth E, Funovics J, Muhlbacher F, et al. Metabolic disorders in severe abdominal sepsis: Glutamine deficiency in skeletal muscle. *Clin Nutr* 1982; 1: 25–41.

Cynober L, Moore FA (eds): Nutrition and Critical Care.
Nestlé Nutrition Workshop Series Clinical & Performance Program, Vol. 8, pp 75–98,
Nestec Ltd.; Vevey/S. Karger AG, Basel, © 2003.

Lipids and the Critically Ill Patient

Philip C. Calder

Institute of Human Nutrition, School of Medicine, University of Southampton,
Southampton, UK

Lipid Metabolism in the Critically Ill Patient

Lipid metabolism is altered in the critically ill patient as a result of changes in the status of hormones and other mediators [for reviews see, 1–3]. Enhanced mobilization of adipose tissue triacylglycerol stores is characteristic of the metabolic response to severe stress. This process is promoted by catecholamines and inflammatory cytokines, such as tumor necrosis factor (TNF)-α and interleukin (IL)-1, and is exaggerated by the decreased insulin sensitivity of adipose tissue. The release of fatty acids from adipose tissue is frequently in excess of energy requirements. Those fatty acids not oxidized may be re-esterified into triacylglycerols in the liver and packaged into very low-density lipoproteins (VLDLs). Hepatic triacylglycerol production is increased in critical illness and this can lead to lipid deposition (steatosis) in the liver. Nevertheless, hepatic triacylglycerol output (as VLDLs) is also increased in critical illness. In some conditions (e.g. trauma or after surgery) triacylglycerol clearance is not impaired (or may even be increased) and so plasma triacylglycerol concentrations remain normal (or may even be decreased). However, in some conditions (e.g. sepsis), the activity of adipose tissue lipoprotein lipase is suppressed by inflammatory cytokines (e.g. TNFα and IL-1) and insulin resistance, and so triacylglycerols are not efficiently cleared from the circulation. Thus, hypertriacylglycerolemia occurs in such patients. VLDLs can bind endotoxin and target it for degradation in liver parenchymal cells. Thus, the increase in VLDL concentration may be, in part, a protective mechanism. The plasma cholesterol concentration is decreased in stress conditions, with the concentrations of both low- (LDLs) and high-density lipoproteins (HDLs) being decreased. This decrease occurs despite increased hepatic cholesterol production. The decreased HDL concentration appears to be as a result of enhanced catabolism, while the decreased LDL concentration may be due to increased sequestration and retention in subendothelial spaces. The composition of LDL and HDL is changed in stress conditions, and this might change the properties of these lipoproteins [for reviews see, 2, 3].

A Role for Lipids in Nutritional Support of the Critically Ill Patient

In the meta-analysis of total parenteral nutrition [4], there was a trend towards less complications if lipids were not included in the regimen (p = 0.09 vs. lipids), although inclusion of lipids did not affect mortality. Whether exogenously supplied lipids are, in fact, detrimental to the critically ill patient remains a controversial point, and they are frequently included in nutritional support regimens. Lipids provided enterally undergo normal intestinal metabolism with the fatty acids appearing in circulating chylomicrons. Infused lipid emulsions acquire apolipoproteins from circulating lipoproteins and follow the pathway of chylomicron metabolism. It is important that the lipids used in critically ill patients provide essential fatty acids and fat-soluble vitamins and that the component polyunsaturated fatty acids (PUFAs) be adequately protected against peroxidation by including sufficient α-tocopherol. The lipids contained in emulsions used in nutritional support have traditionally been based on soybean oil, which is rich in the n-6 fatty acid linoleic acid (18:2 n-6). Nutritional support has traditionally been aimed at supplying substrates to meet energy demands and providing building blocks for wound healing and tissue repair, and in the process helping to prevent body wasting. Critically ill patients may be at risk of compromised immunity, resulting in decreased resistance to infection. Furthermore, it is now realized that some patients show an early hyperinflammation than might be damaging to the host. Thus, nutritional support is now aimed at providing substrates to support the immune system and nutrients (and other factors) that can modulate the inflammatory state. It is in these two areas that fatty acids are thought to offer great opportunity for improvement in patient outcome.

Polyunsaturated Fatty Acids, Inflammation and Immunity

Biosynthesis of Polyunsaturated Fatty Acids
There are two main families of PUFAs, the n-6 (or omega-6) and the n-3 (or omega-3) families. Mammalian cells cannot synthesize n-6 or n-3 PUFAs de novo, because they lack the δ-12 and δ-15 desaturase enzymes (found in most plants) for insertion of a double bond at the n-6 or n-3 position (fig. 1). The n-6 and n-3 fatty acids are essential substrates for many of the major

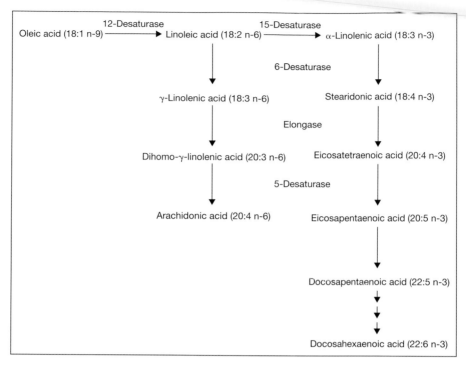

Fig. 1. Outline of the pathway of biosynthesis of polyunsaturated fatty acids.

regulatory lipids in the body and as they cannot be synthesized in the body, they must be obtained from the diet. The commonly consumed PUFAs are linoleic acid (18:2 n-6) and α-linolenic acid (18:3 n-3). Once consumed these fatty acids can be converted to the longer chain, more unsaturated derivatives (fig. 1). Thus linoleic acid is converted to arachidonic acid (ARA; 20:4 n-6) and α-linolenic acid is converted to eicosapentaenoic acid (EPA; 20:5 n-3) and docosapentaenoic acid (22:5 n-3; fig. 1). There is some controversy about the extent to which docosahexaenoic acid (DHA; 22:6 n-3) can be synthesized from EPA in humans. EPA, docosapentaenoic acid and DHA are termed long-chain n-3 PUFAs. These fatty acids are found in oily fish and in the preparations known as fish oil.

Arachidonic Acid as a Substrate for Synthesis of Bioactive Mediators
The principal functional role for 20-carbon PUFAs is as substrates for synthesis of the family of bioactive mediators known as eicosanoids, which include prostaglandins (PGs), thromboxanes (TXs), leukotrienes (LTs), lipoxins, and hydroxyeicosatetraenoic acids (fig. 2). Although several 20-carbon PUFAs are able to serve as precursors of eicosanoids, ARA is usually

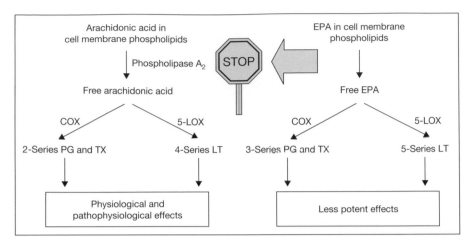

Fig. 2. Basis of the anti-inflammatory effects of eicosapentaenoic acid. COX = Cyclooxygenase; EPA = eicosapentaenoic acid; LOX = lipoxygenase; LT = leukotriene; PG = prostaglandin; TX = thromboxane.

the principal substrate for their synthesis. This is because the membranes of most cells contain large amounts of ARA, compared with other potential eicosanoid precursors (including EPA). ARA in cell membranes can be mobilized by various phospholipase enzymes, most notably phospholipase A_2, and the free ARA can subsequently act as a substrate for the enzymes that synthesize eicosanoids (fig. 2). Metabolism of ARA by cyclooxygenase (COX) enzymes gives rise to the 2-series PG and TX (fig. 2). There are two isoforms of COX: COX-1 is a constitutive enzyme and COX-2 is induced in inflammatory cells as a result of stimulation and is responsible for the markedly elevated production of PG which occurs upon cellular activation. Metabolism of ARA by the 5-lipoxygenase (5-LOX) pathway gives rise to hydroxy and hydroperoxy derivatives and the 4-series LT, LTA_4, B_4, C_4, D_4 and E_4 (fig. 2).

Eicosanoids act as mediators in their own right (e.g. PGE_2 causes pain), modify the responses to other mediators (e.g. PGE_2 potentiates the pain caused by bradykinin) and act as regulators of other processes, such as platelet aggregation, blood clotting, smooth muscle contraction, leukocyte chemotaxis, inflammatory cytokine production, and immune function. The effects of eicosanoids on inflammation and immunity have attracted much attention in recent years [5]. The effects of PGE_2 and LTB_4 have been studied most widely. PGE_2 has a number of proinflammatory effects including inducing fever, increasing vascular permeability and vasodilation and enhancing pain and edema caused by other agents such as bradykinin and histamine. PGE_2 suppresses production of $TNF\alpha$ and IL-1 and so in these respects is anti-inflammatory. PGE_2 suppresses lymphocyte proliferation and natural killer cell activity and inhibits production of IL-2 and interferon

(IFN)-γ, and so in these respects PGE_2 is immunosuppressive. PGE_2 also promotes immunoglobulin (Ig) E production by B lymphocytes; IgE is a mediator of allergic inflammation. TXA_2 promotes platelet aggregation, leukocyte adhesion, and smooth muscle contraction. LTB_4 increases vascular permeability, enhances local blood flow, is a potent chemotactic agent for leukocytes, induces release of lysosomal enzymes, enhances generation of reactive oxygen species, and enhances production of TNFα, IL-1, and IL-6. In all of these respects LTB_4 is proinflammatory. In inflammatory conditions increased rates of production of ARA-derived eicosanoids are found and elevated levels of certain eicosanoids are found in blood and tissues from patients with inflammatory disorders, burns and critical illness. Interestingly, recent studies have shown that PGE_2 inhibits 5-LOX, so preventing the generation of the inflammatory 4-series LTs [6]. Furthermore, PGE_2 was found to induce generation of the 15-LOX product lipoxin A_4, a known inflammation 'stop signal' [6]. Thus, although PGE_2 does possess distinct proinflammatory actions, it is involved in mediating the resolution of inflammation through effects on the generation of other eicosanoids.

Alternatives to n-6 Polyunsaturated Fatty Acids for Use in Critically Ill Patients

Although most standard lipid emulsions for use in critically ill patients are based upon soybean oil, there is a view that an excess of n-6 PUFAs should be avoided since this could contribute a state where physiological processes become dysregulated. However, while there are some studies that indicate that provision of emulsions rich in n-6 PUFAs is detrimental to the host (e.g. impairing immune function), there are other, similar studies showing no such impairment [for references see, 7]. Nevertheless, nutritional support regimens containing alternative types of fatty acids are being sought. One alternative is to reduce the amount of n-6 PUFA-containing oil by partly replacing it with medium-chain triglycerides (MCTs; i.e. triacylglycerols containing fatty acids of carbon chain length 6–12). This approach will not be further discussed here. A second approach is to replace part of n-6 PUFA-rich oil in emulsions designed for parenteral use with olive oil, which is rich in the n-9 monounsaturated fatty acid oleic acid (18:1 n-9). This approach is currently under investigation and will not be discussed further here. The third approach is to replace part of n-6 PUFA-rich oil with fish oil, which contains long-chain n-3 PUFAs.

Eicosapentaenoic Acid as an Arachidonic Acid Antagonist

When fish oil is provided, EPA is incorporated into cell membrane phospholipids, partly at the expense of ARA. Thus, there is less ARA available for eicosanoid synthesis. In addition, EPA inhibits the oxidation of ARA by COX. Hence, fish oil decreases production of PGs like PGE_2, of thromboxanes like TXA_2 and of LTs like LTB_4. This has been demonstrated many times in cell culture, animal feeding and healthy volunteer studies. Thus, n-3 PUFAs can potentially reduce platelet aggregation, blood clotting, smooth muscle contraction, and leukocyte chemotaxis, and can modulate inflammatory cytokine production and immune function (fig. 2).

In addition to inhibiting metabolism of ARA, EPA is able to act as a substrate for both COX and 5-LOX (fig. 2), giving rise to derivatives which have a different structure to those produced from ARA (i.e. 3-series PGs and TXs and 5-series LTs). Thus, the EPA-induced suppression in the production of ARA-derived eicosanoids is accompanied by an elevation in the production of EPA-derived eicosanoids. The eicosanoids produced from EPA are considered to be less biologically potent than the analogues synthesized from ARA, although the full range of biological activities of these compounds has not been investigated. The reduction in generation of ARA-derived mediators which accompanies fish oil consumption has lead to the idea that fish oil is anti-inflammatory (fig. 2). Additionally, recent studies suggest that metabolism of EPA by COX gives rise to a novel series of eicosanoids that are anti-inflammatory in nature [8].

The isolated, perfused rabbit lung has been used as a model to study the pathophysiological effects of ARA- and EPA-derived eicosanoids. Infusion with *Escherichia coli* hemolysin was shown to induce vasoconstriction/ hypertension, mediated by TXB_2, and vascular permeability/leakage, mediated by 4-series LTs [9, 10]. Inclusion of free ARA in the perfusate increased TXB_2 and 4-series LT generation, arterial pressure and vascular leakage. In contrast, inclusion of EPA decreased TXB_2 and 4-series LT generation, arterial pressure and vascular leakage and increased generation of TXB_3 and 5-series LTs [9, 10]. Perfusion of isolated rabbit lungs with a fish oil-containing emulsion markedly attenuated the vascular inflammatory reaction (hypertension) induced by calcium ionophore [11]. Compared with perfusion with a soybean oil-rich emulsion, fish oil decreased the concentration of LTC_4 in the perfusate by >50% and increased the concentration of LTC_5 from barely detectable (<10 pg/ml) to a concentration very similar to that of LTC_4 (approximately 150 pg/ml) [11]. These observations indicate that n-3 PUFAs can significantly inhibit the acute inflammatory responses induced, or at least marked, by production of ARA-derived eicosanoids.

n-3 Polyunsaturated Fatty Acids and Inflammatory Cytokines

Although the action in antagonizing ARA metabolism is a key anti-inflammatory effect of n-3 PUFAs, these fatty acids have other effects that might occur downstream of altered eicosanoid production or might be independent of this [12]. Cell culture, animal feeding and healthy human volunteer studies have demonstrated that n-3 PUFAs can decrease the production of TNFα, IL-1β, IL-6 and tissue factor by stimulated monocytes, macrophages, osteoblasts, chondrocytes and/or endothelial cells [for review see, 16]. Endotoxin was used most often as the cell stimulus in these studies.

Fish Oil and Animal Models of Endotoxemia and Sepsis

The importance of a hyperinflammatory response, characterized by overproduction of TNFα, IL-1β, IL-6 and IL-8, in the progression of trauma patients towards sepsis is now recognized. Enhanced production of ARA-derived eicosanoids, such as PGE_2, is also associated with trauma and burns. The inflammatory effects of infection can be mimicked by administration of endotoxin, which causes an elevation in circulating concentrations of inflammatory cytokines. The ability of n-3 PUFAs to decrease production of inflammatory cytokines and eicosanoids suggests that fish oil might be a useful agent to aid the control of endotoxemia and the so-called systemic inflammatory response syndrome (SIRS).

Fish oil feeding to rats resulted in a markedly altered profile of post-endotoxin circulating eicosanoids (e.g. less PGE_2, TXB_2 and 6-keto-$PGF_{1\alpha}$) and of eicosanoid generation by isolated alveolar macrophages (40% less LTB_4 and over 10 times more LTB_5) [13, 14]. Mice fed fish oil and then injected with endotoxin had significantly lower plasma TNFα, IL-1β and IL-6 concentrations than mice fed safflower oil [15]. Fish oil-containing parenteral nutrition significantly decreased serum TNFα, IL-6 and IL-8 concentrations in burned rats [16]. Fish oil feeding in guinea pigs or rats or fish oil infusion in guinea pigs enhanced survival following endotoxin challenge [for references see, 15]. Fish oil feeding decreased endotoxin-induced metabolic perturbations (fever, acidosis, hypotension, anorexia, weight loss) in guinea pigs and/or rats [for references see, 15]. Fish oil (or EPA) improved heart and lung function and decreased lung edema in endotoxic rats [14, 17, 18] and pigs [19].

Total parenteral nutrition using fish oil as the lipid source was found to prevent the endotoxin-induced reduction in blood flow to the gut and to reduce the number of viable bacteria in mesenteric lymph nodes and liver following exposure to live bacteria [20]. Fish oil did not, however, decrease bacterial translocation across the gut and the authors concluded that fish oil must have improved bacterial killing. Fish oil administration prior to exposure to live pathogens decreased mortality of rats compared with vegetable oil [21]. More recently, fish oil infusion after induction of sepsis by cecal ligation and puncture in rats was shown to decrease mortality (and PGE_2 production) compared with vegetable oil [22]. Intragastric administration of fish oil into chow-fed rats prior to cecal ligation and puncture improved survival compared with vegetable oil or saline infusion [23].

Studies of Fish Oil-Containing Parenteral Nutrition in Patients

Parenteral nutrition supplemented with fish oil has been shown to affect circulating inflammatory mediator concentrations and/or the capacity of leukocytes to produce inflammatory mediators in various patient groups. For example, infusion of a fish oil-containing lipid emulsion into postoperative patients resulted in an increased capacity of stimulated blood leukocytes to generate LTC_4 6 days after operation [24]. Fish oil infusion was also found to decrease the production of TXB_2 and to increase the production of TXA_3 by platelets from patients after surgery [25]. In another study, patients received either a MCT-long-chain triacylglycerol mix or this mix also containing fish oil for 5 days following surgery [26]. Patients in the fish oil group received 3 g (days 1 and 2) and 6 g (days 3, 4 and 5) n-3 PUFAs/day. Neutrophils from patients infused with fish oil produced less LTB_4 and significantly more LTB_5 at postoperative days 6 and 10. Plasma $TNF\alpha$ (days 6 and 10) and IL-6 (day 10) concentrations were lower in patients receiving fish oil [26]. This study did not report clinical outcomes. Recently the results of three further studies with parenteral fish oil administration have become available [27–29]. In the first of these, patients received total parenteral nutrition that included an 8% soybean oil plus 2% fish oil emulsion (controls received a 10% soybean oil emulsion) for 5 days following surgery [27]. Patients in the fish oil group received 0.2 g fish oil/kg body weight/day; it is not clear from the fatty acid compositions of the emulsions provided exactly how much n-3 PUFAs this would equate to. There were no differences between groups with respect to the concentrations and/or activities of a range of coagulation factors, the function of platelets, and complications. Another study compared the effects of lipid emulsions on lymphocyte functions in patients following large bowel surgery [28]. Patients received lipid-free total parenteral nutrition or parenteral nutrition including 10% soybean oil or 8.3% soybean oil plus 1.7% fish oil for 5 days postoperatively. The amount of fish oil provided was 0.1 g/kg body weight for the first day and 0.2 g/kg body weight for days 2–5; this equated to about 3 g long-chain n-3 PUFAs/day based on a 70-kg body weight. Blood lymphocyte numbers and functions were measured before surgery and at days 3 and 6 after surgery. Although surgery affected blood lymphocyte numbers, there were no differences between the groups with respect to the numbers of total lymphocytes, T cells, B cells, CD4+ lymphocytes, CD8+ lymphocytes or natural killer cells in the circulation at any of the time points. Furthermore, there were no differences between the groups with respect to lymphocyte proliferation stimulated by a mitogen. In contrast, ex vivo IL-2 production was increased in the fish oil group, and the decline in ex vivo IFN-γ production after surgery was prevented by fish oil [28]. Thus, this study indicates that, in these patients, parenteral fish oil does not impair cell-mediated immune responses, and may even preserve or improve them. Weiss et al. [29] infused 10% fish oil on the day before surgery and on days 1–5 after surgery into patients undergoing abdominal surgery. On postoperative days 4 and 5 the patients also received standard total parenteral nutrition, which included 50 g fat/day. Control patients received the same regimen apart from the fish oil infusions. White cell count, the serum concentrations of C-reactive protein and $TNF\alpha$, and neutrophil respiratory burst activity were not different between groups, although they were affected by surgery. $TNF\alpha$ production by endotoxin-stimulated whole blood tended to be lower at postoperative day 5 in the fish oil group, but the difference did not reach significance. The serum IL-6 concentration was significantly lower in the fish oil group at days 0, 1 and 3 after surgery. In contrast, monocyte expression of human leukocyte antigen-DR, which is involved in antigen presentation, was preserved in the fish oil group but declined at days 3 and 5 after surgery in the control group [29]. No differences in infection rates or mortality between the groups were observed. Postoperative stay in the intensive care unit tended to be shorter in the fish oil group (4.1 vs. 9.1 days) as did total hospital stay (17.8 vs. 23.5 days). Postoperative stay on the medical wards was significantly shorter in the fish oil group [29]. These studies indicate the potential for significant modification of the inflammatory and immune changes induced by surgery by infusion of n-3 PUFAs in the form of fish oil. However, larger studies are needed to evaluate the effects on complication rates, hospital stay and mortality.

Studies of Fish Oil-Containing Enteral Nutrition in Patients

A large number of studies incorporating fish oil into enteral formulae have been conducted in intensive care and surgical patients. The majority of these trials have used the commercially available product IMPACT® which contains arginine, nucleotides and n-3 PUFAs. n-3 PUFAs make up about 10% of the fatty acids in IMPACT, and it contains about 3 g n-3 PUFAs/l. A comprehensive meta-analysis of 15 randomized, controlled studies using IMPACT or Immun-Aid® (also rich in arginine, RNA and n-3 PUFAs) has been performed [30]. This analysis confirmed significant reductions in infection rate, number of ventilator days and length of hospital stay, but not in overall mortality. Table 1 lists the studies of enteral nutrition involving n-3 PUFAs that have reported immune and/or inflammatory outcomes. A number of studies have reported circulating lymphocyte numbers and subsets and circulating immunoglobulin concentrations and most report little difference in these compared with the control group. Some studies have reported aspects of immune function such as phagocytosis, respiratory burst, lymphocyte proliferation, human leukocyte antigen DR expression on monocytes and cytokine production; several of these studies report some significant improvements in the these functions in patients given IMPACT compared with the control group. The most frequently reported outcomes of these types are those related to inflammatory cytokines, which is perhaps not surprising given their role in progression to SIRS. One study has reported lower spontaneous production of TNFα and IL-6 by diluted whole blood after several days of IMPACT administration [30]. Several studies report lower circulating concentrations of IL-6 in the IMPACT group, while there are also reports of lower circulating TNFα concentrations (for references see table 1).

Table 1. Summary of studies employing enteral nutrition including fish oil that have reported immune or inflammatory outcomes

Ref	Type No. of patients	Formula studied	Immune/inflammatory outcomes	Effects of formula with fish oil on immune/inflammatory outcomes	Comments
31	Burns (av. 40% BSA)	50:50 Fish oil:safflower oil vs. 50:40:10 MCT:corn oil: soybean oil vs. 70:30 soybean oil:MCT	Lymphocyte count Bacterial killing by neutrophils	None None	↓ Wound infections, infectious episodes and length of hospital stay (expressed as percent of original BSA burn) in fish oil group No effect on mortality
32	ICU (trauma, surgery, sepsis)	IMPACT vs. Standard	Lymphocyte proliferation	↑At days 3 and 7	No effect on length of hospital stay or mortality
33	Cancer surgery	IMPACT vs. Standard	Complement C3 Circulating lymphocyte and subset numbers HLA-DR expression on monocytes Lymphocyte proliferation	None None None ↑ At day 7	↓ Number of patients with infectious/ healing complications in IMPACT group No effect on mortality
34	Cancer surgery	IMPACT vs. Standard	Circulating IgG and IgM Circulating lymphocyte subsets IFN-γ production by stimulated lymphocytes	IgG ↑ at day 16; IgM ↑ at days 7 and 10 Number of T cells, helper T cells and B cells ↑ at days 7, 10 and 16 ↑ At day 16	

35	Cancer surgery	IMPACT vs. Standard	PGE$_2$ production by endotoxin stimulated cells	Time-dependent ↓ by up to 60%	↓ Infections and length of hospital stay
36	Cancer surgery	IMPACT vs. Standard	Spontaneous or mitogen-stimulated production of:		
			IL-1α	None	
			IL-1β, IL-2	↑ At day 16 (+mitogen)	
			IL-2R	↑ At days 7 and 10 (+mitogen)	
			IL-6	↓ At days 3 and 7 (spontaneous)	
			TNFα	↓ At day 7 (spontaneous)	
37	Cancer surgery	IMPACT vs. Standard vs. low-fat TPN	Circulating IgA, IgG, IgM	None	
			Circulating complement C3	None	
			Circulating TNFα, IL-1, IL-6, sIL-2R	None	
			Leukocyte counts and subset numbers	Some	
			Phagocytosis by monocytes and neutrophils	↑ At days 8–10 for monocytes	
38	Cancer surgery	IMPACT vs. Standard vs. TPN	Circulating IgA, IgG, IgM	None	No effect on percent infected patients but ↓ infection score ↓ Length of hospital stay
			Circulating complement C3	None	
			Circulating sIL-2R	↑ At day 8	

(continued overleaf)

Table 1. (continued)

Ref	Type No. of patients	Formula studied	Immune/inflammatory outcomes	Effects of formula with fish oil on immune/inflammatory outcomes	Comments
			Circulating IL-6	↓ At day 8	
			Circulating lymphocytes and subset numbers	None	
			Phagocytosis by monocytes	↑ At days 4 and 8	
			DTH response	↑ At day 8	
39	Trauma	IMPACT vs. Standard	Circulating C-reactive protein	↓ At day 4	No effects on infection rate, length of hospital or ICU stay or mortality
			Circulating lymphocytes and subset numbers	None	
			IL-2R expression on lymphocytes	None	
			HLA-DR expression on monocytes	↑ At day 7	
40	Cancer surgery	IMPACT vs. Standard	Circulating C-reactive protein and IL-6	↓ At days 1 and 8	↓ Number of antibiotic days, percent infected patients and length of hospital stay
41	Cancer surgery	IMPACT vs. Standard	Circulating IgA, IgG, IgM	None	
			Circulating complement C3	None	
			Circulating sIL-2R	↑ At days 1, 4 and 8	

		Circulating IL-6	↓ At days 1, 4 and 8	
		Circulating sIL-1R	↓ At days 4 and 8	
		DTH response	↑ At days 1, 4 and 8	
42	Cardiac bypass surgery	IMPACT vs. Standard (from ≥5 d pre-operatively)	Circulating IL-6	↓ Immediately before and during surgery	No effect on time on ventillator or length of ICU or hospital stay
		Monocyte HLA-DR expression	None	
		DTH response	↑ At admission	
43	Cancer surgery	Nutrison vs. Standard	Circulating C-reactive protein	↓ At day 8	
		Circulating lymphocytes and subset numbers	↑ Total lymphocytes and percent T cells, T helper cells, NK cells at day 8, ↓ Cytotoxic T cells at day 8	
		Circulating IL-1, IL-2	None	
		Circulating TNFα, IL-6	↓ At day 8	
		Circulating PGE$_2$	None	
		Neutrophil phagocytosis	↑	
		Neutrophil respiratory burst	↑	

BSA = Body surface area; DTH = delayed-type hypersensitivity; HLA = human leukocyte antigen; ICU = intensive care unit; IFN = interferon; Ig = immunoglobulin; IL = interleukin; MCT = medium-chain triglyceride; NK = natural killer; PG = prostaglandin; R = receptor; TNF = tumor necrosis factor; TPN = total parenteral nutrition.

Although many of these observations fit with the effects of n-3 PUFAs that might be predicted based upon studies in cell culture, animals and healthy humans, and could be used as evidence of the efficacy of n-3 PUFAs in the trauma and postoperative settings, the complex nature of the formulae prevents such a clear interpretation. The effects could be due to any one of the specified nutrients (i.e. arginine, RNA, n-3 PUFAs) or to the combination of these nutrients. Indeed, the positive outcomes from the use of IMPACT and Immun-Aid have often been used as evidence for the benefit of arginine in these settings.

One other recent trial performed in patients with moderate and severe acute respiratory distress syndrome has used an enteral preparation apparently differing only in lipid source from the control (32% canola oil + 25% MCT + 20% borage oil + 20% fish oil + 3% soy lecithin vs. 97% corn oil + 3% soy lecithin) [44]. However, as well as the difference in fatty acid composition between the formulae, the n-3 PUFA-rich formula contained more vitamin C and E than the control and contained β-carotene, taurine and carnitine, which the control did not. Patients received about 7 g EPA, 3 g DHA, 6 g γ-linolenic acid, 1.1 g vitamin C, 400 IU vitamin E and 6.6 mg β-carotene per day for up to 7 days. By 4 days the numbers of leukocytes and neutrophils in the alveolar fluid had significantly declined in the fish oil + γ-linolenic acid group and were lower than in the control group. Furthermore, arterial oxygenation and gas exchange were improved in the treatment group. Patients in the treatment group had a decreased requirement for supplemental oxygen, reduced time on ventilation support, and shorter length of intensive care unit stay (12.8 ± 1.1 vs. 17.5 ± 1.7 days). Total length of hospital stay also tended to be shorter (29.4 ± 2.6 vs. 34.6 ± 3.3 days). Fewer patients in the treatment group developed new organ failure (4/51 vs. 13/47). Mortality was 19% in the control group and 12% in the treatment group, but this was not a significant difference. Nevertheless, this study suggests the efficacy of n-3 PUFAs (in combination with γ-linolenic acid, MCT, antioxidant vitamins, taurine and carnitine) in this group of patients.

Concluding Statement

Inflammation is a normal part of host defense. However, excessive or inappropriate inflammation is a component of a range of acute and chronic human diseases, including the systemic inflammatory response to trauma, injury and infection. Inflammation is characterized by the production of inflammatory cytokines, ARA-derived eicosanoids, other inflammatory mediators (e.g. platelet-activating factor) and adhesion molecules. n-3 PUFAs decrease the production of inflammatory cytokines and eicosanoids. They act both directly (e.g. by replacing ARA as an eicosanoid substrate and inhibiting ARA metabolism) and indirectly (e.g. by altering the expression of inflammatory genes through effects on transcription factor activation [12]). Thus, n-3 PUFAs are potentially potent anti-inflammatory agents. As such, they may be of therapeutic use in a variety of acute and chronic inflammatory settings. Evidence of their clinical efficacy is strong in some settings (e.g. in rheumatoid arthritis) but generally weak in others (e.g. in asthma). An emerging application is in critically ill patients. At the levels that have been used parenterally or enterally they do not appear to exert any adverse effects. Parenteral nutrition including n-3 PUFAs appears to preserve immune function better than standard total parenteral nutrition and appears to partly prevent some aspects of the inflammatory response. There may be some clinical benefit from these effects. n-3 PUFAs are a component of enteral formulae (e.g. IMPACT, Immun-Aid) that have been examined in a number of clinical trials. There is a lack of consistency in many of the immune and inflammatory outcomes from these studies. However, several studies do report maintenance of immune function and a decreased capacity for production of some inflammatory cytokines. Unlike the studies using parenteral nutrition, it is not possible to ascribe these effects to n-3 PUFAs, since the formulae contain several other 'immunonutrients'. Nevertheless, theses studies support the inclusion of n-3 PUFAs in such formulae.

References

1. Hardardottir I, Grunfeld C, Feingold KR. Effects of endotoxin and cytokines on lipid metabolism. *Curr Opin Lipidol* 1994; 5: 207–15.
2. Khovidhunkit W, Memon RA, Feingold KR, Grunfeld C. Infection and inflammation-induced proatherogenic changes of lipoproteins. *J Infect Dis* 2000; 181: S462–S72.
3. Carpentier YA, Scruel O. Changes in the concentration and composition of plasma lipoproteins during the acute phase response. *Curr Opin Clin Nutr Metab Care* 2002; 5: 153–8.
4. Heyland DK, MacDonald S, Keefe L, Drover JW. Total parenteral nutrition in the critically ill patient: A meta-analysis. *JAMA* 1998; 280: 2013–19.
5. Tilley SL, Coffman TM, Koller BH. Mixed messages: Modulation of inflammation and immune responses by prostaglandins and thromboxanes. *J Clin Invest* 2001; 108: 15–23.
6. Levy BD, Clish CB, Schmidt B, Gronert K, Serhan CN. Lipid mediator class switching during acute inflammation: Signals in resolution. *Nat Immunol* 2001; 2: 612–9.
7. Calder PC, Sherrington EJ, Askanazi J, Newsholme EA. Inhibition of lymphocyte proliferation in vitro by two lipid emulsions with different fatty acid compositions. *Clin Nutr* 1994; 13: 69–74.
8. Serhan CN, Clish CB, Brannon J, Colgan SP, Gronert K, Chiang N. Anti-microinflammatory lipid signals generated from dietary n-3 fatty acids via cyclooxygenase-2 and transcellular processing: A novel mechanism for NSAID and n-3 PUFA therapeutic actions. *J Physiol Pharmacol* 2000; 51: 643–54.
9. Grimminger F, Wahn H, Kramer HJ, Stevens J, Mayer K, Walmrath D, Seeger W. Differential influence of arachidonic acid vs. eicosapentaenoic acid on experimental pulmonary-hypertension. *Am J Physiol* 1995; 268: H2252–H9.
10. Grimminger F, Wahn H, Mayer K, Kiss L, Walmrath D, Seeger W. Impact of arachidonic acid versus eicosapentaenoic acid on exotoxin-induced lung vascular leakage: Relation to 4-series versus 5-series leukotriene generation. *Am J Respir Crit Care Med* 1997; 155: 513–9.
11. Breil I, Koch T, Heller A, Schlotzer E, Grunert A, van Ackern K, Neuhof H. Alteration of n-3 fatty acid composition in lung tissue after short-term infusion of fish oil emulsion attenuates inflammatory vascular reaction. *Crit Care Med* 1996; 24: 1893–902.

12. Calder PC. Dietary modification of inflammation with lipids. *Proc Nutr Soc* 2002; 61: 345–58.

13. Utsunomiya T, Chavali SR, Zhong WW, Forse RA. Effects of continuous tube feeding of dietary fat emulsions on eicosanoid production and on fatty acid composition during an acute septic shock in rats. *Biochim Biophys Acta* 1994; 1214: 333–9.

14. Sane S, Baba M, Kusano C, Shirao K, Andoh T, Kamada T, Aikou T. Eicosapentaenoic acid reduces pulmonary edema in endotoxemic rats. *J Surg Res* 2000; 93: 21–7.

15. Sadeghi S, Wallace FA, Calder PC. Dietary lipids modify the cytokine response to bacterial lipopolysaccharide in mice. *Immunology* 1999; 96: 404–10.

16. Hayashi N, Tashiro T, Yamamori H, Takagi K, Morishima Y, Otsubo Y, Sugiura T, Furukawa K, Nitta H, Nakajima N, Suzuki N, Ito I. Effects of intravenous omega-3 and omega-6 fat emulsion on cytokine production and delayed type hypersensitivity in burned rats receiving total parenteral nutrition. *JPEN J Parenter Enteral Nutr* 1998; 22: 363–7.

17. Mancuso P, Whelan J, DeMichele SJ, Snider CC, Guszcza JA, Karlstad MD. Dietary fish oil and fish and borage oil suppress intrapulmonary proinflammatory eicosanoids biosynthesis and attenuate pulmonary neutrophil accumulation in endotoxic rats. *Crit Care Med* 1997; 25: 1198–206.

18. Mancuso P, Whelan J, DeMichele SJ, Snider CC, Guszcza JA, Claycombe KJ, Smith GT, Gregory TJ, Karlstad MD. Effects of eicosapentaenoic and gamma-linolenic acid on lung permeability and alveolar macrophage eicosanoid synthesis in endotoxic rats. *Crit Care Med* 1997; 25: 523–32.

19. Murray MJ, Kumar M, Gregory TJ, Banks PL, Tazrlaar HD, DeMichele SJ. Select dietary fatty acids attenuate cardiopulmonary dysfunction during acute lung injury in pigs. *Am J Physiol* 1995; 269: H2090–H7.

20. Pscheidl E, Schywalsky M, Tschaikowsky K, Boke-Prols T. Fish oil-supplemented parenteral diets normalize splanchnic blood flow and improve killing of translocated bacteria in a low-dose endotoxin rat model. *Crit Care Med* 2000; 28: 1489–96.

21. Barton RG, Wells CL, Carlson A, Singh R, Sullivan JJ, Cerra FB. Dietary omega-3 fatty acids decrease mortality and Kupffer cell prostaglandin E2 production in a rat model of chronic sepsis. *J Trauma* 1991; 31: 768–74.

22. Lanza-Jacoby S, Flynn JT, Miller S. Parenteral supplementation with a fish oil emulsion prolongs survival and improves lymphocyte function during sepsis. *Nutrition* 2001; 17: 112–6.

23. Johnson JA, Griswold JA, Muakkassa FF, Meyer AA, Maier RV, Chaudry IH, Cerra F. Essential fatty acids influence survival in stress. *J Trauma* 1993; 35: 128–31.

24. Morlion BJ, Torwesten E, Lessire A, Sturm G, Peskar BM, Furst P, Puchstein C. The effect of parenteral fish oil on leukocyte membrane fatty acid composition and leukotriene-synthesizing capacity in postoperative trauma. *Metabolism* 1996; 45: 1208–13.

25. Roulet M, Frascarolo P, Pilet M, Capuis G. Effects of intravenously infused fish oil on platelet fatty acid phospholipid composition and on platelet function in postoperative trauma. *JPEN J Parenter Enteral Nutr* 1997; 21: 296–301.

26. Wachtler P, Konig W, Senkal M, Kemen M, Koller M. Influence of a total parenteral nutrition enriched with ω-3 fatty acids on leukotriene synthesis of peripheral leukocytes and systemic cytokine levels in patients with major surgery. *J Trauma* 1997; 42: 191–8.

27. Heller AR, Fischer S, Rossel T, Geiger S, Siegert G, Ragaller M, Zimmermann T, Koch T. Impact of n-3 fatty acid supplemented parenteral nutrition on haemostasis patterns after major abdominal surgery. *Br J Nutr* 2002; 87: S95–S101.

28. Schauder P, Rohn U, Schafer G, Korff G, Schenk H-D. Impact of fish oil enriched total parenteral nutrition on DNA synthesis, cytokine release and receptor expression by lymphocytes in the postoperative period. *Br J Nutr* 2002; 87: S103–S10.

29. Weiss G, Meyer F, Matthies B, Pross M, Koenig W, Lippert H. Immunomodulation by perioperative administration of n-3 fatty acids. *Br J Nutr* 2002; 87: S89–S94.

30. Beale RJ, Bryg DJ, Bihari DJ. Immunonutrition in the critically ill: A systematic review of clinical outcome. *Crit Care Med* 1999; 27: 2799–805.

31. Gottsclich MM, Jenkins M, Warden GD, Baumer T, Havens P, Snook JT, Alexander JW. Differential effects of 3 enteral dietary regimens on selected outcome variables in burn patients. *JPEN J Parenter Enteral Nutr* 1990; 14: 225–36.

32. Cerra FB, Lehman S, Konstantinides N, Konstantinides F, Shronts EP, Holman R. Effect of enteral nutrient on in vitro tests of immune function in ICU patients: A preliminary report. *Nutrition* 1990; 6: 84–7.

33. Daly JM, Lieberman, Goldfine J, Shou J, Weintraub F, Rosato EF, Lavin P. Enteral nutrition with supplemental arginine, RNA, and omega-3 fatty acids in patients after operation: Immunologic, metabolic, and clinical outcome. *Surgery* 1992; 112: 56–67.
34. Kemen M, Senkal M, Homann H-H, Mumme A, Dauphin A-K, Baier J, Windeler J, Neumann H, Zumtobel V. Early postoperayive enteral nutrition with arginine-ω-3 fatty acids and ribonucleic acid-supplemented diet versus placebo in cancer patients: An immunologic evaluation of Impact®. *Crit Care Med* 1995; 23: 652–9.
35. Daly JM, Weintraub FN, Shou J, Rosato EF, Lucia M. Enteral nutrition during multimodality therapy in upper gastrointestinal cancer patients. *Ann Surg* 1995; 221: 327–38.
36. Senkal M, Kemen M, Homann H-H, Eickhoff U, Baier J, Zumtobel V. Modulation of post-operative immune response by enteral nutrition with a diet enriched with arginine, RNA, and omega-3 fatty acids in patients with upper gastrointestinal cancer. *Eur J Surg* 1995; 161: 115–22.
37. Schilling J, Vranjes N, Fierz W, Joller H, Gyurech D, Ludwig E, Marathias K, Geroulanos S. Clinical outcome and immunology of postoperative arginine, ω-3 fatty acids, and nucleotide-enriched enteral feeding: A randomized prospective comparison with standard enteral and low calories/low fat iv solutions. *Nutrition* 1996; 12: 423–9.
38. Braga M, Vignali A, Gianotti L, Cestari A, Profili M, Di Carlo V. Immune and nutritional effects of early enteral nutrition after major abdominal operations. *Eur J Surg* 1996; 162: 105–12.
39. Weimann A, Bastian L, Bischoff WE, Grotz M, Hansel M, Lotz J, Trautwein C, Tusch G, Schlitt HJ, Regel G. Influence of arginine, omega-3 fatty acids and nucleotide-supplemented enteral support on systemic inflammatory response syndrome and multiple organ failure in patients after severe trauma. *Nutrition* 1998; 14: 165–72.
40. Braga M, Gianotti L, Radaelli G, Vignali A, Mari G, Gentilini O, Di Carlo V. Perioperative immunonutrition in patients undergoing cancer surgery. *Arch Surg* 1999; 134: 428–33.
41. Gianotti L, Braga M, Fortis C, Soldini L, Vignali A, Colombo S, Radaelli G, Di Carlo V. A prospective, randomised clinical trial on perioperative feeding with an arginine-, omega-3 fatty acid-, and RNA-enriched enteral diet: Effect on host response and nutritional status. *JPEN J Parenter Enteral Nutr* 1999; 23: 314–20.
42. Tepaske R, te Velthuis H, Oudemans-van Straaten M, Heisterkamp SH, van Deventer SJH, Ince C, Eysman L, Keseciogu J. Effect of preoperative oral immune-enhancing nutritional supplement on patients at risk of infection after cardiac surgery: A randomised placebo-controlled trial. *Lancet* 2001; 358: 696–701.
43. Wu GH, Zhang YW, Wu ZH. Modulation of postoperative immune and inflammatory response by immune-enhancing enteral diet in gastrointestinal cancer patients. *World Rev Gastroenterol* 2001; 7: 357–62.
44. Gadek JE, DeMichele SJ, Karlstad MD, Pacht ER, Donahoe M, Albertson TE, Van Hoozen C, Wennberg AK, Nelson J, Noursalehi M, the Enteral Nutrition in ARDS Study Group. Effect of enteral feeding with eicosapentaenoic acid, γ-linolenic acid, and antioxidants in patients with acute respiratory distress syndrome. *Crit Care Med* 1999; 27: 1409–20.

Discussion

Dr. Planas Vila: It is now a reality that fish oil lipid emulsion is superior to long-chain triacylglycerol (LCT) or medium-chain triglyceride (MCT) LCT because, in MCT LCT, the amount of n-6 fatty acid is lower than in LCT alone but the ratio of n-3 to n-6 fatty acid is the same. My question is should we be concerned about the auto-oxidation of n-3 fatty acids of fish oil in very ill patients?

Dr. Calder: By oxidation you presumably mean peroxidation, the damaging oxidation that occurs because of the larger number of double bonds in n-3 fatty acids. Yes, I think that is a worry and it is a worry if one is recommending fish oil for oral administration or for parenteral administration. I think we have therefore to ensure that there is appropriate antioxidant protection and monitoring of both the products and the individual. I think that is perhaps the one concern about n-3 fatty acids.

Dr. Planas Vila: Because another possibility is a lipid emulsion with a mix of fish oil and also with olive oil.

Dr. Calder: One of the benefits of olive oil is that it is rich in oleic acid which only has a single double bond, and is therefore much more resistant to peroxidation than n-6 or n-3 fatty acids. In addition olive oil, as you would most certainly know, as a material naturally contains high levels of antioxidants, so I think there are two sides to the apparent benefit of olive oil.

Dr. De Bandt: To prolong the point on peroxidation, there was recently some controversy about the role of vitamin E supplementation and the importance of vitamin E with regard to the huge amount of fish oil supplied and the different responses to fish oil according to the presence or not of vitamin E.

Dr. Calder: I certainly think that in animal studies and in healthy human studies with very large amounts of fish oil being given, some of the effects reported are probably due to lipid peroxidation because of insufficient vitamin E. So I think the vitamin E n-3 polyunsaturated fatty acid balance is an important one, but we don't really know what that balance should be very precisely. Muggli [1] has calculated the vitamin E requirement according to the number of fatty acid double bonds and his equation seems to work alright in terms of inclusion of n-3 in foodstuffs, but I haven't seen anything about that in terms of clinical nutrition. But it is an important point for us to keep in mind.

Dr. Baracos: I have a question about dose. Could you comment, I wonder if dose is getting a patient to swallow a certain amount or dose is equal to achieving a certain level of n-3 fatty acids in phospholipids in a certain cell, and whether you can actually perfuse a concentrated priming dose to achieve such a level and then back off to a maintenance dose. I guess one of the reasons I think about this is I would like to know how much sushi I have to eat to keep it up, and also because I have tried to feed this as very big fish oil capsules to patients with advanced cancer and they find it hard to swallow. Then there are the enteral nutrition products, at least the ones I am experienced with come in attractive flavors like chocolate, hazelnut, soybean, and they also have the additional burden that the concentration of the n-3 fatty acid in the enteral formula comes along with a big piece of baggage which is the rest of the nutrients in that enteral formula, that is to say that those n-3 fatty acids are quite dilute as delivered in enteral formulae. So whatever the dose is, you have got to tell me which is the right one.

Dr. Calder: I am not going to tell you the right one. But you raise a number of important points. So far people have really worked, and I am talking about studies in healthy volunteers here, with the concept that more is better. But the curve that I showed suggested that it is not necessarily the case; there is probably a threshold. Many people, in fact most people, have not been concerned about the status of the cells that they are studying, merely about the amount of fish oil or n-3 fatty acids that the people they are studying are taking. But I personally think it is important to be clear about the status of the target cells that one is studying. So if you are interested in inflammation or immune function you have got to look in those cells and look at the n-3 fatty acid status or eicosapentaenoic acid (EPA) status. There is a linear dose-response relationship between the oral supply of EPA and the concentration of EPA in these cells, so you can sort of do a dose-response curve and see where you are. Now your second point is really related to how you get the amount that you might want to get into people. And it is true that in most fish oil capsules available only 30% of the fatty acids are long-chain n-3 fatty acids, so 70% of the fatty acids are not n-3. So this is a dilute form of supplementation. There are products available that are more highly enriched in n-3 fatty acids. But again if you want to supply a gram of long-chain n-3 fatty acids you have got to give people 3 of the typical capsules per day. If you want to supply 10 g you have got to give them 30 of the typical capsules a day. People are not going to do that, and they can't afford to do it. In addition there is the problem of taste that you have highlighted and also the problem of nausea because above a certain level of consumption of this stuff people feel nauseous. If you are talking about public health nutrition, which you are not, there is really an alternative: eating oily fish a few times a week. In terms of clinical nutrition, obviously there is the problem with enteral nutrition of gastrointestinal upset and other sorts of things, and I don't know how people are going to get around that with the doses that are required.

Dr. Berger: I would like to ask a bit more about this dose question. There was a nice trial carried out in Canada in burn patients. Garrel et al. [2] and his team studied major burns in 3 groups: standard enteral feed with 30% fat, and 2 low-fat groups both with 15% fat but 1 had fish oil. Those groups with reduced fat had the same reduction in infectious complications and so on. There was absolutely no difference between these 2 groups. What was interesting was the reduction in total fat, and here we are talking about actually increasing the amount of fat, which is against cardiovascular recommendations and so on.

Dr. Calder: There is a major debate about the importance of the amount of fat versus the type of fat in public health nutrition, and some people actually don't think that the amount of fat is such a problem because the difficulty then is that people eat carbohydrates [3]. So the type of fat is important rather than the absolute amount. If for example people are eating 100 g fat/day and they are recommended to take 3 fish oil capsules/day, that isn't a major burden in terms of the amount of fat, but the recommendation in public health terms is not to take capsules but to eat fish instead of eating steak.

Dr. Berger: But in the critically ill the amount is important.

Dr. Calder: Yes I know that in clinical nutrition the amount of fat is a key issue and I think you have highlighted that when you are looking at extremes, which you can do in clinical nutrition but not so much in public health nutrition. Yes, the amount of fat is probably very important. Now one would imagine that against the background of lower fat, n-3 fatty acids would be more important but perhaps the effect of lowering fat is greater than the effect of n-3 fatty acids at the dose that was used in that study.

Dr. Déchelotte: I would like to raise an issue about the kinetic effects of fish oil on the immune response and cytokine production. Most of the studies I am aware of were performed in peripheral blood cells after 5–7 days of supplementation of fish oil, and it seems also from clinical studies in patients that there is a need for at least 5 days either pre- or postoperatively to achieve any influence on leukotriene or prostaglandin production. Do you think that this time could be shorter in other tissues, maybe in the gut especially which is the route we use to provide fish oil, then we could achieve some earlier modulation in the gut before anything is to be seen.

Dr. Calder: In studies on healthy volunteers you are right that rather prolonged periods of supplementation have actually been looked at. The shorter studies are 3 weeks in duration, and probably the maximal change in fatty acid composition has occurred at 3 weeks, but it probably takes 2–3 weeks with oral supplementation. People haven't looked at the functional effects during that sort of loading period. So time is important and of course in the clinical arena one can't play so much with time. However, studies using infusion of fish oil-containing parenteral nutrition show effects or differences between groups that are apparent reasonably early on, within a matter of a few days [4]. Recent data from some groups [5] are suggesting that the incorporation of fatty acids provided intravenously can be very quick into some targets, for example into the endothelium. So it may be that there is very quick incorporation into some pools, and by looking at circulating white blood cells we are just not picking that up.

Dr. Déchelotte: But what about enterocytes?

Dr. Calder: I think one of the advantages with something like enterocytes is the rapid rate of turnover. So when there is increased availability of particular fatty acid substrates there is the possibility of their incorporation.

Dr. McClain: Do you think that fish oils are equally protective for all cell types and organs? The reason I am asking this is that if you want to induce experimental liver injury, you give fish oils along with some other toxin such as ethanol.

Dr. Calder: There is a problem: I think that some particular situations and processes where there is liver damage are particularly sensitive to n-3 fatty acids, and you know you can kill animals with liver disease by giving them fish oil. So I think that is a problem.

Dr. McClain: It is a worry in intensive care unit (ICU) patients, where the liver is one of the first organs damaged during multiple organ failure.

Dr. Calder: Obviously it is a worry, one hopes that people who are involved in this research in the clinical arena are looking at that and are concerned about it. I haven't seen anything from enteral or parenteral studies that has indicated a problem there. But you are right that there may be differences between tissues, certainly there are differences between people.

Dr. Neu: Is there a difference between the inflammatory response that you see between preformed docosahexaenoic acid (DHA) and fish oils?

Dr. Calder: I think you are asking what is the active ingredient in fish oil, which is a mix of fatty acids? That is not absolutely clear; people have tried to differentiate between EPA and DHA and there are several papers reporting that each of those is the active fatty acid, so that is unclear. If they work through antagonism of arachidonic acid metabolism then I would put my money on EPA because DHA is not a good substrate for cyclooxygenase and lipoxygenase.

Dr. Neu: This is of major interest right now in pediatrics because many of the formula companies in Europe and Japan have actually started to add DHA to the formulas, and now in the United States we are seeing thousands of babies that have been treated with DHA-containing formulas, and I don't think we really know the mechanism of potential beneficial effects here and it is a preformed fatty acid that they are adding.

Dr. Calder: The idea there is that the DHA is important for brain and eye development and therefore preterm and perhaps term infants have a requirement for DHA to be supplied. You are right that people who have been looking at brain and visual development have not been looking at any other physiological system, so they don't know the potential difficulties or problems within that area.

Dr. Herndon: I would like to come back to a question from Dr. Berger. I don't quibble that fish oils are better than linoleic acid but the question that I would pose to each individual performing a clinical trial is that they do kinetic studies in the body to demonstrate what contribution these exogenously delivered oils have towards total fat economy. Endogenous lipolysis occurs to such a huge extent throughout the hospital course that the primary fat source is from endogenous fat. That amount of endogenous fat can't be handled by the liver as it is, and so no excess fat should be given to the liver except perhaps minimal essential fatty acids for neurological development in neonates.

Dr. Calder: I can't comment. I think n-3 fatty acids have been included in a range of enteral formulae that have been used for a long period of time now in trials and in normal application. I am not aware of reports of adverse effects related to the n-3 content of those products.

Dr. Herndon: I think specifically those studies looked at whole body fat kinetics and they have not looked at the liver. They have had naïve outcomes and naïve results.

Dr. Calder: The authors are somewhere in the room.

Dr. Herndon: I will be happy to discuss it with them.

Dr. Déchelotte: Going with protein metabolism and fish oil we have rather little data in comparison to the immunological and inflammatory parameters in this field. Barber et al. [6] presented very nice studies in pancreatic cancer patients with high doses of n-3 fatty acids showing a reduction in cachexia and an improvement in some protein levels and even perhaps some reduction in the proteasome activity. Do you think we could expect something of this kind in ICU patients?

Dr. Calder: I think you are right that the studies of Barber et al. have used very high doses and I think these are probably the studies that Dr. Baracos was referring to earlier on. The mechanism of action that they identified is a downregulation of proinflammatory cytokine production thereby decreasing the drive on muscle proteolysis, liver acute phase protein synthesis, and so on. So it fits within the context of what I have been talking about, but you are right that they used very high doses although from the top of my head I can't remember what the doses were.

Dr. Déchelotte: Would you expect fish oil to have any direct effect on muscle proteasomes, for instance, regardless of its being mediated by less cytokine response?

Dr. Calder: A lot of recent studies have shown in experimental systems the effects of n-3 fatty acids on many cell-signaling systems including kinases and so on, and that perhaps relates to the work on NFκB and other transcription factors. Certainly they may be active on signaling pathways that lead to activation of many intracellular events including protein degradation, but I haven't seen anything specific on proteasomes.

Dr. McClave: Not all the immune formulas have fish oil, some have MCT oil, and my question is, my understanding of the n-6 contents in the membrane is that they represent long-term ingestion and they don't change very dynamically, very quickly. Are we doing anything by switching out the amount of fat with MCT or is there any immune modulation that is not going to displace the n-6.

Dr. Calder: Immunologically not very much has been shown with MCTs. I think they were seen as an alternative for a simple way of decreasing the amount of n-6 fatty acids available without really increasing the total fat burden because of their ready oxidation. You are right that it is quite difficult to change the n-6 fatty acid content of cell membranes and there are actually only 2 ways to change the arachidonic acid content, and that is to either give arachidonic acid or to give long-chain n-3 fatty acids and they have opposing action. In fact you can change the linoleic acid content of the diet over quite a wide range but you won't change the arachidonic acid content. I think the very first slide I showed of mouse macrophages taken from animals that were fed for 10 weeks on lots of things, coconut oil, olive oil, vegetable oil, the arachidonic acid content was exactly the same.

Dr. Moore: I have had a long interest in acute lung injury and something that trauma surgeons see is fat embolism syndrome. In an early report Dr. Holman described that about 10% of the people with fat embolism syndrome did not have long bone fractures and he attributed this to the fact that they were administering exogenous Intralipid which was coming out of solution. Subsequently other people have correlated this 'creaming effect' with C-reactive protein levels, meaning that if a patient is stressed we should not infuse a lot of Intralipid. So the first question: do you think that happens? Second question: if it does come out of solution, two ways in which you could adversely affect somebody would be to clog up the reticuloendothelium system or the fat globules can cause a fat embolism syndrome in which nobody really knows what happens but it somehow causes acute bone injury. I wonder what your thoughts are.

Dr. Calder: There is only one aspect of your question that I can comment on which is that there is a very long history of studies with Intralipid showing this clogging up of the reticular endothelium system in animals and humans administered Intralipid [7]. I think this was one of the earliest indications of the need for a modification of the profile or the amount of lipid provided. So I think clearly historically it has been documented that it happens, as you suggest, with Intralipid, and it may be that modification of the lipid profile of emulsions can counter that because it can make the particle more readily hydrolyzed at the endothelium wall in various places. Actually MCTs, as you probably know, have the effect of increasing the ability of particles to be hydrolyzed, so that would be an advantage for MCTs over n-6.

Dr. Rosenfeld: My question is about infantile respiratory distress syndrome (IRDS) patients. Some of these patients are septic, and recent work recommending the administration of fish oil to these patients improved the outcome. But I am worried about septic patients who may have more harm than good with the fish oil with immunosuppression and more peroxidation. I would like to hear your comment about that.

Dr. Calder: In adult respiratory distress syndrome (ARDS), there is a particular study which many of you may know by Gadek et al. [8]. I had two slides of that study but I had to take those out along with about 30 other slides to keep to the time allocated like every other speaker. In that study there was enteral provision of fish oil along with some other active ingredients including γ-linolenic acid, taurine, and some antioxidants like β-carotene. They quite clearly showed significant differences from the standard enteral regimen in terms of many of the cellular and clinical markers they were looking at, but not in mortality. I think that study seems to have quite an important impact on people's view about the inclusion of fish oil in patients with ARDS. There is the problem that we already highlighted of this sort of predisposition to lipid peroxidation, and one of the things about the Gadek study was that it included additional antioxidants which are very clearly specified in the article. So I think that this is an important area which they have covered. You highlight the potential for immunosuppression. Certainly if you give animals very high levels of fish oil you get immunosuppression. There are studies in healthy humans that are suggestive of immunosuppression with high levels of fish oil but with insufficient antioxidant protection. The recent studies that I showed you on the parenteral administration of fish oil, at least in the short-term, are in fact suggestive of the opposite: that n-3 fatty acids maintain immune function in postsurgical patients. I think those studies are quite clean and they were just looking at the inclusion of n-3 fatty acids. They did not have all these other things like arginine and so on that are included in the enteral formulae. So the parenteral studies suggest that in the short-term there is no immunosuppression and there may be a protection of immune function.

Dr. Kudsk: There was a comment made before about the slow uptake of the oils into membranes and that it may be quicker than you suspect. I remember a study by Kenler et al. [9] that was published in the *Annals of Surgery* in which they gave fish oil capsules daily preoperatively and within 5 days they found significant increases incorporated in the red blood cell membranes.

Dr. Calder: Yes you are right, you can get them into membranes within days but the maximum incorporation takes a matter of weeks and for red blood cells longer because of the long half-life. But you are right, you can get them into cells reasonably quickly.

Dr. Kudsk: I am curious about the potential mechanism of action. One purpose is the suppression of the PG2 series, and it has been thought that it may be the primary action. There have been studies in critically ill patients where prostaglandin synthesis inhibitors and COX2 inhibitors have been ineffective generally in altering outcome in critically ill patients. Couldn't that argue that there may be some other mechanism that we haven't explored?

Dr. Calder: I agree with you completely. I personally don't believe that these fatty acids work primarily as, lets say, COX antagonists. I believe that they have effects on cell signaling in their own right, and I think that many of the studies I showed show direct actions of fatty acids in cell culture systems on gene expression. There are these studies on NFκB, on the IκB activation state and IκB phosphorylation, and so on. So I think they have effects on cell-signaling pathways that have nothing to do with eicosanoids. Nevertheless I think eicosanoids at the moment allow us to explain the potential but I think the reality is that they are working in a different way.

Dr. Nitenberg: I want to go back to the study by Gadek et al. [7], I think we have to be very cautious with this study because it was not an intent-to-treat study. 140 patients entered the study, but only 86 were analyzed, so I think the conclusions are not so clear. The second point is how to use these products in ICU patients. In septic patients because, as you have shown, the first part of the patient is probably in the first position and, maybe if we accord some value to the bone classification, it is then in the marked position which is the mixed inflammatory status. So according to the potential value of fish oil, do you think we have to give this type of oil only for the first 5 days, for 10 days, for 30 days, to stop for a while, to come back after? It is very difficult in clinical practice.

Dr. Calder: What I didn't show on the slide, although it was redrawn from the original, is that these authors suggested a role for n-3 fatty acids throughout because of the potential to decrease the early inflammation and prevent the later immunosuppression. There is evidence for the first of these: I showed you data on tumor necrosis factor, IL-1 and IL-6. There is actually little evidence for the second. We and others have looked for increased IL-10 and TGF-β production and not seen it [10]. So I think the original idea of these authors that n-3 fatty acids should play a role throughout may not be entirely correct, but we have to do something to try to find the answer to your question. But it may be that there is a role for them early on and then we stop and move over to some other form of support.

Dr. McClave: Along the lines of this same comment I would be more worried about the arginine timing with these curves, that you hold back on the arginine in the first part and then start giving it in the second part.

Dr. Planas Vila: I am talking about lipid emulsions in critically ill patients, and in reality in general we find more hyperglycemia than hypertriglyceridemia in these patients, and when we find hypertriglyceridemia it is generally in patients who simultaneously receive another kind of lipid, such as glopophol, along with lipid emulsions. But if we administer lipid emulsions, we can safely administer 30–40% of nonprotein calories and control hypertriglyceridemia because I think for these patients it is worse to have hyperglycemia, and we have hyperglycemia every day in critically ill patients. It is a reality that in the lipid emulsions that have been used until now, LCT or MCT LCT, the amounts of n-6 fatty acids are too high, but really I am more afraid of hyperglycemia in this kind of patient.

References

1. Muggli R. Polyunsaturated fatty acids and requirements of vitamin E. *Fett Wissenschaft Technol/Fat Sci Technol* 1974; 96: 17–9.
2. Garrel DR, Razi M, Lariviere F, et al. Improved clinical status and length of care with low-fat nutrition support in burn patients. *JPEN J Parenter Enteral Nutr* 1995; 19: 482–91.
3. Sanders TAB. High fat versus low fat diet in human diseases. *Curr Opin Clin Nutr Metab Care,* 2003, in press.
4. Wachtler P, Konig W, Senkal M, et al. Influence of total parenteral nutrition enriched with omega-3 fatty acids on leukotriene synthesis of peripheral leukocytes and systemic cytokine levels in patients after major surgery. *J Trauma* 1997; 42: 191–8.

5. Dupont IE, Scruel O, Lontre JF, Carpenter YA. Fish oil-containing lipids emulsions induce rapid incorporation of n-3 fatty acids into endothelial cell phospholipids. *Clin Nutr* 2001; 20 (suppl 3): 7–8.
6. Barber MD, Fearon KCH, Tisdale MJ, et al. Effect of a fish oil-enriched nutritional supplement on metabolic mediators in patients with pancreatic cancer catexia. *Nutr Cancer* 2001; 40: 118–24.
7. Koga Y, Swanson VL, Hayes DM. Hepatic 'intravenous fat pigment' in infants and children receiving lipid emulsion. *J Pediatr Surg* 1975; 10: 641–8.
8. Gadek JE, DeMichele SL, Karlstad MD, et al. Effect of enteral feeding with eicosapentaenoic acid, gamma-linolenic acid, and antioxidants in patients with acute respiratory distress syndrome. Enteral Nutrition in ARDS Study Group. *Crit Care Med* 1999; 27: 1409–20.
9. Kenler AS, Swails WS, Driscoll DF, et al. Early enteral feeding in postsurgical cancer patients. Fish oil structured lipid-based polymeric formula versus a standard polymeric formula. *Ann Surg* 1996; 223: 316–33.
10. Sadeghi S, Wallace FA, Calder PC. Dietary lipids modify the cytokine response to bacterial lipopolysaccharide in mice. *Immunology* 1999; 96: 404–10.

Cynober L, Moore FA (eds): Nutrition and Critical Care.
Nestlé Nutrition Workshop Series Clinical & Performance Program, Vol. 8, pp. 99–117,
Nestec Ltd.; Vevey/S. Karger AG, Basel, © 2003.

Key Vitamins and Trace Elements in the Critically Ill

Mette M. Berger and René L. Chioléro

Surgical ICU and Burns Centre, CHUV, Lausanne, Switzerland

Introduction

Trace elements and vitamins are essential components of nutrition (unless specified, vitamins and trace elements will hereafter be designated globally as micronutrients). Trace elements are metals and metalloids present in the body at fairly constant concentrations. Trace elements act as a structure of enzymes or as cofactors, and frequently they exert electron transfer functions. Their absence causes reproducible structural or biochemical deficits, and they are associated with specific biochemical alterations. These alterations can be prevented or corrected by the intake of the deficient element alone. Vitamins are organic substances required in minute amounts, and they are not synthesized by the body (or not in sufficient quantities). Vitamins are cofactors in the different metabolic steps of enzymes, carbohydrate, protein, and lipid metabolism.

Micronutrients are involved in the prevention of nutritional deficiencies, immune humoral and cellular defense, regulation of gene expression during the acute phase response, antioxidant defense, and prevention of chronic diseases. Most micronutrients have been discovered due to acute nutritional deficiencies causing specific diseases, such as ascorbic acid and scurvies, zinc and delayed wound healing and dwarfism, selenium and skeletal myopathy, and iron and anemia.

Micronutrient deficiency in the general population is infrequent, but inadequate intake is widespread as shown by a series of epidemiological studies carried out over the last 2 decades [1–3]. Due to changes in nutrient composition and in eating habits, a large proportion of the population does not ingest the recommended intakes for micronutrients such as iron, selenium, zinc, and vitamins B and C. Inadequate intakes are considered to contribute to the development of cardiovascular diseases, cancer and ageing in the general population [4, 5]. There is growing evidence that micronutrient deficiencies occur in the critically ill patient, particularly in sepsis, major burns, and conditions with ischemia-reperfusion. A previously compromised status will rapidly be unbalanced by acute disease, and the related increased demands on the body.

Key micronutrients in critically ill patients will be those that are directly or indirectly involved in metabolic support, as well as in antioxidant and immune defense. In the following their roles will be detailed.

Systemic Responses of the Critically Ill

Critically ill patients differ from noncritically ill in many respects. Outcome is influenced by the life-threatening conditions they suffer: such patients are dependent on artificial, technical and metabolic support, which the noncritically ill rarely are. The metabolic consequences of their diseases are extensive. They are generally hypermetabolic and subsequently have increased nutritional requirements [6]. In addition the wound healing process of surgical patients increases the general and specific nutrient requirements. Many patients have abnormal vitamin and trace element losses due to their disease or injury. For example, septic patients have high vitamin A urinary excretion [7]; trauma patients lose zinc and selenium through their drains, and burn patients lose major amounts of copper, selenium, and zinc with their cutaneous exudates [8, 9].

Most critically ill patients exhibit intense inflammatory and acute phase responses which cause major changes to endocrine and immune systems, and to metabolic regulations with resistance to nutrition. The acute phase response is associated with increased production of cytokines and other mediators, with subsequent reorientation of hepatic protein synthesis, redistribution of micronutrients to different organs and tissues, and their displacement from the circulating compartment. Activation of the nuclear transcription factor κB (NFκB) is a key step in the development of the full-blown inflammatory picture [10]. The acute phase response is also associated with a major increase in free radical production. The production of ROS and nitric oxide (NO) species is particularly enhanced in conditions, such as acute respiratory failure, sepsis, acute renal or hepatic failure, pancreatitis, major trauma and burns, and organ transplantation (table 1). An acute inflammatory response constitutes a serious risk factor for the development of organ dysfunction and failure in critically ill patients.

Table 1. ICU conditions at risk of endogenous antioxidant depletion

Condition	⇑ ROS production ⇑ degradation products	Vitamin and trace elements at risk or depleted
Acute illness	Lipoperoxides, plasma redox status [a]	Vitamin B1 [19] Ascorbic acid [b]
Acute coronary syndrome	TBARS [c]	Selenium [d]
Acute renal failure	TBARS [e]	Selenium, ascorbic acid, and β-carotene [f] Copper, Selenium [Berger et al, unpublished data]
Acute liver failure/cirrhosis	Lipoperoxides [g]	Zinc [h, i]
ARDS	Lipoperoxides [j, k]	Vitamin E [k]
Brain injury	Lipoperoxides [l–n]	Copper, Zinc [o, 27]
Burns	TBARS [22, 24, p, q]	Selenium [8, r] Copper, Zinc [9, 23, s, t] Vitamin C [u] Vitamin E [p]
Myocardial ischemia	Lipoperoxides [v]	Vitamin E, Selenium [w]
Organ transplantation (heart, kidney, liver, lung)	NO mediated vascular responses [x]	Copper [y], Selenium [z], Zinc [aa]
Pancreatitis	Lipoperoxides [bbc]	Selenium [cc],
Sepsis	Ethane, TBARS [42]	Vitamin A [dd], Selenium [21, ee], Glutathione [42]
Stroke (ischemic)	Lipoperoxides [ff]	Selenium [gg]
Trauma	[hh]	Selenium, Zinc [ii, 25]

a. Alonso de Vega JM, et al.: Crit Care Med 2000; 28:1812–1814.
b. Schorah CJ, et al.: Am J Clin Nutr 1996; 63:760–765.
c. Andican G, et al.: Clinical Chemistry & Laboratory Medicine 2001; 39:234–238.
d. Poltronieri R, et al.: Cardioscience 1992; 3:155–160.
e. Richard MJ, et al.: Biol Tr Elem Res 1993; 39:149–159.
f. Metnitz GH, et al.: Acta Anaesthesiol Scand 2000; 44:236–240.
g. Britton RS, & Bacon BR. : Hepato-gastroenterology 1994; 41:343–348.
h. Riordan SM,& Williams R.: New Engl J Med 1997; 337:473–479.
i. Marchesini G, et al.: Hepatology 1996; 23:1084–1092.
j. Richard C, et al.: Crit Care Med 1990; 18:4–9
k. Reddy KV, et al.: Nutrition 1998; 14:448–451.
l. Hall ED, & Braughler JM.: Free Rad Biol Med 1989; 6:303–313
m. Inci S, et al.: Neurosurgery 1998; 43:330–335
n. Willson RL.: Proc Nutr Soc 1987; 46:27–34.
o. Chan PK.: J Neurotrauma 1992; 9:S417–S423.
p. Mingjian Z, et al.: Burns 1992; 18:19–21.
q. Demling RH,& LaLonde C.: J Trauma 1990; 30:69–74.
r. Boosalis MG, et al.: Burns 1986; 12:236–240.
s. Sampson B, et al.: Ann Clin Biochem 1996; 33:462–464.
t. Shakespeare PG.: Burns 1982; 8:358–364.
u. Lund CC, et al.: Arch Surg 1946; 55:557–583.
v. Lapenna D, et al.: Ann Thorac Surg 1994; 57:1522–1525.
w. Gaziano JM.: Nutrition 1996; 12:583–588.
x. Berkenboom G, et al.: Cardiovascular Research 1997; 33:650–654
y. Singer P, et al.: Transplant Proc 2000;32:701
z. Hussein O, et al.: Transplantation 1997; 63:679–685.
aa. Chin SE, et al.: Am J Clin Nutr 1992; 56(1):164–8.
bb. McCloy R.: Digestion 1998; 59 (Suppl 4):36–48.
cc. Schoenberg MH, et al.: Am J Clin Nutr 1995; 62:1306S–1314S.
dd. Stephensen CB, et al.: Am J Clin Nutr 1994; 60:388–392.
ee. Forceville X, et al.: Crit Care Med 1998; 26:1536–1544.
ff. Imai H, et al.: Stroke 2001; 32:2149–2154.
gg. Yamaguchi T, et al.: Stroke 1998; 29:12–17.
hh. Waxman K: New Horizons 1996; 4:153–160.
ii. Berger MM, et al.: J Trauma 1996; 40:103–109.

(alphabetic references only appear in the present table, numeric references are quoted in the text)

Antioxidation and Immunity: Role of Micronutrients

Free radicals are atoms or molecules containing one or more unpaired electrons: they are unstable and strive to restore parity. They are also called ROS and their production occurs under normal aerobic metabolism. NO species are a normal byproduct of endothelial metabolism. ROS are mainly produced by leukocytes and by the respiratory mitochondrial chain. ROS are required for cell signalling, and for bacterial defense. In the normal subject the endogenous antioxidant defenses balance the ROS production. Antioxidants are substances, which inhibit or delay oxidation of a substrate while present in minute amounts [11]. Endogenous antioxidant defenses are both enzymatic (e.g. superoxide dismutase, glutathione peroxidases (GSHPx), catalase) and nonenzymatic (e.g. uric acid, glutathione, bilirubin, thiols, albumin, and nutritional factors, including vitamins and trace elements). The enzymes act in cascades and depend on trace elements for structure and activity. Nutritional antioxidants act through different mechanisms: (1) they directly neutralize free radicals; (2) they reduce the peroxide concentrations and repair oxidized membranes; (3) they quench iron to decrease ROS production, and (4) via lipid metabolism, short-chain free fatty acids and cholesteryl esters neutralize ROS [12]. Most antioxidants interact and contribute to their respective regeneration.

In clinical settings 'oxidative stress' has been defined either by direct evidence of increased ROS and NO production, respectively, of increased byproducts of lipid peroxidation (e.g. increased thiobarbituric acid reactive substances (TBARS)), or by determination of low antioxidant defense (losses or low circulating levels). Table 1 shows conditions in which such changes have been observed in the critically ill. In addition it shows which micronutrients have been shown to be deficient and at risk of depletion in the various conditions.

Immunity is frequently compromised in the critically ill patient. Immune defense is closely linked to antioxidant defense: membrane fluidity and integrity (vitamin E), genomic changes (selenium), and cell replication (zinc) are essential for immunity but depend on appropriate antioxidant control. The leukocyte membranes are constituted by saturated and unsaturated fatty acids that may be oxidized, and consequently destroyed by the ROS. The subsequent loss of fluidity of the membrane is associated with an alteration in lymphocyte function [13]. Selenium has a key function in antioxidant defense such as the electron carrier properties in GSHPx, which is essential for the immune defense. Selenium supplements have been shown to modulate NFκB expression under various circumstances, including HIV infection [14]. In animal and human trials selenium supplements have been shown to reduce the incidence of hepatitis B [15]. This is explained by the action of the viral genome. Selenium inhibits the activity of the reverse RNA transcriptase required for viral replication [16], an effect which is probably mediated by

GSHPx. The increased virulence of the Coxsackie B3 virus in selenium-deficient mice is another example of the impact of the antioxidant status on the stability of the viral genome [17], as the viral phenotype can be modified by the selenium status [18].

The B vitamin group contributes indirectly to antioxidant defense through the intermediary metabolism. Thiamine (vitamin B_1) is the coenzyme of carbohydrate decarboxylation reactions. Thiamine deficiency is very frequent in critically ill patients [19]. Riboflavin (vitamin B_2) is constitutive of flavine adenine dinucleotide and is an electron carrier in the oxidation and reduction reactions of the flavine coenzymes in the mitochondrial respiratory chain. Vitamin PP (B_3 = niacin) is converted in the tissues to nicotinamide adenine dinucleotide (NAD$^+$; involved in hydrogen transport) and NAD phosphate (NADP$^+$; fatty acid synthesis and pentose cycle). NAD$^+$ and NADP$^+$ play important roles in the antioxidant spiral, providing electrons for the reduction of oxidized glutathione.

In healthy subjects with adequate nutritional status, endogenous antioxidants including vitamins and trace elements are able to neutralize normal ROS production. But about 1% of the ROS production escapes antioxidant control and contributes to ageing phenomena. In the critically ill, the unstable equilibrium is lost in most pathologies (table 1). Under such stress conditions, an imbalance results from enhanced free radical production combined with depletion of the endogenous antioxidants through losses, redistribution, and inadequate intake. This contributes to worsening of acute illnesses and to the development of organ failure due to the side effects of the persistence of an intense systemic inflammatory response syndrome (SIRS).

Supplementation Trials in the Critically Ill

Before considering trace element and vitamin supplementation, a distinction should be made between the previous diets and the provision of immunomodulating diets. The latter diets have been used extensively during the last decade. Various diets on the market contain 'immunomodulating substrates' (e.g. glutamine, arginine, n-3 fatty acids, nucleotides) and variable amounts of antioxidant micronutrients, bringing uncertainty as to what has caused the changes. But while immunomodulating diets have been associated with increased mortality in critically ill patients [20], this has never been shown to occur with micronutrient supplements alone. Therefore the latter may be considered as safe.

Research on antioxidant supplementation in the critically ill has focused mainly on five micronutrients: vitamins C and E, copper, selenium and zinc. table 2 summarizes the available trials. Surprisingly, retinol has so far not been investigated in the critically ill. In 42 critically ill patients with SIRS due

Table 2. Studies on micronutrient supplementation in critically ill patients

Trial	Patient category	Type of study	Patient number	Micronutrients	Endpoint
Angstwurm et al. [21], 1999	Sepsis	PRCT	42	Selenium	Renal failure Mortality
Berger et al. [22], 1995	Major burns	Prospective consecutive series	10	Copper, selenium, zinc	Length of stay
Berger et al. [23], 1998	Major burns	PRCT	20	Copper, selenium, zinc	Infections
Berger et al. [40], 2002	Major burns	PRCT	20	Copper, selenium, zinc	Tissue levels
Tanaka et al. [24], 2000	Major burns	Randomized by month of admission	37	Ascorbic acid	Resuscitation fluid volume and retention
Berger et al. [26], 2001	Trauma	PRCT	32	Selenium, α-tocopherol	Thyroid function Organ failure
Porter et al. [25], 1999	Major trauma	PRCT	18	NAC, ascorbic acid, α-tocopherol, selenium	Infections
Preiser et al. [41], 2000	Critically ill	PRCT	37	Vitamin A, ascorbic acid, α-tocopherol	Ex vivo LDL tolerance to oxidative stress
Young et al. [27], 1996	Traumatic brain injury	PRCT	68	Zinc	Neurological outcome
Ortolani et al. [42], 2000	Septic shock	PRCT	30	N-acetyl cysteine, glutathione	Ethane breath, TBARS plasma

PRCT = Prospective randomized controlled trial; NAC = N-acetyl cysteine; LDL = low-density lipoprotein; TBARS = thiobarbituric acid reacting substance.

to an infectious disease, selenium supplementation for 9 days was associated with a significant reduction in acute renal failure (3/21 patients versus 9/21, $p = 0.035$), and a nonsignificant reduction in mortality [21]. In major burns, copper, selenium and zinc supplements amounting to 6–8 times the RDA intakes were associated with reduced lipid peroxidation and a reduction in infectious complications [22, 23]. In the same trial the interleukin-6 levels were lower in the supplemented patients after 24 h of trace element supplementation including 350 μg/day selenium [23]. Mega doses of ascorbic acid, provided during the first 24 h of resuscitation in patients with major burns, reduced fluid requirements by about 30% [24] by reducing alterations in capillary permeability. Providing N-acetylcysteine, selenium and vitamins C and E or placebo to 18 trauma patients was associated with a decrease in infectious complications (8 versus 18) and fewer organ dysfunctions (0 versus 9) [25]. A trial using selenium in combination with vitamin E, or placebo in 32 patients with major trauma was associated with a normalization of thyroid function (triiodothyronine and thyroxin concentrations in particular) [26], with significant changes in antioxidant status in the supplemented patients [26a]. In severe brain injury, zinc supplements (20 mg for 2 weeks) were associated with improved neurological recovery [27]. The reinforcement of the antioxidant defenses is argued to be the mechanism leading to the clinical benefits observed in these trials.

Supplementation Strategies

The aims of supplementation can be summarized as follows: (1) to provide basic nutritional support, the increased nutritional requirements related to hypermetabolism and wound healing; (2) to prevent or correct deficiencies [9], and (3) to modulate the acute phase and immune responses by reinforcement of the endogenous antioxidant defenses. While classical, this sequence 1–3 ought to be reversed in the critically ill, starting with antioxidant reinforcement.

Micronutrients: Basic Nutritional and Antioxidant Requirements

There are changing paradigms regarding the methods to establish micronutrient requirements in the general population. Making universal recommendations among the different ecological, anthropological, and geographical settings appears futile as lower than normal body stores may be adaptive [28]. Establishing requirements is even more difficult in the critically ill. There are still gaps in our knowledge regarding the bases of

Table 3. Recommended daily intakes (RDIs) for intravenous (i.v.) administration according to the American Medical Association in comparison with nutritional micronutrient recommendations for the general population (RDA) [39] and in sick patients (FDA) [29], and examples of doses used in clinical trials in critically ill patients

Micronutrient	RDI for i.v. use [43, 44]	Oral RDA [45] %	i.v. FDA 2000 [29] mg	Doses used in critically ill trials
Copper	0.5–1.5 mg	45	–	Burns: 2.0–5.0 mg Liver disease: 5.0 mg
Selenium	30–60 µg	70	–	Burns: 350 µg SIRS sepsis: 300–900 µg
Zinc	2.5–4 mg	25	–	Burns: 35 mg Liver cirrhosis: 10–20 mg
α-Tocopherol	10 mg	100	10	100 mg to 3 g
Ascorbic acid	100 mg	160	200	1–110 g
Niacin	40 mg	250	40	–
Thiamine	3 mg	300	6	100–200 mg

The recommended i.v. doses of trace elements are proportionally lower than i.v. vitamin doses compared with the oral RDA, which shows the concern about trace element toxicity.

nutrient requirements. Moreover trace elements are inorganic, with a potential for accumulation: the fear of toxicity has delayed the recognition of increased requirements. The American Food and Drug Administration has recently recognized that vitamin requirements are increased during acute illness, particularly in critically illness [29], but this upgrading process has still not been completed for trace elements (table 3).

Available tools for the assessment of requirements include balance studies and depletion-repletion trials. These approaches have pitfalls, and losses are always underestimated. Nutrient requirements are defined as the amount required to replace endogenous losses or to maintain appropriate concentrations in the circulating compartment. Generally the latter does not reflect the status and the tissue and organ levels. The circulating levels only reflect the flow between the various organs. Moreover, estimating requirements from losses fails to consider homeostatic adjustments in nutrient metabolism. The functional approach, which is closer to metabolism and includes assessment of enzymatic activities depending on micronutrients (e.g. selenium and GSHPx, or zinc and alkaline phosphatase), requires the definition of other appropriate endpoints (only those for Se and Zn are defined), yet is not available in the critically ill [30].

Which doses should then be supplied? In general population intervention trials using nutritional doses close to the RDAs have achieved a reduction in infectious morbidity [31, 32]. But the RDAs are by definition not designed for the critically ill. There is actually no consensus as to which quantities should be proposed and whether the doses are the same in all critically ill patient categories. There is growing evidence that the micronutrients required for nutritional and antioxidant purposes should be considered separately.

Timing

Clinical trials in burns suggest that early intervention determines the antioxidant impact [21–24]. The most important decreases in circulating levels of micronutrients and the most important losses are observed early on during the first 2 weeks of the acute disease, during which the largest increases in ROS production occur. Therefore micronutrient supplements with antioxidant objectives should be supplied early in the course of disease, while nutritional requirements should be covered separately, and may be started later, when nutritional support is required.

Single versus Combined Micronutrient Provision

The advantage of providing a single nutrient is the possibility of investigating its effects and determining the dose required to achieve an action. Indeed multi-supplementation trials have the same disadvantage as immunonutrition trials: it would be interesting to know which of the single micronutrients is responsible for benefits or harm. The disadvantage of single nutrient trials is that as micronutrients function as a network, providing increased amounts of a single component may generate an imbalance. The rationale underlying the use of a combination of micronutrients instead of single elements is based on the observation of the biochemical properties of the endogenous antioxidant network [33]. Micronutrients depend on each other for regeneration in a continued spiral. In a few trials, selenium has been used alone, but there is a risk of increasing the internal imbalance by doing so, especially with large amounts.

Route of Delivery

The intravenous route is the only one that guaranties bioavailability in the circulating compartment, avoiding the absorption problems and the liver first-pass effect. The clinical trials that have used the enteral route in the critically ill are few (burns [34], trauma [25]). This is explained by the unpredictable

107

absorption in the critically ill [35], and the difficulty in guarantying full enteral delivery very early on during the course of acute illness. The large variability of enteral micronutrient absorption in healthy subjects is increased in the critically ill, for instance hemodynamic failure, bowel ischemia, bowel edema due to a local inflammatory response and fluid resuscitation [36] may compromise absorption. Vitamin E absorption is reduced in critically ill compared to healthy volunteers [37]. In addition many micronutrients compete for enteral absorption, such as copper and zinc, selenium and copper, and many others. These interactions may compromise the therapeutic intervention as observed for copper and zinc during a supplementation trial carried out in burned children, where enteral supplementation failed to correct copper and zinc deficiency [34]. Moreover, providing micronutrients by the enteral route after bowel surgery does not increase the circulating levels [38]. Therefore, to achieve systemic antioxidant effects, the intravenous route remains the only predictable one.

Monitoring of Intervention
There are actually no clinical laboratory determinations available that can be used as targets during antioxidant supplementation. Therefore such micronutrient treatments remain empirical for the moment.

Perspectives

There is increasing evidence that micronutrients play a major role in the nutritional and metabolic management of the critically ill. Early in the course of disease, their antioxidant properties modulate the inflammatory response and immunity, and later on, they are essential components of nutritional support. Future clinical trials should be performed in large patient populations to determine their effects in the prevention of remote organ failure and infectious complications.

Conclusions

Some vitamins and trace elements are particularly important in the critically ill patient, mainly thiamine, α-tocopherol, ascorbic acid, copper, selenium, and zinc. The key micronutrients are those that are involved in antioxidant and immune function as well as in the carbohydrate metabolism. Based on actual knowledge, patients that may benefit from early large micronutrient supplementation include subjects presenting an intense inflammatory response, and those who have demonstrable large micronutrient losses like major burns, patients on renal replacement therapy or with abnormal intestinal losses (diarrhea, fistulae, aspirations), as well as those who have deficient clearances of metabolic end products due to hepatic and renal failure. Further research is required to determine the clinical endpoints and laboratory tests for clinical settings.

References

1. Hercberg S, Preziosi P, Galan P, Deheeger M, Papoz L, Dupin H. Apports nutritionnels d'un échantillon représentatif de la population du Val-de-Marne: III. Les apports en minéraux et vitamines. *Rev Epidém Santé Publ* 1991; 39: 245–61.
2. Rayman MP. Dietary selenium: Time to act. *BMJ* 1997; 314: 387–8.
3. Hercberg S, Preziosi P, Galan P, Faure H, Arnaud J, Duport N, et al. 'The SU.VI.MAX Study': A primary prevention trial using nutritional doses of antioxidant vitamins and minerals in cardiovascular diseases and cancers. SUpplementation on VItamines et Mineraux AntioXydants. *Food Chem Toxicol* 1999; 37: 925–30.
4. Hercberg S, Galan P, Preziosi P, Roussel AM, Arnaud J, Richard MJ, et al. Background and rationale behind the SU.VI.MAX study: A prevention trial using nutritional doses of a combination of antioxidant vitamins and minerals to reduce cardiovascular diseases and cancers. *Int J Vitam Nutr Res* 1998; 68: 3–20.
5. Fairfield KM, Fletcher RH. Vitamins for chronic disease prevention in adults: Scientific review. *JAMA* 2002; 287: 3116–26.
6. Chioléro R, Revelly JP, Tappy L. Energy metabolism in sepsis and injury. *Nutrition* 1997; 13: S45–S51.
7. Stephensen CB, Alvarez JO, Kohatsu J, Hardmeier R, Kennedy JI Jr, Gammon RB. Vitamin A is excreted in the urine during acute infection. *Am J Clin Nutr* 1994; 60: 388–92.
8. Berger MM, Cavadini C, Bart A, Blondel A, Bartholdi I, Vandervale A, et al. Selenium losses in 10 burned patients. *Clin Nutr* 1992; 11: 75–82.
9. Berger MM, Cavadini C, Bart A, Mansourian R, Guinchard S, Bartholdi I, et al. Cutaneous zinc and copper losses in burns. *Burns* 1992; 18: 373–80.
10. Flohé L, Brigelius-Flohé R, Saliou C, Traber MG, Packer L. Redox regulation of NF-kappa B activation. *Free Radic Biol Med* 1997; 22: 1115–26.
11. Halliwell B, Gutteridge JMC. The antioxidants of human extracellular fluids. *Arch Biochem Biophys* 1990; 280: 1–8.
12. Parke DV. Nutritional antioxidants in disease prevention: mechanisms of action. In: Basu T, Temple N, Garg M, eds. *Antioxidants in human health and disease*. Wallingford: Cabi, 1999; 1–13.
13. Bendich A. Immunological role of antioxidant vitamins. In: Basu T, Temple N, Garg M, eds. *Antioxidants in human health and disease*. Wallingford: Cabi, 1999; 27–42.
14. Makropoulos V, Bruning T, Schulze-Osthoff K. Selenium-mediated inhibition of transcription factor NF-kappa B and HIV-1 LTR promoter activity. *Arch Toxicol* 1996; 70: 277–83.
15. Yu SY, Zhu YJ, Li WG. Protective role of selenium against hepatitis B virus and primary liver cancer in Qidong. *Biol Trace Element Res* 1997; 56: 117–24.
16. Schrauzer GN, Sacher J. Selenium in the maintenance and therapy of HIV-infected patients. *Chem Biol Interact* 1994; 91: 199–205.
17. Beck MA, Kolbeck PC, Shi Q, Rohr LH, Morris VC, Levander OA. Increased virulence of a human enterovirus (Coxsackievirus B3) in selenium-deficient mice. *J Infect Dis* 1994; 170: 351–7.
18. Levander OA, Beck MA. Interacting nutritional and infectious etiologies of Keshan disease – Insights from Coxsackie virus B-induced myocarditis in mice deficient in selenium or vitamin E. *Biol Trace Element Res* 1997; 56: 5–21.
19. Cruickshank AM, Telfer ABM, Shenkin A. Thiamine deficiency in the critically ill. *Intens Care Med* 1988; 14: 384–87.

20. Heyland DK, Novak F, Drover JW, Jain M, Su X, Suchner U. Should immunonutrition become routine in critically ill patients? A systematic review of the evidence. *JAMA* 2001; 286: 944–53.
21. Angstwurm MWA, Schottdorf J, Schopohl J, Gaertner R. Selenium replacement in patients with severe systemic inflammatory response syndrome improves clinical outcome. *Crit Care Med* 1999; 27: 1807–13.
22. Berger MM, Chioléro R. Relations between copper, zinc and selenium intakes and malondialdehyde excretion after major burns. *Burns* 1995; 21: 507–12.
23. Berger MM, Spertini F, Shenkin A, Wardle C, Wiesner L, Schindler C, et al. Trace element supplementation modulates pulmonary infection rates after major burns: A double-blind, placebo-controlled trial. *Am J Clin Nutr* 1998; 68: 365–71.
24. Tanaka H, Matsuda T, Miyagantani Y, Yukioka T, Matsuda H, Shimazaki S. Reduction of resuscitation fluid volumes in severely burned patients using ascorbic acid administration. *Arch Surg* 2000; 135: 326–31.
25. Porter JM, Ivatury RR, Azimuddin K, Swami R. Antioxidant therapy in the prevention of organ dysfunction syndrome and infectious complications after trauma: Early results of a prospective randomized study. *Am Surg* 1999; 65: 478–83.
26a. Berger MM, Baines M, Wardle CC, Cayeux C, Henry H, Shenkin A, et al. Influence of early trace element and vitamin E supplements on the plasma antioxidant status after major trauma: A controlled trial. *Nutr Res* 2001; 21: 41–54.
26. Berger MM, Reymond MJ, Shenkin A, Rey F, Wardle C, Cayeux M, Schindler C, Chioléro RL. Influence of selenium supplements on the post-traumatic alterations of the thyroid axis – a prospective placebo-controlled trial. Intensive Care Med 2001; 27: 91–100.
27. Young B, Ott L, Kasarskis E, Rapp R, Moles K, Dempsey RJ, et al. Zinc supplementation is associated with improved neurologic recovery rate and visceral protein levels of patients with severe closed head injury. *J Neurotrauma* 1996; 13: 25–34.
28. Solomons NW, Ruz M. Trace element requirements in humans – An update. *J Trace Elem Exp Med* 1998; 11: 177–95.
29. FDA. Parenteral multivitamin products; Drugs for human use; Drug efficacy study implementation; Amendment. *Federal Register* 2000; Vol 65: No 77.
30. King J. The need to consider functional endpoints in defining nutrient requirements. *Am J Clin Nutr* 1996; 63: S983–S4.
31. Bogden JD, Bendich A, Kemp FW, Bruening KS, Skurnick JH, Denny T, et al. Daily micronutrient supplements enhance delayed hypersensitivity skin responses in older people. *Am J Clin Nutr* 1994; 60: 437–47.
32. Chandra RK. Effect of vitamin and trace-element supplementation on immune responses and infection in elderly subjects. *Lancet* 1992; 340: 1124–7.
33. Grimble RF. Interactions between nutrients, pro-inflammatory cytokines and inflammation. *Clin Sci* 1996; 91: 121–30.
34. Pochon JP, Klöti J. Zinc and copper replacement therapy in children with deep burns. *Burns* 1979; 5: 123–6.
35. Berger MM, Berger-Gryllaki M, Wiesel PH, Hurni M, Revelly JP, Tappy L, et al. Gastrointestinal absorption after cardiac surgery. *Crit Care Med* 2000; 28: 2217–23.
36. Kinski MP, Milner SM, Button B, Dubick MA, Kramer GC. Resuscitation of severe thermal injury with hypertonic saline dextran: Effects on peripheral and visceral edema in sheep. *J Trauma* 2000; 49: 844–53.
37. Seeger W, Ziegler A, Wolf HRD. Serum alpha-tocopherol levels after high-dose enteral vitamin E administration in patients with acute respiratory failure. *Intens Care Med* 1987; 13: 395–400.
38. Berger MM, Goette J, Stehle P, Cayeux MC, Chiolero R, Schroeder J. Enteral absorption of a solution with high dose antioxidants and glutamine early after upper gastrointestinal surgery. *Clin Nutr* 2002; 21 (suppl): 17.
39. Elia M. Changing concepts of nutrient requirements in disease: Implications for artificial nutritional support. *Lancet* 1995; 345: 1279–84.
40. Berger MM, Baines M, Wardle CA, Cayeux MC, Chiolero R, Shenkin A. Trace element supplements modulate tissue levels, antioxidant status and clinical course after major burns – Preliminary results. *Clin Nutr* 2002; 21 (suppl): 66.

41. Preiser JC, Van Gossum A, Berré J, Vincent JL, Carpentier Y. Enteral feeding with a solution enriched with antioxidant vitamins A, C, and E enhances the resistance to oxidative stress. *Crit Care Med* 2000; 28: 3828–32.
42. Ortolani O, Conti A, Raffaele De Gaudio A, Moraldi E, Cantini Q, Novelli G. The effect of glutathione and N-acetylcysteine on lipoperoxidative damage in patients with early septic shock. *Am J Respir Crit Care Med* 2000; 161: 1907–11.
43. Shils ME, Burke AW, Greene HL, Jeejeebhoy KN, Prasad AS, Sandstead HH. Guidelines for essential trace element preparations for parenteral use. *JAMA* 1979; 241: 2051–4.
44. American Medical Association. Department of Foods and Nutrition. Multivitamin preparations for parenteral use. A statement by the Nutrition Advisory Group. *JPEN J Parenter Enteral Nutr* 1979; 3: 258–62.
45. Subcommittee on the 10th edition on RDAs. *Recommended dietary allowances*, 10th ed. New York: National Academy Press, 1989.

Discussion

Dr. Martindale: Thank you, that was a wonderful review. What do you do in your intensive care unit (ICU) for vitamin C with the provocative data like those of Tanaka et al. [1] out there?

Dr. Berger: We need more information and some of the next data are probably going to come from Stuttgart in Germany where Biesalsky's team has started investigating what is going on in the endothelium. It is too early to use such amounts yet. But the intervention lasts 24 h, and only 24 h: no deleterious effects have been observed, such as kidney stones, oxalate formation or any of those, no prooxidative lesions. We are watching these developments with very high interest.

Dr. Martindale: To follow up on the same question, I heard him saying that this mechanism involves membrane stabilization, avoiding alterations in the intracellular volume; which then is the catabolic response?

Dr. Berger: Yes exactly, you maintain hydration through the decrease in nitrosylation of the membrane. That is the actual hypothesis. So as soon as you alter cell hydration, you have a catabolic response.

Dr. Cynober: When I look at your figure with the zinc losses in burns, I notice that the urinary losses compared to others were very low, and I remember old studies on trace elements which indicated that in burn injury, there was an important decrease in copper reabsorption by the kidney [2]. Therefore my question is, what is typical for trace elements after major trauma, is it the zinc figure with low elimination in urine or copper with very high renal elimination?

Dr. Berger: Actually these amounts were considered very important and correspond to what Cuthbertson et al. [3] found. You have an increased excretion of zinc at the end of the first week and we found exactly the same patterns of excretion. If I had shown you the copper figure, you would see that copper is actually excreted very little in urine, but excretion essentially occurs by the biliary route and the cutaneous route in burns. The copper balance in burn trials were difficult to carry out also because copper has a slow intestinal transit early after injury, so the balances were not completely correct for copper as late losses occurred in the feces. At the intestinal level there is competition for absorption. It was actually attempted to give it enterally to children in a trial carried out in Zürich in 1978 and 1979 [4]. This trial showed that there was a competition and that both copper and zinc could not be increased when given together by the enteral route. Either you give copper or you give zinc, but then you have a corresponding decrease in the other's absorption.

Dr. Bozzetti: Could you better specify which patients should receive this supplementation? From your presentation I see that you have extensively studied burn patients, then you have shown the results of other critically ill patients, but I have some difficulty defining which the critically ill patients are. I mean, you can define critically ill patients as the patients who are in a critically ill condition really, but also the patients who are admitted to the critical care unit, and you have some elective surgery, surgical patients, so which are the patients for whom such a supplementation is advised?

Dr. Berger: Thank you for this question, which is a very important one. What we actually define as a critically ill patient who would receive an antioxidant cocktail, as we call it, in our unit, includes emergency patients admitted for acute respiratory failure, severe sepsis or septic shock, organ transplant, major trauma, major burns, pancreatitis. But we would not consider giving it to a patient just coming to us after elective surgery: those patients would not come to our unit anyway. But a patient in failure or organ failure would be an indication to give it, but you have to have organ failure, not just requiring monitoring.

Dr. Labadarios: On what evidence have you arrived at or do you recommend these doses? If you look at thiamine, it is almost the amounts that we used to treat Wernicke's encephalopathy. Now I know we give a lot of glucose wrongly, but one would like to know the background to our recommendation. The second part of the question: the administration of vitamin C in daily doses exceeding 500 mg has been reported to have prooxidant properties [5, 6]. And the third part of the question: there are things that one needs to understand. Your second slide was actually showing tremendous losses in thermally injured patients which one understands. But I understood from your presentation that within 1 or 2 days in other types of injury you actually lose a lot of these micronutrients. Where do they go?

Dr. Berger: I am starting with the last question. Actually we have also made balance trials in critically ill trauma patients: they have also negative trace element balances. We have just completed a trial in patients with any condition requiring continuous renal replacement therapy. They are in negative selenium and copper balance. We have learned from these balance studies that whenever you have drains, whenever you have a therapy which will draw biological fluids from the patient, you have micronutrient losses, and frequently at that time you are just not providing these patients with any supplement: they are in a phase in which they just require more. We know that the deficiency itself comes on the top of a frequently suboptimal status before the acute hit. So in addition you threaten the status. As far as I know, nobody knows how large the stores are but we do know that there is increased stress to the patient who is critically ill. Now why these doses? Those doses are not my invention, they are those I found in the literature. I haven't shown all the references, but lets take the example of thiamine. An article from the Netherlands shows clearly that acutely critically ill patients have very low thiamine activity [7]. The depression is correlated with outcome: this team recommended 100–200 mg/day for at least 3 days, to just compensate the depression and cope with our glucose infusions we just infuse some glucose to all our patients, and we don't know where they are standing with the thiamine status. Another nice article published from an Emergency Department in London [8], in alcoholic and nonalcoholic patients, shows that about 30% of them were deficient in vitamin B. So our emergency patients are just deficient and the critically ill too, for reasons which vary, depending on the condition. α-Tocopherol has been used in many trials and has been given up to 3 g/day [9], and this has been shown to have no deleterious effect when given by the enteral route. I haven't indicated the route here but the route is perhaps of importance. These are doses which have been recommended for the burn and trauma patients and exist since the 1940s [10], and they have not been reassessed since nor have they been contradicted since. For selenium, different trials [11, 12] have shown selenium deficiency: ours was based on a balance study. We also conducted a balance study in major trauma, showing trace element deficiencies [13].

Dr. Bozzetti: There is the question of prooxidant damage that we may be doing to these people and that is really the question behind the two regarding tocopherol and ascorbic acid. I heard what you said and I accept what you said and I would probably do the same as you, the question though is when we say it is free of side effects. Very often we don't know what side effects we are looking for, so I don't know how we can actually arrive at the conclusion that they are safe.

Dr. Berger: The 1,000 mg vitamin C/day? You are totally right, it is very important to consider the potential side effects of something, and that was what I alluded to when I said don't give one single agent because you may end up in trouble and we don't know. This one has been built for burns and is also based on a trial by Schorah et al. [14] which showed that within 48 h after acute injury you are below 25% of the lowest reference value in these patients, so it is a repletion. The things here should not be considered for continued supplementation. What we have decided in our unit for the moment is to give such things for 5 days and there are no deleterious effects shown for such short supplementation periods. I agree with you, we don't have anything we can follow-up on.

Dr. McClain: These are intravenous doses?

Dr. Berger: Yes, except for tocopherol given enterally.

Dr. McClain: One of the things you get with some of these metals, like zinc, in low doses is deficiency: There is nice work in a biochemical journal showing that if you give very high levels you can actually induce zinc deficiency.

Dr. Berger: Yes these things do exist. Lets come back to the doses. I was not precise enough, but these doses are provided on the top of multivitamin and multitrace element daily supplements because you should just give the full cocktail. So the doses indicated in my presentation are the quantities you top up on: something in the concept we have developed in Lausanne. The trials with zinc, and you can go back to Chandra [15], showing that if you give more than 50 mg/day for prolonged periods of time you have a decreased immune response. So clearly we do risk deleterious side effects, as there is a true dose-response curve. The 20- to 30-mg zinc/day dose has never to my knowledge been associated with deleterious effects when given for periods of less than 2 months.

Dr. McClain: In the Chandra study the dose is given orally. Basically 3 mg of zinc would keep a person in stable balance on home total parenteral nutrition, so 15 mg of zinc orally is the same as 3 mg intravenously. I actually did a study giving 12 mg/day i.v. and then switching over to 30 mg/day orally. So I think you have to be careful about how much you are giving.

Dr. Berger: You are perfectly right, I was quoting your trial exactly for the reason that you gave it over a prolonged period of time, and in our unit these doses have not been given for very long except in burn patients who receive 30 mg zinc for 3 weeks. Supplementation should not proceed for ages, that is for sure. Critically ill patients should not be continued on such high stress doses, as the stress is initial. We have done the trials in burn patients, and we now have experience with 3 weeks of 35 mg i.v. We are watching the immune response and we have observed no deleterious effects. Our patients had 40–90% body surface area burns, but that is the only category where we would continue with such high doses for prolonged periods because the patients have persistent losses from the skin surface if not surgically covered by skin grafts.

113

Dr. Allison: Under pressure from the chairman you rather rushed through the last bit about the effect of salt and water on gastrointestinal function, which is an area of interest to us. I wonder if you could just sort of review that and elaborate on the influence of fluid resuscitation on edema, and the effect this had on absorption. Are you saying that this impairs trace element absorption for a significant period of time?

Dr. Berger: I don't have definite evidences. I am just observing that during resuscitation things occur which have an impact at least on sugar absorption, and we know there is edema related to fluid resuscitation, and this occurs in hemorrhagic trauma as in burns, and this trial just nicely showed the edema in these areas. So you know that during shock you have alterations in cell energetics and the absorption of trace elements and vitamins is not a passive one. So as soon as you have edema you are likely to have altered absorption, and this may explain that when you give such doses orally, enterally, early you cannot count on a perfect absorption. It does not mean that the gut does not use it, but perhaps it is just not available in the blood, and that is also something we saw in our patients with gastrointestinal surgery. We were not able to maintain glutathione peroxidase activity despite 300 µg selenium/day for 5 days, and this we do easily by the intravenous route in both trauma and burn patients who are much more severely stress patients, but they are getting 300 µg i.v. So I hypothesize that without being able to prove it.

Dr. Allison: We have heard very little about salt and water today, which are the major problems in these patients and that is very interesting.

Dr. Ribeiro: I have two questions. First, a practical question. If your patients receive parenteral nutrition do you mix everything within the solution or do you give it intermittently?

Dr. Berger: We are doing quite a lot of research on it and as parenteral nutrition is only 15% of our nutrition days we just give it separately, and we have a continuous separate micronutrient infusion. We don't give it as a bolus but this is running for a 12-hour period. We have stability problems, so we give two small 100-ml sodium chloride solutions, one containing the trace elements and the other containing the vitamins.

Dr. Ribeiro: Are you worried about the degradation of vitamins?

Dr. Berger: Of course, the vitamins are protected from light, whereas there is no problem with the trace elements, they are not degraded.

Dr. Ribeiro: You mentioned that elderly people present low levels of some micronutrients. Do they eat less or do they absorb less?

Dr. Berger: As far as I know there are no data showing lower absorption in these patients, and in our trial with major surgery we had 80-year-old patients, and they just behaved like the others. What we all know with nutrition is that elderly patients tend to eat less and that their intake is simply lower.

Dr. Rosenfeld: You don't mention chromium in your key cocktail. There is concern about hyperglycemia in critically ill patients. It is important for glucose control and cytochrome oxidase. Isn't it time to look more for chromium supplementation?

Dr. Berger: We included it there, but there are not enough data. These have not yet been published, so in this table I just used the data which we know about. But you are absolutely right and chromium should probably be included. There are unresolved toxicity concerns with this trace element. Probably just providing the multitrace element products which contain 20–40 µg/day i.v. should at least decrease the issue of the problem, but here we went for 400 µg/day enterally. So yes, we should probably include chromium but the data are still not strong enough.

Dr. Nitenberg: You know that there is a controversy and some debate in the literature about what is called the antioxidant paradox, and I think we discussed that before. Do you agree with the fact that the only thing we have to do now is to correct the deficiencies of the patients and not to overload patients with the so-called antioxidant products? That was my first question, and I think it is very difficult to achieve this goal. My second question is about the other micronutrients you have not discussed, mainly about iron deficiency because there is also a debate in the literature about the risks and benefits of iron supplementation. Could you comment on these two points?

Dr. Berger: It is very important to address these issues. Regarding burns, what we have been doing is basing our supplementation doses on balances. We knew we were just actually repleting acute depletion, but we do not know what the balances are for quite a few conditions. I only have balance trials in burns, trauma and now renal replacement therapy. These balances are very difficult to carry out in burn patients and in the critically ill in general, so there won't be many of these. We know that our patients are probably below the requirements when they start [16]. We have evidence of low levels of many micronutrients which can reflect redistribution as I said as deficiency. I think that at the present stage we know that we can reinforce antioxidant defenses and this is rather easy to measure when you measure plasma glutathione peroxidase: if you can restore its activity, then you should probably not go beyond the delivered selenium dose. Really if we continue much above the normal requirements for a prolonged period, we should have something to measure, because we don't know what we are doing, especially we don't know what we are doing by providing one single micronutrient. I am very worried about the trials which are giving $1,000 \mu g$ of selenium for 2 or 3 weeks, or even more, because we have evidence from the general population that we may have an inhibition of thioredoxin reductase with these large doses [17]. So there is evidence against the theory that more is better. The doses I have been talking about are those which have not been shown to have deleterious effects, whether on endocrine aspects or whatever: the duration of supplementation is of importance too. We have, I think, to tackle this progressively and try to discover the optimal replacement doses. What I mean is that there are proposals for discussion. I don't think we have a definitive answer yet, and more is not necessarily better. Then regarding iron: yes there is worry in those patients with an acute phase response and those with infection. Iron is required for quite a few metabolic steps, for electron transfer and so on, but it is also the main initiator of the prooxidative reaction. Iron also has catalase antioxidant effects. It is prooxidant when free. Our sick patients have a large proportion of free iron, and the free iron is the worry. And we also know that quite a few bacteria including *Pseudomonas* very quickly develop channels to incorporate just the free iron that they need for proliferation. So the current consensus, and this has been investigated in children with malnutrition, is that during the acute malnutrition phase you should be very cautious with a large supplementation and you should not give doses which are intended for correction of anemia, but just the basic thing. If you look at the trace element-containing products which are on the market, they just have this minimal level of iron, and everybody is very much worried about increasing that without clearly knowing exactly what to do. So as soon as the acute phase is fading you can probably increase the supplementation dose without any problem.

Dr. Labadarios: The WHO recommendations that you just referred to regarding malnourished children, are a little bit stronger than that, because they actually say don't give iron for the first 14 days of the patient's management course, am I right?

Dr. Berger: Yes you are right.

Dr. Déchelotte: Coming back to glutathione, I am pretty convinced that selenium will help to get back some reduced glutathione by glutathione reductase or peroxidase action, but oxidized glutathione is really lost, it passes well from cell membranes so maybe selenium will not be able to get it back. So don't you think that there is a need together with selenium to have some glutathione precursors such as glutamine or cysteine?

Dr. Berger: There is a very nice trial by Ortolani et al. [18] in septic patients, providing N-acetylcysteine, N-acetylcysteine plus glutathione versus placebo showing that you can reinforce much better if you give a combination. Now that there is free glutathione, and these groups are important to the body, we should also head in that direction. So I fully agree with you, but this was just next to the pure topic on vitamins and trace elements, but I think we should add cysteine to it, clearly.

Dr. De Bandt: If you associate micronutrients with n-3 fatty acids do you think that you have to decrease your supply in order to prevent the paradoxical effects of micronutrients?

Dr. Berger: I think it has to be investigated, as there are no data yet.

Dr. Calder: I think if one is going to give n-3 fatty acids you need the appropriate lipid-soluble antioxidants present, but the exact level or ratio between them isn't known.

References

1. Tanaka H, Matsuda T, Miyagantani Y, et al. Reduction of resuscitation fluid volumes in severely burned patients using ascorbic acid administration. *Arch Surg* 2000; 135: 326–31.
2. Boosalis MG, McCall JT, Solem LD, et al. Serum copper and ceruloplasmin levels and urinary copper excretion in thermal injury. *Am J Clin Nutr* 1986; 44: 899–906.
3. Cuthbertson DP, Fell GS, Smith CM, Tilstone WJ. Metabolism after injury. 1: Effects of severity, nutrition, and environmental temperature on protein potassium, zinc, and creatine. *Br J Surg* 1972; 59: 925–31.
4. Pochon JP, Klöti J. Zinc and copper replacement therapy in children with deep burns. *Burns* 1979; 5: 123–6.
5. Podmore ID, Griffiths HR, Herbert KE, et al. Vitamin C exhibits pro-oxidant properties. *Nature (Lond)* 1998; 392: 559.
6. Levine M, Dhariwal KR, Welch RW, et al. Determination of optimal vitamin C requirements in humans. *Am J Clin Nutr* 1995; 62 (suppl): 1347S–56S.
7. Cruickshank AM, Telfer AB, Shenkin A. Thiamine deficiency in the critically ill. *Intens Care Med* 1988; 14: 384–7.
8. Jamieson CP, Obeid OA, Powell-Tuck J. The thiamin, riboflavin and pyridoxin status of patients on emergency admission to hospital. *Clin Nutr* 1999; 18: 87–91.
9. Seeger W, Ziegler A, Wolf HR. Serum alpha-tocopherol levels after high-dose enteral vitamin E administration in patients with acute respiratory failure. *Intens Care Med* 1987; 13: 395–400.
10. Lund CC, Levenson SM, Green RW, et al. Ascorbic acid, thiamine, riboflavin and nicotinic acid in relation to acute burns in man. *Arch Surg* 1946; 55: 557–83.
11. Berger MM, Cavadini C, Bart A, et al. Selenium losses in 10 burned patients. *Clin Nutr* 1992; 11: 75–82.
12. Boosalis MG, Solem LD, Ahrenholz DH, et al. Serum and urinary selenium levels in thermal injury. *Burns* 1986; 12: 236–40.
13. Berger MM, Cavadini C, Chioléro R, Dirren H. Copper, selenium, and zinc status and balances after major trauma. *J Trauma* 1996; 40: 103–9.
14. Schorah CJ, Downing C, Piripitsi A, et al. Total vitamin C, ascorbic acid, and dehydroascorbic acid concentrations in plasma of critically ill patients. *Am J Clin Nutr* 1996; 63: 760–5.
15. Chandra RK. Excessive intake of zinc impairs immune responses. *JAMA* 1984; 252: 1443–6.

16. Hercberg S, Preziosi P, Galan P, et al. Apports nutritionnels d'un échantillon représentatif de la population du Val-de-Marne. III: Les apports en minéraux et vitamines. *Rev Epidém Santé Publ* 1991; 39: 245–61.
17. Brätter P, Negretti de Brätter VE. Influence of high dietary selenium intake on the thyroid hormone level in human serum. *J Trace Elem Med Biol* 1996; 10: 163–6.
18. Ortolani O, Conti A, Raffaele de Gaudio A, et al. The effect of glutathione and N-acetylcysteine on lipoperoxidative damage in patients with early septic shock. *Am J Respir Crit Care Med* 2000; 161: 1907–11.

Cynober L, Moore FA (eds): Nutrition and Critical Care.
Nestlé Nutrition Workshop Series Clinical & Performance Program, Vol 8, pp 119–129,
Nestec Ltd.; Vevey/S. Karger AG, Basel © 2003

What Is the Goal of Nutrition in the Intensive Care Unit?

S.P. Allison

Clinical Nutrition Unit, University Hospital, Nottingham, UK

Introduction

It is difficult to give a simple answer to this question for a number of reasons. Firstly, because the major determinants of outcome on the ICU are the severity of the disease, coincident cardiorespiratory pathology, sepsis and organ failure. Nutritional support is therefore likely to have only a modest effect on survival although it may have an important role in accelerating recovery. On the other hand, prolonged periods of starvation are deleterious, as is excessive or inappropriate nutrition. Secondly, as pointed out by Griffiths et al. [1] in their studies on glutamine supplementation, it is important to follow the whole course of the patient's illness before, during and after the intensive care unit (ICU) episode, through convalescence to full recovery (fig. 1), since the patients pre-ICU condition and treatment during ICU stay may influence subsequent events. Our goals must therefore be long- as well as short-term. Thirdly, the ICU population is not only heterogeneous within each institution, but also varies from center to center. In a recent paper by Van Den Berghe et al. [2], 63% of the population studied were patients recovering from cardiac surgery. In our own ICU there are none. Berger et al. [3] have a high proportion of burned patients in their practice. Another unit may contain a high proportion of patients recovering from major abdominal surgery or even, in some American series, of gunshot wounds. The patient ventilated for 24–48 h for status asthmaticus suffers not one jot from being starved during their stay. In contrast, the catabolic patient ventilated for 1–2 weeks intuitively needs feeding to minimize a huge loss of lean mass. The average length of stay in many ICUs may be 3–4 days, but this average conceals a wide range.

119

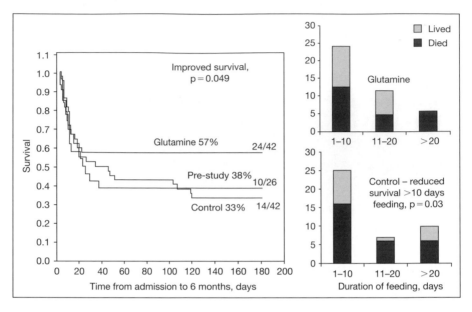

Fig. 1. Six-month outcome of critically ill patients given glutamine-supplemented parenteral nutrition during their ICU stay. From Griffiths et al. [1].

I will therefore try to approach this subject by taking all these factors into account and setting goals for nutritional treatment that are realistic and relevant. Since our normal nutrition in everyday life is inseparable from the ingestion of fluid and electrolytes, I make no apology for including some aspects of this under the nutritional banner.

Finally, it is one thing to set goals and another to recommend measurements for use in clinical practice, as opposed to research programs, to define how well these goals have been achieved. I will, however, make some attempt to do this. While distinguishing between routine postoperative recovery and true critical illness – not always made clear in some systematic reviews – I shall nonetheless include some aspects of nutrition after major surgery. I shall also consider the whole of the patient's journey through their illness, since, as I have argued above, it is misleading and illogical to consider the period of critical care in isolation.

Protein Energy Malnutrition

The normal anthropometric measurements of body mass index, mid arm circumference and triceps skinfold thickness may be relevant to the initial identification of this problem which adversely affects outcome from critical

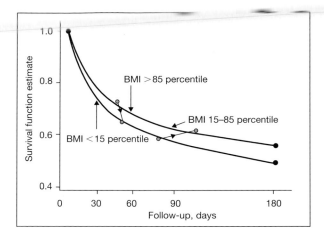

Fig. 2. Multiple organ failure survival and body mass index (BMI) showing outcome with BMI <15th percentile compared with >75th percentile. Outcome can be improved by raising the BMI above the 15th percentile towards the 85th percentile. Conversely, outcome is worsened if the BMI is allowed to fall excessively. From Galanos et al. [4].

illness during and after ICU stay (fig. 2) [4]. They are, however, poor short-term measures of nutritional success, since increases in their values are likely to reflect gains in fluid from excess salt and water retention or gains in fat from excess calories, concealing a diminished lean mass. Restoration of lost lean mass awaits return to normal oral intake and mobility and takes many weeks or months to achieve. On the other hand, as Sakurai et al. [5] has stated: 'The goal of nutritional management of critically ill patients is to promote wound healing and resistance to infection while preventing persistent loss of muscle protein since survival of critically ill patients is inversely correlated with loss of lean mass.'

It must therefore be a goal of nutrition to minimize the loss of muscle mass during ICU stay, while recognizing that the combination of immobility and the catabolic response to injury will defeat any attempt to achieve meaningful positive nitrogen balance. Although there is a correlation between muscle mass and muscle strength, renutrition may have immediate and short-term effects on muscle function before any change in mass is achieved [6, 7]. I recognize, of course, that one cannot measure voluntary muscle strength while the patient is sedated on a ventilator, but it can be measured post-ICU as can the rate of subsequent physical rehabilitation as we showed in our fractured femur study many years ago [8]. It may also be useful to measure muscle function by direct stimulation as described by Pichard and Jeejeebhoy [9], although this is more a research than a standard clinical procedure. However, since the respiratory muscles suffer just as much as the limb

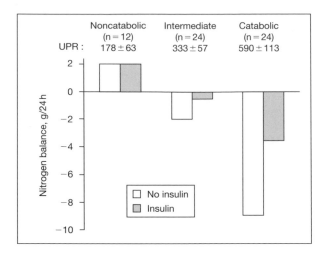

Fig. 3. Nitrogen balance (g/24 h) in burns with and without insulin according to the degree of initial catabolism. UPR = Urea production rate (mmol/24 h; mean ± SD). From Woolfson et al. [14].

muscles from wasting [10–12] – and in surgical patients we have shown a good correlation between muscle strength and peak flow [13] as did Hill [6] – earlier weaning from the ventilator as well as the length of ICU stay are relevant end points of nutritional support. This example relating to muscle illustrates the greater importance of improved function as a short-term goal of nutrition in critical illness than the more static anatomical measures of tissue mass. Can we improve on the protein-conserving effect of standard nutrition by the use of special substrate formulae or by the use of adjunctive hormone therapy? I think we probably can – indeed we were the first to show the beneficial effects of insulin in this respect during the 1970s (fig. 3) [14]. Campbell [15] described the problem clearly in a recent review: 'In the severely septic and injured patient, an improvement of nutritional status or increase of lean body mass by nutritional support alone is likely to be impossible. The most one can hope for is to slow the rate of decline. If lean body mass is to be maintained, it is likely that pharmacological methods will have to be found for doing so.'

Children

Babies and small children have special problems of growth and brain development – clearly pediatricians have the goal to maintain such growth although it may be difficult to maintain this at a normal rate during acute illness. As I have no experience of pediatric practice. I merely mention this as an important goal.

Survival

All other factors being equal, nutrition is likely to have only a small impact on survival, this effect will probably be more marked in those with more prolonged illness. Survival, however, needs to be measured in terms of 3–6 months post-ICU and not just during ICU stay (fig. 2) [4]. It is therefore reasonable to hope that some improvement in overall survival is a realistic goal, at least in some patients. This is likely to be more marked when comparing some nutrition against none at all, but may also be a feature of the use of improved nutritional formulae or of adjunctive therapy.

Inflammation and Immune Response

Protein energy deficit is associated with an impaired immune response and an increased infection rate. Different substrate mixes may also modify the initial inflammatory response and the subsequent reduction in immune function, as others will describe in this meeting. We may therefore include modification of inflammation and improved resistance to infection among the reasonable aims of nutrition therapy. A number of studies have used infection rates and antibiotic use to assess clinical outcome of nutrition support [16]. Laboratory measures of cytokine levels and immune function are largely research tools.

Wound Healing

The healing of wounds from surgery and accidental trauma or the taking of skin grafts in burns are impaired by prior malnutrition but particularly correlate with recent and current nutritional intake [17]. Mineral and micronutrient supplementation may also be important, as Berger et al. [3] have shown. Improved healing is therefore an important goal and clearly observable.

Avoidance of Complications

It is axiomatic that the techniques of feeding, whether enteral or parenteral, should not pose a greater risk than benefit to the patient. It should be the goal of ICU doctors to reduce such complications to negligible levels as shown by good nutrition teams [18]. Such problems as aspiration, bloating and diarrhea from enteral feeding or infectious and mechanical complications of feeding lines can largely be avoided.

Hyperalimentation, i.e. giving large amounts of carbohydrate calories in an attempt to bludgeon protein catabolism into reverse, was shown to increase demands for gas exchange, making ventilatory support more difficult. It also caused fatty liver, abnormal liver function and increased adipose tissue. Problems of the refeeding syndrome were also exacerbated. It should be our goal to avoid the consequences of such excess, reserving increased intake for the anabolic convalescent period when the patient is able to utilize higher protein and energy intake for restoration of lost tissue.

Fluid and Electrolytes

Some overexpansion of the interstitial compartment of the extracellular space may be, to some extent, an inevitable consequence of adequate acute resuscitation with sodium-containing fluids. Even normal subjects are slow to clear a salt and water load [19] and this is greatly exacerbated by the response to injury [20]. There is a tendency, however, to give excessive amounts of salt in maintenance fluids after the period of resuscitation, resulting in unnecessary overload with consequent edema and dilutional hypoalbuminemia [21]. Sitges-Serra et al. [22] and others have described the increased pulmonary and other complications caused by this and we have shown [23], as did Mecray et al. [24] in 1937, that even modest saline overloads of 3 kg are sufficient to inhibit a return of gastrointestinal function and the use of the gut for nutritional purposes. I even wonder, rather mischievously perhaps, whether some of the ill effects of parenteral nutrition in the Veterans' Administration [25] and other studies, were due to the salt and water load rather than to the nutritional substrates. In enteral nutrition it is difficult to cause such overload simply because the rate of administration is limited by the tolerance of the gut. Moore and Shires [26] summarized the problem of fluid balance admirably: 'The objective of care is restoration to normal physiology and normal function of organs with a normal blood volume, functional body water and electrolytes. This can never be achieved by inundation.'

I would make a plea, therefore, for including a consideration of fluid and electrolyte balance in any nutritional prescription and for the restoration of normal balance as soon as possible to avoid the ill effects of cumulative overload.

Gastrointestinal Function

Although the role of gut atrophy and bacterial translocation are more clearly established in animal studies than in human clinical work, it seems a reasonable goal to introduce some enteral feeding (combined with parenteral if necessary) at the earliest possible stage with the aim of preserving gut function and perhaps the function of gut-associated lymphatic tissue.

Preoperative Care

A proportion of the ICU population usually consists of patients recovering from major elective surgery. Ljungqvist et al. [27] have shown clearly the advantages of bringing patients to surgery in a metabolically fed state and the improved outcome from a carbohydrate drink 2 h preoperatively. It is also advantageous to give a period of nutritional support preoperatively of 7–10 days in those with prior weight loss >10% [28]. Providing fluid overload is avoided, the goals of such treatment are improved physiological function and fewer complications postoperatively.

Cost Effectiveness

A reduction in length of ICU and hospital stay, reduced investigation and treatment costs, and more rapid return to a productive life may all follow if

Table 1. Goals of nutritional support in the ICU and clinical measurement of outcome

Goal	Clinical measurement
Survival	In ICU and 3–6 months after ICU

Muscle function	After ICU
	  Handgrip dynamometry
	  Peak flow
	In ICU
	  Ventilator weaning
	  Time on ventilator

Muscle mass	Inspection Anthropometry
Immune function	Infection rate Antibiotic rate
Gastrointestinal function	Symptoms Gastric emptying and aspirate
Growth (in children)	Length/height and weight Growth velocity Head circumference
Wound healing	Inspection
Rate of rehabilitation	Time to achieve physical goals Time to return to normal function and quality of life
Complications, infections and other	Inspection and recording
General and economic	Length of ICU stay Length of hospital stay Drug and other costs Costs of complications

the above goals are achieved. This may appeal to managers and budget holders, particularly when we are asking for more resources for nutritional care!

Conclusion

We may therefore summarize (table 1) the goals of nutritional care in critically ill patients by emphasizing its role in the preservation of function and achieving a more rapid recovery from illness, with fewer complications from either the illness or its treatment. Preservation of muscle mass and function and of immune resistance to infection are major goals. In some cases, improvements in survival may be expected, but these are likely to be modest compared with effects on the rate of recovery. In assessing outcome, we must consider the whole course of the patient's illness in which the ICU stay may be an episode, recognizing that management in the ICU may influence subsequent outcome.

References

1. Griffiths RD, Jones C, Allan Palmer TE. Six month outcome of critically ill patients given glutamine supplemented parenteral nutrition. *Nutrition* 1997; 13: 295–302.
2. Van Den Berghe G, Wouters P, Weeks F, Werwaest C, Bruyninckx F, Schetz M, Vlasselaers D, Ferdinande P, Lauwers P, Bouillon R. Intensive insulin therapy in critically ill patients. *N Engl J Med* 2001; 1359–67.
3. Berger MM, Spertini F, Shenkin A, Reymond J, Schindler C, Tappy L, Wiesner L, Menoud V, Cavadini C, Cayeux C, Wardle CA, Gaillard RC, Chioléro L. Clinical, immune and metabolic effects of trace element supplements in burns: A double-blind placebo-controlled trial. *Clin Nutr* 1996; 15: 94–6.
4. Galanos AN, Pieper CF, Kussin PS, Winchell MT, Fulkerson WJ, Harrell FE Jr, Teno JM, Layde P, Connors AF Jr, Phillips RS, Wenger NS. Relationship of BMI to subsequent mortality among seriously ill hospitalized patients. *Crit Care Med* 1997; 25: 1962–8.
5. Sakurai Y, Aarland A, Herndon DN, Chinkes DL, Pierre E, Jguyenm TT, Patterson BW, Wolfe RR. Stimulation of muscle protein synthesis by longterm insulin infusion in severely burned patients. *Ann Surg* 1995; 22: 283–94.
6. Hill GL. Body composition research: Implications for the practice of clinical nutrition. *JPEN J Parenter Enteral Nutr* 1992; 16: 197–218.
7. Jeejeebhoy KN. Bulk or bounce – The object of nutritional support. *JPEN J Parenter Enteral Nutr* 1988; 12: 539–49.
8. Bastow MD, Rawlings J, Allison SP. Benefits of supplementary tube feeding after fractured neck of femur: A randomised controlled trial. *Br Med J* 1983; 287: 1589–92.
9. Pichard C, Jeejeebhoy KN. Muscle dysfunction in malnourished patients. *Q J Med* 1988; 260: 1021–45.
10. Kelsen SG, Ference M, Kapoor S. Effects of prolonged undernutrition on structure and function of the diaphragm. *J Appl Physiol* 1985; 58: 1354–9.
11. Lewis MI, Sieck GC, Fournier M, Belman MJ. Effect of nutritional deprivation on diaphragm contractility and muscle fibre size. *J Appl Physiol* 1986; 60: 596–603.
12. Lewis MI, Sieck GC. Effect of acute nutritional deprivation on diaphragm structure and function. *J Appl Physiol* 1990; 68: 1938–44.
13. Hillman TE, Hornby ST, Lobo DN, Stanga Z, Rowlands BJ, Allison SP. Relationships between structural and functional measures of nutritional status in a normally nourished population. *Clin Nutr* 2001; 20 (suppl 3): 37.

14. Woolfson AMJ, Heatley RV, Allison SP. Insulin to reduce protein catabolism after injury. N Engl J Med 1979; 300: 14–7.
15. Campbell IT. Limitations of nutrient intake. The effect of stressors: trauma, sepsis and multiple organ failure. Eur J Clin Nutr 1999; 53 (suppl 1): 143.
16. Kudsk KA, Minard G, Groce MA, Brown RO, Lowrey TS, Pritchard FE, Dickerson RN. A randomized trial of isonitrogenous enteral diets after severe trauma. An immune-enhancing diet reduces septic complications. Ann Surg 1996; 224: 531–43.
17. Windsor JA, Knight GS, Hill GL. Wound healing response in surgical patients: Recent food intake is more important than nutritional status. Br J Surg 1988; 75: 135–7.
18. Allison SP. The uses and limitations of nutritional support. Clin Nutr 1992; 11: 319–30.
19. Lobo DN, Stanga Z, Simpson JAD, Anderson JA, Rowlands BJ, Allison SP. The dilution and redistribution effects of rapid 2 litre infusions of 0.9% (w/v) saline and 5% (w/v) dextrose on haematological parameters and serum biochemistry in normal subjects: A double-blind crossover study. Clin Sci 2001; 101: 173–9.
20. Moore FD. The Metabolic Care of the Surgical Patient. Philadelphia: Saunders, 1959.
21. Lobo DN, Bjarnason K, Field J, Rowlands BJ, Allison SP. Changes in weight, fluid balance and serum albumin in patients referred for nutritional support. Clin Nutr 1999; 18: 197–201.
22. Sitges-Serra A, Arcas G, Guirao X, Garcia-Domingo M, Gil MH. Extracellular fluid expansion during parenteral refeeding. Clin Nutr 1992; 11: 63–9.
23. Lobo DN, Bostock KA, Neal KR, Perkins AC, Rowlands BJ, Allison SP. Effect of salt and water balance on recovery of gastrointestinal function after elective colonic resection: A randomised controlled trial. Lancet 2002; 359: 1812–18.
24. Mecray PM, Barden RP, Ravdin IS. Nutritional edema: Its effect on the gastric emptying time before and after gastric operations. Surgery 1937; 1: 53–64.
25. Veterans Affairs Total Parenteral Nutrition Study Group. Perioperative total parenteral nutrition in surgical patients. N Engl J Med 1991; 325: 525–32.
26. Moore FD, Shires JT. Moderation. Ann Surg 1967; 166: 300–1.
27. Ljungqvist O, Nygren J, Thorell A. Modulation of postoperative insulin resistance by preoperative carbohydrate loading. Proc Nutr Soc 2002; 61: 329–36.
28. Satyanarayana R, Klein S. Clinical efficacy of perioperative nutrition support. Curr Opin Clin Nutr Metab Care 1998; 1: 51–8.

Discussion

Dr. Peeters: I have heard that we should be more humble in our goals when treating an intensive care unit (ICU) patient. We used to make him better, now we try to keep him in a steady state. We set our goals on long-term as I understood, which is very good, and which is explained by the fact that we probably could not achieve our short-term goals. I think here is an important factor that comes into the game, that is the psychological stress that you have to take into account when you look at long-term goals, certainly in burn patients this might come into the discussion. Again the last thing that I remember very well is that we are going back to the basics and trying to look again at salt and water, something that has been forgotten for several years. This lecture is open to discussion.

Dr. Chioléro: I have a question concerning patient populations since clearly in the ICU we have trauma, septic and postoperative patients. I think this is an important point since when we go from goals to nutritional support, we clearly have to use different solutions and different regimens as highlighted for example by the metaanalysis of Heyland et al. [1] on immunonutrition which could harm some specific populations and be good in others. So how can we be a bit more specific in our goals?

Dr. Allison: I think this is a gradual process, there is no getting away from planning proper studies, and we are not going to fix this one in a short period of time. I think there are certain groups of patients who are better studied than others, I think we know a great deal about burns and cardiac surgery. Some of the others are less well known, and I think we just have to plan careful studies in the future and look at each one in isolation, not necessarily by throwing cocktails of this and that at people but carefully looking at each substrate at different stages and building up a picture over the next 10 years. Getting this funded is part of the problem. Of course if these were some cardiac drugs then a company could afford to pay a million dollars to fund an enormous study but these kinds of nutritional studies are not going to yield enormous financial benefits. Now I think there is genuine difficulty about obtaining proper studies at the national or international levels through the EU to solve this sort of common place question.

Dr. Bozzetti: Congratulations on your very clear and excellent presentation. I would like to come back briefly to the paper of Van Den Berghe et al. [2] that you reported and which was recently published in the *New England Journal of Medicine*. I would like to have your opinion about the interpretation of this study. I want to stress that the control group maintained a median glucose level of about 153 mg/dl, that is a value lower than that able to impair the host defense, which is roughly about 200 mg/dl. So my question is: was the mechanism of the beneficial effect of intensive insulin therapy in this study different from the simple prevention of hyperglycemia-associated infections?

Dr. Allison: I think this is the great question of that study. I think the great value of that study was that it showed for the first time that a drug or a hormone, which we know has perhaps some desirable biological effects, actually has a beneficial effect on outcome in contrast to the growth hormone studies, for example. Although we discussed yesterday how there are perhaps groups in whom growth hormone will be beneficial, there are others in whom it will not, particularly children in the former instance. So I don't think we know the answer. We know from the work of Bistrian [3] and others that hyperglycemia predisposes to infection. We know in studies of diabetic patients undergoing myocardial infarction that controlling the blood sugar very tightly has a beneficial effect on outcome; but of course insulin does other things, it affects protein, it affects fat metabolism and it affects salt and water metabolism as well. Following the effect on salt and water excretion in burn patients I actually did a study on patients with severe heart failure, some of whom where about to undergo cardiac surgery, and one showed the same effect of insulin on severe heart failure with abrupt and rapid excretion of salt and water. There is a recent review by Parsonage in one of the heart journals in which he looked systematically at the effect of insulin on cardiac output, and then beneficial cardiovascular effects. So in the Van Den Berghe study [2], with 63% of the patients being post-cardiac surgery, I would expect the insulin to have more effects on that group of patients than just control of the blood sugar, although I accept that control of blood sugar is desirable. Perhaps we need to design a study where you control blood sugar by restricting carbohydrate and then you give carbohydrate plus insulin to the other group so that you have 2 groups comparable in blood sugar control, and see whether there is any difference between them. I think like all good studies, it suggests further studies.

Dr. Douglas: I just wanted to make a comment about the work that we have undertaken in Edinburgh, and we have actually found that in patients 3 months after discharge from intensive care, a third remained nutritionally depleted. Furthermore we found that handgrip dynamometry, our tool for assessing function, is actually very poor in this population, and the reason for that is anticipated to be critically ill initiated neuropathy. Do you have any suggestion on how we can further assess the function of these patients at this time?

Dr. Allison: That is a very good question. I suppose we can employ, or perhaps we need to design quality-of-life scores. We tend to take quality-of-life measurements off the shelf, like going [illegible] out, we take it ready-made and we try to adapt it from one situation to another. Maybe we need quality-of-life scores that are appropriate to particular patient groups. I would have thought that some measure of the ability to fulfill physical tasks hence the Ancel Keys study, which is perhaps the great classic of nutritional depletion in normal subjects. They employed a kind of fitness score in carrying out a number of physical tasks. I think that the mood score issue is an important one. This is one we use very regularly on our patients. I don't have a really clear-cut answer to your question. I think that what you say also reflects on the article by Beattie et al. [4] in postoperative patients, whereas Hessov showed that giving nutritional supplements after discharge from hospital increased the weight by 2 or 3 kg at 3 months, but had no effect on function. However he was looking at a well-nourished population. When Beattie et al. selected out those who had been depleted subsequent to their acute illness and gave it to them, they found not only anthropometric improvements but also functional improvements. I don't know whether anybody else has any suggestions for assessing these patients after discharge, 3 months down the line, and how they do it. We heard a bit about the burns yesterday but does anybody else have any thoughts about that?

Dr. Peeters: I think it is very difficult to make the assessment when you just take into account the somatic situation of a patient and my own work in burn patients showed me through the years that quality of life is a very important topic for the patient, maybe much more important in survival, and I think that over the last 10 years we have put our interest more in this field. I think it is not so important that you keep the patient alive, I think that you have to take into account the quality of life that they will have afterwards, which is a very difficult question that will probably not be answered today, but I think the psychological situation of the patient is as important as his somatic situation.

Dr. McClave: This is more of a comment than a question really. The goals that I think about are the concept that we can attenuate the stress response, that we can strike and do several changes in major strategies that would set them on a different curve in the stress response. If you attenuate the stress response usually there are fewer complications: in head injury there is a faster return of cognitive function, the patients get out of the hospital sooner, sometimes you effect survival, and the question to ask as a nutritionist is what are the other tools, we have to do that. I think Dr. Berger showed yesterday how an antioxidant cocktail during the N phase, certainly getting enteral feeding going early, attenuates the stress response, and the question whether there are other things like paying attention to anxiety, controlling pain, maybe the salt and water inundation you are talking about, is an additional stress or so. Paying attention to these strategies that put them on a different stress curve is important. After the stress is gone, attacking the pick of the curve is kind of fruitless, it is setting their course ahead of time.

Dr. Allison: I think this is a crucial point and maybe nutritional support is an old-fashioned term. What we should be talking about is integrated nutrition and metabolic care because I find it totally impossible to prescribe nutrition to a patient for whom I don't have a comprehensive understanding of everything else that is going on, and indeed some degree of control, either direct or indirect, through agreement with colleagues. What you say reflects the fact that over the last 30 years the energy expenditure of these patients described in the literature has dropped dramatically due to such factors as earlier surgery in burns, control of infection and pain and anxiety. Without integrating our nutritional and metabolic care with all these other things, we just fly blind. So I think you make a very important point, maybe we should rather talk about integrated nutrition rather than nutritional support.

Dr. Rosenfeld: You point out that water and salt balance in critically ill patients is related to the amount of sodium these patients receive. But we have been following patients who were not given huge amounts of sodium and after starting nutritional support these patients developed a hyperosmolar state, increasing urea too. We hypothesized that these patients are not able to excrete all the osmolar amount, the osmolar charge nutritional support is giving to these patients. So high amounts of proteins must be metabolized and generate high amounts of osmolar charge. We think these patients can't excrete this osmolar charge and so they develop a hyperosmolar state. We stopped the nutritional support for 5 or 7 days, increased the amount of water and they returned to a normal osmolar state, and we gave these patients less protein and they didn't develop a hyperosmolar state anymore.

Dr. Allison: I think you make an important point. Many studies in the literature have shown that giving critically ill patients more than 0.2 or 0.25 g nitrogen/kg/day merely increases urea production. You also make the point about water. Unfortunately I think some people don't distinguish between the salt-containing fluids necessary to correct the volume and to resuscitate in the acute phase and the maintenance fluids necessary to maintain what Bernard beautifully called the volume obligatoire. If you give them salt and water you don't increase the urine volume unless you are correcting volume depletion. All you do is put them into more and more cumulative sodium balance. It is not just sodium, I think chloride is the hidden villain in this. We don't understand the excretion of chloride quite so well as we understand that of sodium. Certainly there are probably advantages of Ringer lactate over saline in this respect, you excrete the sodium from Ringer lactate more readily than you do from saline. So I think that what you are emphasizing here is the interplay between fluid and electrolyte balance and the substrate you are giving, and the fact that you cannot consider any prescription for nutritional support without also considering the sodium, water, potassium, chloride and all the rest. It is part of the integrated nutrition approach.

Dr. Bouletreau: You made a very important point. Certainly in some studies like the Griffiths et al. [5] study, which is long-term, nutritional support had a very long-term effect on survival. I am still a little bit surprised and I wonder why a very short amount has such a striking effect in the very long term. It is very different from the Beattie et al. [4] study in which they give long-term supplementations. Do you think this improvement in lean body mass, which is always modest in these patients, could be the only reason, or what other reasons could be evoked?

Dr. Allison: I don't think it is the lean body mass but I don't know what it is either. I don't know if anybody else has got any idea, whether you are causing some kind of enzyme induction or gene expression. This is one of the great puzzles: why does the patient with the short-term cytokine and neuroendocrine storm develop a catabolic process which goes on for weeks, and why some intervention has an effect weeks later, I have no idea.

Dr. Nitenberg: I don't know how it is in the States or in Britain for ICU patients especially, but I know how it is in France because it is my work. The problem is not to convince myself or my colleagues working on nutrition that nutrition is important for patients. My problem is to convince other teams, then other ICU workers that nutrition is important for the patients. And when I want to convince my coworkers in France that it is important, they always ask me the same question: what is the benefit for the patients. This is the only key question that we have to answer. I think we have many studies in which we can prove that there is an improvement in mood, that there is an improvement in metabolic parameters, and there is an improvement in immunological parameters. OK, that is good. When you are dealing with mechanical ventilation you can show that there is an improvement in PO_2, an improvement in frequency, but the only amelioration that is important for ventilation is that when, for example for low tidal volumes, you reduce the length of ventilation then you reduce the morbidity of ventilation. I think it is exactly the same problem in the ICU. We have to show that. So I do think that, especially with modern management and especially when we are speaking about immunonutrition or pharmaconutrition, we have to do exactly the same as we are doing with drugs and with maybe ventilatory support or the use of catecholamines for example. So don't you think that we have to focus only on outcome parameters such as length of stay in the hospital, not in the ICU. Because everybody knows that the patient only comes out of the ICU when he/she is better, when the anguish of the doctor is not too high, when you have some room, in other words. It is very difficult to measure this and perhaps also to measure the infectious parameter mortality, because mortality is I think a more important value than medical economical parameters because if you are dying you don't care about medical economical amelioration, you want to survive. For example I come back to what Dr. Bouletreau said about the Griffith study. The Griffith study is fantastic. However, when you look carefully at the survival of the patients in the long-term you can see that 2 patients died, 1 from pulmonary embolism and 1 from pulmonary myocardial infarction. I can't imagine that death is related to the 5-day use of glutamine 6 months earlier, it is very difficult to accept that. If I compare this with the results obtained recently by Déchelotte et al. [6], for example, in the same kind of study with glutamine, there is an improvement in early infection and no improvement in late survival. So you can't shake the statistics bottle and pick out what you want to explain the results and systematically put away the other results. Could you comment on this long provocative sentence?

Dr. Allison: I agree with everything you have said. I think at the bottom line we could say that for the patient who is in the ICU because of asthma and is out in 24–48 h, nutrition is irrelevant. The patient with major burns, inhalation problems, on a ventilator for 2, 3, even 4 weeks sometimes, may not survive without feeding. They just waste away and die. I challenge my colleagues to quote me any control trials of ventilation in respiratory failure where you allocate some to be ventilated and some not? Can you quote me any controlled trials of hemodialysis in renal failure where you let the creatinine go on? The bottom line here is that sooner or later you die from malnutrition if you don't eat and that process is accelerated by injury. If we start from there then we begin to focus and start to play around with the substrates and give them earlier or later, a bit more of this, a bit less of that, does that make a difference? I agree with you that we have to show improved survival even though it might be small but no other measures in the ICU are being asked to produce big changes in survival because we know that any advance gives you a small improvement. The rate of recovery is extremely relevant to the patient and to the cost of the hospital and reducing the complications and so on. But apart from that, we are in agreement really.

Dr. Nitenberg: Isn't it dangerous to make a statement saying a patient coming to the ICU with asthma will be out in 48 h. Perhaps he will be out in 48 h, so maybe you should still take nutrition into account in case if he stays for 4 weeks.

Dr. Allison: You can afford to delay the decision for a day or two for instance, particularly if the referral occurs to me, as it often does, on a Friday evening and the weekend is coming up. I think you can spend the weekend in adjusting the fluid balance, and on Monday I would consider some nutrition.

Dr. Peeters: A very good point is made about the length of stay. In our hospital patients do not leave the ICU on a Friday evening, or on Saturday or Sunday. So when they are staying for 10 days, you add. They stay with about 20% just to keep them over the weekend. I think a patient who dies in the ICU makes a very important contribution to the economics of health care. It is a bit cynical

Dr. Cynober: To continue this debate. Perhaps there is a problem of semantics and credibility because when you claim a goal is to reduce the length of stay at the hospital, people can think that these nutrition people have very important drugs to enable a reduction in the stay. In fact, perhaps the true message is to limit the increase in length of stay related to malnutrition or inappropriate nutrition, because I cannot imagine that even with pharmacological nutrition you have an absolute effect even on the primary pathology which is responsible for the hospitalization.

Dr. Allison: Absolutely. We can be asking too much of nutritional support. I think, on a philosophical note, we should remember that colleagues talk about natural recovery, and maybe it is natural to have starvation. What they forget is that most of the patients coming to the ICU would have died without critical care. Our response to illness was never designed to allow us to overcome severe illness. Nature is the statistician which allows us to overcome minor injuries but if we are holding up the tribe with a severe injury we are designed to die. So in the ICU we are looking at patients who are designed by nature to die. We are starting from a zero position, and therefore to talk about some kind of natural response being appropriate after 5 days in the ICU is nonsense. We are dealing with a totally unnatural situation where we have to explore the complexity of it and try to intervene in a way which produces better outcome.

Dr. Chioléro: Another aspect concerns the patient who should not receive nutritional support, is able to have a short starvation resuming oral feeding after some days. What is your view on ICU and starvation assignment?

Dr. Allison: I don't know. You can detect early changes, starvation for 48–72 h produces significant physiological changes. For example your thermoregulatory capacity is impaired by starvation from over 48 h. I think what we don't understand is whether short periods of starvation are clinically significant or not. They may be, particularly in the perioperative context. Early oral intake after elective surgery may be a very important issue, but I have tried to keep away from that because I regard the ICU patients by definition as unable to eat normally. If we get into normal eating I could go on for another 20 min.

Dr. Peeters: Thank you very much. I think the issue was, do we have to feed patients or not. I think maybe we should reverse the question to those who don't agree that you have to feed them. Perhaps they have to prove that you don't have to feed them, although some living beings don't need to be fed, you can go into hibernation and you are not fed for several months.

References

1. Heyland DK, Novak F, Drover JW, et al. Should immunonutrition become routine in critically ill patients? A systemic review of evidence. *JAMA* 2001; 286: 944–53.
2. van den Berghe G, Wouters P, Weekers F, et al. Intensive insulin therapy in the critically ill patients. *N Engl J Med* 2001; 345: 1359–67.
3. Bistrian BR. Hyperglycemia and infection: Which is the chicken and which is the egg? *JPEN J Parenter Enteral Nutr* 2001; 25: 180–1.
4. Beattie AH, Prach AT, Baxter JP, Pennington CR. A randomized controlled trial evaluating nutritional supplements *postoperatively* in malnourished surgical patients. *Gut* 2000; 46: 813–8.
5. Griffiths RD, Jones C, Palmer TE. Six-month outcome of critically ill patients given glutamine-supplemented parenteral nutrition. *Nutrition* 1997; 13: 295–302.
6. Déchelotte P, Bleichner G, Hasselmann M, et al. O-4: Improved clinical outcome in ICU patients receiving analyl-glutamine (Dipeptiven®) supplemented total parenteral nutrition (TPN). A French double-blind multicenter study. *Clin Nutr* 2002; 21: 1.

Cynober L, Moore FA (eds): Nutrition and Critical Care.
Nestlé Nutrition Workshop Series Clinical & Performance Program, Vol. 8, pp 133–149,
Nestec Ltd., Vevey/S. Karger AG, Basel, © 2003

Enteral versus Parenteral Nutrition: Alterations in Mechanisms of Function in Mucosal Host Defenses

Nicholas A. Meyer and Kenneth A. Kudsk

Department of Surgery, University of Wisconsin – Madison, Madison, Wisc., USA

Parenteral nutrition has significantly advanced the survival of patients who sustain major loss to the GI tract or prolonged delayed ability to take oral or tube feedings. However, there is accumulating evidence that the processing of nutrients via the gastrointestinal (GI) tract maintains an important immunologic defense mechanism, the mucosal associated lymphoid tissue (MALT), which functions as the primary source of specific immunity at all mucosal surfaces. Investigation of trauma patients reveals that parenteral nutrition is associated with a significantly higher incidence of pneumonia, intra-abdominal abscess, and possibly multiple organ dysfunction, than enteral nutrition [1–4]. This chapter describes the mounting evidence supporting the current clinical trend to aggressively pursue nutritional delivery via the GI tract.

Parenteral Nutrition

Parenteral versus Enteral Nutrition: Clinical Data
Total parenteral nutrition (TPN) is extremely concentrated in order to deliver the necessary amount of nutrients within a volume that is tolerated by patients. The high osmolar load requires delivery into a large, central vein where the high flux of blood rapidly dilutes the concentrated nutrient solution. Although the use of central venous catheters themselves present a source of infectious complications, clinical evidence shows an increase in both intra-abdominal abscess formation and pneumonia in studies comparing parenteral feeding to enteral feeding or to starvation.

Supported by National Institutes of Health grant R01 GM53439.

In early studies of this phenomenon, Moore and Jones [1] randomized moderately to severely injured patients to either enteral feeding or intravenous dextrose. Parenteral feeding was instituted in the patients who did not tolerate a diet by day 5. The enterally fed group had a significantly lower incidence of infectious complications, primarily intra-abdominal abscess formation. In a follow-up study, patients with similar injuries were randomized to either parenteral formula or protein- and calorie-matched enteral formula advanced to goal rate within 72 h of injury [2]. Patients fed enterally had a significantly lower incidence of infectious complications, primarily pneumonia, with a trend toward a reduction in intra-abdominal abscess. Subsequent research at the University of Tennessee randomized 98 patients to either enteral feeding or to a nitrogen- and calorie-matched parenteral formula including more severely injured patients with extremely high abdominal trauma indices (ATI) and high injury severity scores (ISS) [3]. In this study, patients receiving parenteral feeding had a significantly higher incidence of pneumonia, intra-abdominal abscess formulation and line sepsis. In addition, infected patients fed parenterally sustained significantly more infections. Most of the differences between enterally and parenterally fed patients occurred in the more severely injured patients (ATI ≥ 25 or ISS ≥ 20).

Specific nutrients in the enteral formula appear to provide additional protection. Moore et al. [4] demonstrated a significant reduction in intra-abdominal abscess and a lower rate of multiple organ dysfunction syndrome (MODS) in patients randomized to a diet enriched in glutamine (GLN), arginine, n-3 fatty acids, and nucleotides [4]. In a subsequent study of high-risk trauma patients (ATI ≥ 25 and ISS ≥ 20), Kudsk et al. [5] found a significant reduction in intra-abdominal abscess formation in patients receiving the immune-enhancing diet compared to an isonitrogenous, isocaloric standard enteral formula and a markedly reduced incidence of infection compared to patients receiving no feeding at all.

Mechanisms for the Reduced Incidence of Pneumonia and Intra-Abdominal Abscess Formation

Many investigators have studied the potential mechanisms underlying the septic complications associated with TPN and a lack of enteral stimulation. One hypothesis involves bacterial translocation (BT) where lack of intraluminal stimulation leads to a loss of integrity of intestinal mucosal defenses, which in turn allows BT from the intestinal lumen into the gut lymphatic and blood stream to seed distant sites. Most of this work has been done in rats which are extremely sensitive to a lack of enteral feeding where 'gut starvation' produces rapid atrophy in the proximal gut mucosal to approximately to 50–60% of normal. Simultaneously, biliary immunoglobulin A (IgA) levels decrease associated with an overgrowth of aerobic bacteria in the cecum. While protein calorie malnutrition by itself does not increase BT, addition of an extra-intestinal inflammatory focus such as a sterile abscess or zymosan dramatically increases BT to the mesenteric lymph nodes (MLNs), liver, spleen and lung. BT, however, has never been linked to MODS or extra-intestinal infectious complications clinically. Moore et al. [6] sampled portal vein blood in the early post-trauma period and noted no translocation. Positive blood cultures are not uncommon following trauma, but they do not correlate with subsequent infectious complications. Interestingly, laboratory conditions which increase BT are also associated with a reduction in the primary specific immunologic mucosal defense, IgA. Because of the inconsistent findings associated with BT, an alternative mechanism based on the mucosal immune hypothesis provides a better supported explanation for the increases in pneumonia and intra-abdominal abscess associated with lack of enteral feeding.

Mucosal Immunity

Gut-associated lymphoid tissue (GALT) is an integral part of the body's immune system both by providing immunological control of resident intraluminal flora and, as part of the larger MALT, provides protection of distant sites such as the lungs, nasopharynx, mammary glands and genitourinary tract. The afferent limb of GALT consists of Peyer's patches (PP) and MLNs. Intraluminal antigen is taken up by M cells overlying the PP, processed by antigen-presenting cells that then interact with naïve T and B lympho-cytes which enter the PP via interaction with mucosal addressin adhesion molecule-1 (MAdCAM-1). These sensitized cells are distributed via thoracic duct drainage and the vascular system to various submucosal locations where they contribute to the efferent limb of GALT. The lamina propria (LP) of the intestine is one effector site where activated T and B lymphocytes accumulate and produce IgA after conversion of B cells to plasma cells. Polymeric IgA manufactured in the submucosa is transported into the lumen by the overlying epithelial cells which are enriched with the polymeric immunoglobulin receptor, secretory component (SC) [7]. The IgA prevents adherence of bacteria, viruses, and other toxic molecules to the mucosal surface. Multiple animal models demonstrate that IgA levels correlate inversely with bacterial overgrowth, translocation and changes in intestinal permeability. Activated T and B lymphocytes also distribute themselves to other mucosal effector sites where they contribute to local IgA production in a similar fashion. In this manner continued intraluminal antigenic stimulation maintains an immunologic barrier to microbial invasion.

In the mouse, the lack of enteral stimulation quickly leads to a dramatic reduction in PP, LP, and intraepithelial lymphocytes. Within 72 h of stopping enteral feeding, the PP and LP sustain a 55–66% reduction in B and 40%

reduction in T lymphocytes [8]. MAdCAM-1 is partly responsible for this change since MAdCAM-1 direct unsensitized lymphocytes to the PP and sensitized lymphocytes to the LP. Within hours of parenteral nutrition alone, PP MAdCAM-1 expression drops but recovers rapidly with enteral refeeding [9].

The lack of enteral stimulation also affects the balance of cytokines controlling lymphocyte maturation. T-cell subpopulations change with a decrease in the CD4:CD8 ratio. CD4 cells produce interleukin (IL)-4 and IL-10, both of which upregulate IgA production [10]. In mice, parenteral nutrition decreases intestinal IL-4 and IL-10 levels creating an imbalance in favor of the IgA-inhibiting cytokine interferon-γ (INFγ) which is unaffected thereby decreasing IgA production by plasma cells [11]. Since CD4 cells stimulate B cell proliferation, colony expansion, and immunoglobulin secretion, the relative depression in CD4 cells, IL-4 and 10 appears to reduce the stimulatory effects on B cells since levels of IL-4 and IL-10 correlate positively with IgA levels.

The lack of enteral stimulation also decreases epithelial transport of IgA. IgA produced in the LP is normally transported across the epithelium by binding to SC, a protein receptor on the basolateral surface of the mucosal epithelial cell [7]. The IgA-SC receptor complex is transported to the apical surface where the IgA and part of the receptor are cleaved off the cell. TPN depresses the selective transport of IgA into the lumen but does not completely abolish it [12]. Cytokine changes can at least partially explain this effect. SC expression is regulated by IFNγ and IL-4 in a synergistic fashion [13]. Although TPN does not appear to affect intestinal levels of IFNγ, TPN reduces intestinal IL-4. The effect on MALT is lowered IgA production and epithelial transport due to reduced lymphocytes and cytokine alterations. Laboratory studies using the mouse have consistently shown decreases in both intestinal and nasotracheal IgA levels within 3 days of 'gut starvation' with TPN [8, 11, 14].

The decreases in intraluminal IgA induced by a lack of gut feeding and parenteral nutrition may explain the increased incidence of pneumonia seen with parenteral feeding. Mice intranasally immunized against *Pseudomonas aeruginosa* accumulate antigen-specific respiratory mucosal IgA in their respiratory tracts which reduces mortality to an otherwise lethal dose of *P. aeruginosa*. When successfully immunized animals are challenged with a lethal bacterial load 5 days after initiating a parenteral diet, their mortality rate is over 70% higher than chow-fed animals, comparable to the mortality rate of nonimmunized animals [15], reflecting a loss in established antibacterial immunity. A similarly increased susceptibility to viral upper respiratory tract infections has been found. An influenza virus infection well documented to be IgA-mediated, A/PR8, was studied in the mouse model. Previously immunized mice which normally sterilize a second viral dose within hours were fed TPN for 5 days and then challenged with an intranasal virus load. Two days later 50% of the animals receiving TPN continued to shed virus in the respiratory tract compared to none in groups receiving an enteral diet [16].

Peritoneal Protection

Several laboratories have reported differences in the peritoneal response of animals fed parenterally following intraperitoneal sepsis. Lin et al. [17] noted that the number of peritoneal exudative cells (PECs) was significantly reduced in parenterally fed compared to enterally fed mice tract. This reduction in PECs was associated with a blunted intraperitoneal tumor necrosis factor response, an increase in bacterial proliferation, and an augmented vascular inflammatory cytokine response. Recently, our laboratory investigated the response to a sterile peritonitis model using a 1% glycogen solution [18]. A lack of enteral stimulation and TPN significantly reduced the number of polymorphonuclear cells (PMNs), macrophages, and lymphocytes within the peritoneal cavity 4 h after glycogen injection. Interestingly, supplementation of TPN with 2% GLN reversed the TPN-induced peritoneal effects to glycogen peritonitis.

Vascular Inflammatory Responses

The alterations in the mucosa-associated immune system associated with a lack of enteral nutrition may also contribute to noninfectious-mediated multiple organ failure by augmenting inflammatory responses to subsequent stressors. Polymorphonuclear neutrophils are the major effector of the nonspecific immune inflammatory response and their role in organ failure after injury is becoming well established. The vascular bed of the GI tract has the capacity to prime PMNs which, once activated, respond to subsequent insults by causing further tissue destruction. This has been especially well documented in the lungs [19]. PMNs are intrinsically involved in the acute, nonspecific inflammatory response where they adhere to the capillary endothelium, migrate across the endothelial wall and can cause destruction of both invasive microbes and body tissues by releasing destructive enzymes and toxic oxygen radicals. Such nonspecific tissue destruction can contribute to eventual organ failure.

TPN induces priming of PMNs compared to enteral nutrition by recruiting PMNs to the GI tract. Intercellular adhesion molecule-1 (ICAM-1) is the endothelial ligand counterpart of CD11/18 integrins expressed on PMNs. The binding of CD11/18 integrins to ICAM-1 is the basis for PMN margination and triggers the maturation process for PMNs enabling them to pass through the endothelial cell lining and begin the activation process [20]. IFNγ is an important stimulator of ICAM-1 expression while IL-4 and IL-10 are important inhibitors of ICAM-1 expression. Lack of enteral feeding does not alter IFNγ levels, but it reduces gut IL-4 and IL-10 levels [21]. The observed induction of intestinal ICAM-1 expression is consistent with this change in cytokines [22]. P- and E-selectin also influence the PMN-endothelial cell interaction.

These adhesion molecules expressed on the surface of endothelial cells trigger leukocyte rolling along the endothelium of postcapillary venules as a precursor to firm adhesion through CD11/18-ICAM-1 interaction. TPN increases expression of P-selectin in the GI tract and E-selectin in the lungs [23]. The detection of elevated myeloperoxidase (MPO) levels in the GI tract confirm an accumulation of PMNs associated with increased adhesion molecule expression [22]. Both intestinal ICAM-1 and MPO levels return to normal 4 days after reinstitution of an oral diet. Therefore the lack of enteral feeding induces a transient, nonspecific response, with endothelial changes in the intestine and subsequent PMN priming.

This priming is evident when TPN-fed mice are exposed to a second insult. Similar to classic models of hemorrhagic shock with splanchnic hypoperfusion, mice fed parenterally for 5 days were exposed to either 15 min of superior mesenteric artery occlusion and compared to animals fed chow, a complex enteral diet, or TPN formula delivered intragastrically. Within 72 h of this ischemic event, mortality was significantly higher in the parenterally fed group (40%) than in animals fed via the GI tract (mortality 5–10%). When studied 3 h after this ischemic event, there was a significant increase in vascular permeability in the lung and liver of parenterally fed animals compared to the enterally fed groups. Expression of CD11a or CD11b (markers of PMN activation) did not increase any of the groups prior to the ischemic event but, CD11b expression was significantly increased 3 h following ischemia only in circulating PMNs isolated from the parenterally fed group. Using immunohistochemistry, only the lung of animals fed parenterally had elevated levels of activated myeloid cells reflected in increased CD18 expression.

Complexity of the Enteral Diet

Not only the route of nutrition (oral vs. parenteral) but also the complexity of oral nutrition affects the integrity of the mucosal immune system and alters the inflammatory response of intestinal and extra-intestinal organs to a nonseptic insult. In many experiments the above effects were investigated in mice by comparing TPN to standard mouse chow taken ad libitum, a complex (intact protein, carbohydrate and fat) enteral diet which could be delivered isonitrogenously and isocalorically to the parenteral group to control for variable nutritional intake values, and the parenteral formula delivered through a gastric feeding tube instead of intravascularly. In most of the experiments, similar differences were observed between parenterally fed mice and mice fed either chow ad libitum or a complex enteral diet. Therefore it is safe to dismiss a possible difference in calories or protein as driving the immunoregulatory changes that have been associated with parenteral nutrition. The elemental diet (intragastric parenteral formula), completely devoid of complex nutrients and roughage, induced a partial suppression of the MALT when compared to chow but not as severely as seen with complete lack of enteral stimulation.

However, some important differences have been noted when the same formula was used intravenously and intragastrically. Mortality in immunized mice after a bacterial pneumonia challenge was less in mice fed an elemental intragastric diet (57%) than in mice fed parentally (88%), yet significantly greater than in mice fed a complex enteral diet (10%) [24]. However, in the model of viral upper respiratory infection, the elemental diet resulted in intact defenses and no viral shedding [25]. An intragastric, elemental diet decreases lymphocyte mass in the PP, LP, and intraepithelial sites, lowers intraluminal IgA, and depresses levels of intestinal IL-4 but not IL-10 [11, 25, 26]. An intragastric, elemental diet also partially upregulates ICAM-1 expression in the intestine but not to as great an extent as TPN [27]. After an intragastric elemental diet, survival to 15 min of mesenteric ischemia is similar to chow-fed mice, but it decreases survival rates to that of mice given parenteral nutrition when ischemia is extended to 30 min.

The Enteric Nervous System

A complex enteral diet or chow preserves the immune system better than a simple elemental diet. It is likely that complex molecules within the diet stimulate the GALT via neurological and hormonal mediators. Strong evidence supports an interaction between intraluminal stimulation, GALT and the enteric nervous system (ENS). The ENS is densely incorporated in the gut with approximately 2 m of nervous tissue/cm^3 of intestinal tissue [28]. Neuropeptides released by this network regulate gut motility, secretions, growth, immune function and mucosal defenses.

Gastrin-releasing peptide is a neuropeptide produced by the human ENS. Exogenous bombesin (BBS), an analogous peptide obtained from frogs, reverses the TPN-associated GALT atrophy and impairment in respiratory defenses to pneumonia and viral infections. BBS given concurrently with TPN prevented decreases in total lymphocyte yield from PP, LP, and intraepithelial spaces, maintained the CD4/CD8 ratio of T cells in the LP, and returned depressed intraluminal IgA levels to normal [29]. BBS also reversed TPN-associated impairment of IgA-mediated defenses to an upper respiratory tract viral challenge [30] and also improved the drop high mortality rate (21%) of the *Pseudomonas* pneumonia to levels comparable to the chow-fed group (15%) [31]. The reversal of detrimental TPN effects with BBS is not complete, however. ICAM-1 levels elevated by TPN in the small intestine are not affected by BBS nor are IL-10 levels returned to normal [32].

BBS may function directly to stimulate GALT or may act by releasing other GI hormones. Gastrin, cholecystokinin and neurotensin are released in response to BBS and may be involved in preserving GALT. When given concomitantly with TPN in the mouse model, each neuropeptide influenced GALT positively but to varying extent [33]. All three preserved lymphoid cell mass in the PP comparable to chow, but the site of activity was different. Gastrin and cholecystokinin had less effect on the distal small bowel while neurotensin was more effective distally. Intestinal IgA levels associated with each neuropeptide were significantly higher than in animals given TPN alone but not as high as in animals given chow. Immunity to bacterial pneumonia was maintained with cholecystokinin and gastrin but neurotensin appeared to have no effect. Although all three neuropeptides help to preserve GALT when enteral stimulation is lacking, none acting singly reflects the nearly complete resolution of GALT depression seen with BBS administration.

Glutamine

Supplementation of TPN with GLN attenuates many of the detrimental GALT effects. GLN is an important respiratory fuel for the intestinal tract but is not routinely added to TPN because of its instability over time in solution especially with heat sterilization. Addition of GLN to TPN increases cellularity and attenuates atrophy of the intestinal mucosa [34], decreases BT [35] and abrogates alterations in mucosal permeability [36]. Replacing of 2% of the amino acids in TPN with GLN improved total lymphocyte yield in the PP and LP, normalized the CD4/CD8 ratio in the LP and normalized IgA concentrations in the small intestine, nasal tract and lungs [37, 38]. GLN partially preserves upper respiratory immunity both to a viral challenge (A/PR8 virus) [37] and to *Pseudomonas* pneumonia [39]. Intestinal IL-4 levels are maintained comparable to chow diet but not IL-10 levels [32, 38]. As with BBS, GLN reverses some but not all of the effects on nonspecific PMN activation. Elevated ICAM-1 expression associated with TPN is returned to normal when TPN is supplemented with GLN [32]. Survival of mice after intestinal ischemia/reperfusion injury is improved with GLN as well, but is still significantly lower than in animals fed chow [40].

Conclusion

Clinical differences clearly occur in response to the route and type of nutrition. A complex enteral diet maintains mucosal immunity whereas a lack of enteral stimulation quickly leads to impairment of the GALT and common mucosal immune system and predisposes patients to remote infections, pneumonia, and noninfectious multisystem organ failure. Complex enteral nutrition is beneficial and should be pursued orally or by nasoenteric, gastric or jejunostomy tube unless absolutely contraindicated. In those situations where TPN must be used, stimulation of mucosal immunity with hormones such as BBS or GLN may overcome some of the detrimental effects of TPN.

References

1. Moore EE, Jones TN. Benefits of immediate jejunostomy feeding after major abdominal trauma – A prospective, randomized study. *J Trauma* 1986; 26: 874–81.
2. Moore FA, Moore EE, Jones TN, McCroskey BL, Peterson VM. TEN versus TPN following major abdominal trauma – Reduced septic morbidity. *J Trauma* 1989; 29: 916–23.
3. Kudsk KA, Croce MA, Fabian TC, Minard G, Tolley EA, Poret HA, Kuhl MR, Brown RO. Enteral versus parenteral feeding. Effects on septic morbidity after blunt and penetrating abdominal trauma. *Ann Surg* 1992; 215: 503–11.
4. Moore FA, Moore EE, Kudsk KA, Brown RO, Bower RH, Koruda MJ, Baker CC, Barbul A. Clinical benefits of an immune-enhancing diet for early postinjury enteral feeding. *J Trauma* 1994; 37: 607–15.
5. Kudsk KA, Minard G, Croce MA, Brown RO, Lowrey TS, Pritchard FE, Dickerson RN, Fabian TC. A randomized trial of isonitrogenous enteral diets after severe trauma. An immune-enhancing diet reduces septic complications. *Ann Surg* 1996; 224: 531–40.
6. Moore FA, Moore EE, Poggetti R, McAnena OJ, Peterson VM, Abernathy CN, Parsons PE. Gut barrier translocation via the portal vein: A clinical perspective with major torso trauma. *J Trauma* 1991; 31: 629–36.
7. Brandtzaeg P. The role of J chain and secretory component in receptor-mediated glandular and hepatic transport of immunoglobulins in man. *Semin Respir Infect* 1985; 22: 111.
8. Li J, Kudsk KA, Gocinski B, Dent D, Glezer J, Langkamp-Henken B. Effects of parenteral and enteral nutrition on gut-associated lymphoid tissue. *J Trauma* 1995; 39: 44–52.
9. Fukatsu K, Zarzaur BL, Johnson CD, Wu Y, Wilcox HG, Kudsk KA. Decreased MAdCAM-1 expression in peyer patches: A mechanism for impaired mucosal immunity during lack of enteral nutrition. *Surg Forum* 2000; 51: 211–4.
10. Lebman DA, Coffman RL. Cytokines in the mucosal immune system. In: Ogra PL, Lamm ME, McGhee JR, Mestecky J, Strober W, Bienenstock J, eds. *Handbook of mucosal immunology.* San Diego: Academic Press, 1994; 243–9.
11. Wu Y, Kudsk KA, DeWitt RC, Tolley EA, Li J. Route and type of nutrition influence IgA-mediating intestinal cytokines. *Ann Surg* 1999; 229: 662–7.
12. Renegar KB, Kudsk KA, DeWitt RC, Wu Y, King BK. Impairment of mucosal immunity by parenteral nutrition: Depressed nasotracheal influenza-specific secretory IgA levels and transport in parenterally fed mice. *Ann Surg* 2001; 233: 134–8.
13. Phillips JO, Everson MP, Moldoveanu Z, Lue C, Mestecky J. Synergistic effect of IL-4 and IFN-gamma on the expression of polymeric Ig receptor (secretory component) and IgA binding by human epithelial cells. *J Immunol* 1990; 145: 1740–4.
14. Renegar KB, Kudsk KA, DeWitt RC, Wu Y, King BK. Impairment of mucosal immunity by parenteral nutrition: Depressed nasotracheal influenza-specific secretory IgA levels and transport in parenterally fed mice. *Ann Surg* 2001; 233: 134–8.
15. King BK, Kudsk KA, Li J, Wu Y, Renegar KB. Route and type of nutrition influence mucosal immunity to bacterial pneumonia. *Ann Surg* 1999; 229: 272–8.
16. Kudsk KA, Li J, Renegar KB. Loss of upper respiratory tract immunity with parenteral feeding. *Ann Surg* 1996; 223: 629–35.
17. Lin MT, Saito H, Fukushima R. Route of nutritional supply influences local, systemic, and remote organ responses to intraperitoneal bacterial challenge. *Ann Surg* 1996; 223: 84–93.
18. Ikeda S, Kudsk KA, Tho L, Zarzaur BL, Johnson CD. Glutamine improves impaired cellular exudation and polymorphonuclear neutrophil (PMN) phagocytosis induced by TPN following glycogen-induced murine peritonitis. *Shock* 2002; 18: 119–24.
19. Moore EE, Moore FA, Franciose RJ, Kim FJ, Biffl WL, Banerjee A. The post-ischemic gut serves as a priming bed for circulating neutrophils that provoke multiple organ failure. *J Trauma* 1994; 37: 881–7.
20. Carlos T, Harian J. Leukocyte-endothelial adhesion molecules. *Blood* 1994; 84: 2068–101.
21. Fukatsu K, Kudsk KA, Zarzaur BL, Wu Y, Hanna MK, DeWitt RC. TPN decreases IL-4 and IL-10 mRNA expression in lipopolysaccharide stimulated intestinal lamina propria cells but glutamine supplementation preserves the expression. *Shock* 2001; 15: 318–22.
22. Fukatsu K, Lundberg AH, Hanna MK, Wu Y, Wilcox HG, Granger DN, Gaber AO, Kudsk KA. Route of nutrition influences intercellular adhesion molecule-1 expression and neutrophil accumulation in intestine. *Arch Surg* 1999; 134: 1055–60.

141

23. Fukatsu K, Lundberg AH, Hanna MK, Wu Y, Wilcox HG, Granger DN, Gaber AO, Kudsk KA. Increased expression of intestinal P-selectin and pulmonary E-selectin during intravenous total parenteral nutrition. *Arch Surg* 2000; 135: 1177–82.
24. King BK, Kudsk KA, Li J, Wu Y, Renegar KB. Route and type of nutrition influence mucosal immunity to bacterial pneumonia. *Ann Surg* 1999; 229: 272–8.
25. Kudsk KA, Li J, Renegar KB. Loss of upper respiratory tract immunity with parenteral feeding. *Ann Surg* 1996; 223: 629–35.
26. Li J, Kudsk KA, Gocinski B, Dent D, Glezer J, Langkamp-Henken B. Effects of parenteral and enteral nutrition on gut-associated lymphoid tissue. *J Trauma* 1995; 39: 44–52.
27. Fukatsu K, Kudsk KA, Zarzaur BL, Sabek O, Wilcox HG, Johnson CD. Increased ICAM-1 and β2 integrin expression in parenterally fed mice after a gut ischemic insult. *Shock* 2002; 18: 119–24.
28. Debas HT, Mulvihill SJ. Neuroendocrine design of the gut. *Am J Surg* 1991; 161: 243–9.
29. Li J, Kudsk KA, Hamidian M, Gocinski BL. Bombesin affects mucosal immunity and gut-associated lymphoid tissue in intravenously fed mice. *Arch Surg* 130: 1164–9.
30. Janu PG, Kudsk KA, Li J, Renegar KB. Effect of bombesin on impairment of upper respiratory tract immunity induced by total parenteral nutrition. *Arch Surg* 1997; 132: 89–93.
31. DeWitt RC, Wu Y, Renegar KB, King BK, Li J, Kudsk KA. Bombesin recovers gut-associated lymphoid tissue and preserves immunity to bacterial pneumonia in mice receiving total parenteral nutrition. *Ann Surg* 2000; 231: 1–8.
32. Fukatsu K, Lundberg AH, Kudsk KA, Hanna MK, Johnson CD, Wu Y, Wilcox HG, Zarzaur BL. Modulation of organ ICAM-1 expression during IV-TPN with glutamine and bombesin. *Shock* 2001; 15: 24–8.
33. Keith Hanna H, Zarzaur BL Jr, Fukatsu K, Chance DR, Renegar KB, Sherrell C, Wu Y, Kudsk KA. Individual neuropeptides regulate gut-associated lymphoid tissue integrity, intestinal immunoglobulin A levels, and respiratory antibacterial immunity. *JPEN J Parenter Enteral Nutr* 2000; 24: 261–9.
34. O'Dwyer ST, Smith RJ, Hwang TL, Wilmore DW. Maintenance of small bowel mucosa with glutamine-enriched parenteral nutrition. *JPEN J Parenter Enteral Nutr* 1989; 13: 579–85.
35. Burke DJ, Alverdy JC, Aoys E, Moss GS. Glutamine-supplemented total parenteral nutrition improves gut immune function. *Arch Surg* 1989; 124: 1396–9.
36. Li J, Langkamp-Henken B, Suzuki K, Stahlgren LH. Glutamine prevents parenteral nutrition-induced increases in intestinal permeability. *JPEN J Parenter Enteral Nutr* 1994; 18: 303–7.
37. Li J, Kudsk KA, Janu P, Renegar KB. Effect of glutamine-enriched total parenteral nutrition on small intestinal gut-associated lymphoid tissue and upper respiratory tract immunity. *Surgery* 1997; 121: 542–9.
38. Kudsk KA, Wu Y, Fukatsu K, Zarzaur BL, Johnson CD, Wang R, Hanna MK. Glutamine-enriched total parenteral nutrition maintains intestinal interleukin-4 and mucosal immunoglobulin A levels. *JPEN J Parenter Enteral Nutr* 2000; 24: 270–4.
39. DeWitt RC, Wu Y, Renegar KB, Kudsk KA. Glutamine-enriched total parenteral nutrition preserves respiratory immunity and improves survival to a *Pseudomonas* pneumonia. *J Surg Res* 1999; 84: 13–8.
40. Ikeda S, Zarzaur BL, Johnson CD, Fukatsu K, Kudsk KA. Total parenteral nutrition supplementation with glutamine improves survival after gut ischemia/reperfusion. *JPEN J Parenter Enteral Nutr* 2002; 26: 169–73.

Discussion

Dr. Peeters: We have heard a lot of people talk about the fact that you can postpone feeding in an acute insult for, let's say, 2 days when a patient comes to the intensive care unit (ICU) with major burn for instance. But what about those effects that happen in the first 24 h?

Dr. Kudsk: We have looked at this. There are only a couple of areas that you can get into the body to test. I can't take out the intestines of my patients to look and see what their mucosal addressin adhesion molecule expression is or what their IgA level is;

however, I can do a bronchoalveolar lavage (BAL) and look at the levels of IgA within their airways which gives an insight into this system. I studied a group of patients with head injury, they were not fed via the gastrointestinal tract, and they were intubated. We quantitated how much of the fluid we got back was epithelial fluid by performing a microurea technique and then corrected for that. Between 24 and 36 h after injury there are approximately 100,000 units of IgA/cm^2 of epithelial fluid. After another 36 h, this value plummets to about 20% of normal. If we wait another 72 h, the results stay the same. I have data from 2 patients who we then started to feed. In these 2 patients I saw IgA levels gradually increase. It does not prove the concept but there is nothing inconsistent between these findings and the data that I showed you in the animals.

Dr. Cynober: Your hypothesis is that the route of administration makes the difference. We have another interpretation, that the content of total parenteral nutrition (TPN) products is imbalanced and inappropriate and as a matter of fact you showed that when you add glutamine to TPN you have the same effect as enteral nutrition on IL-4 expression, on intracellular adhesion molecule (ICAM) expression which mice develop after gut ischemia. I believe that certainly we have to improve the content of the TPN solution and then to discuss the route of administration.

Dr. Kudsk: I might agree with you except that I have given animals intragastric TPN, which is the same solution they were fed intravenously. When that same solution is fed via the gut it preserves a lot of the mechanisms. There may be an effect of nutrients, but it can't only be the nutrients. We have shown [1] that cholecystokinin, gastrin and bombesin (or gastrin-releasing peptide) are all able to bring this immunity back to normal. So that would argue against it just being a component of the TPN.

Dr. Cynober: But we can discuss your argument that providing TPN intragastrically mimics the effect of the chow diet simply for one reason, most of the TPN products, and probably you use standard products, mimic the content of regular diet given by the enteral route, and the major issue with TPN is that you have a shortage of splanchnic metabolization and rebuilding of a new profile. I am absolutely not surprised that the TPN product is working very well when given by enteral route.

Dr. Kudsk: I think that TPN can be improved. There are products available on the market, at least in Europe now, which show some benefits. I am not saying that this is the only product that can work but I think that there are novel things that can be done to improve immunity. And whatever that defect is, our laboratory has been very successful in showing where the immunologic vulnerability is. It is that the bacteria get into the airway in our intubated patients and are not bound by IgA. This is an explanation which has to be disproved before I am going to give it up.

Dr. Planas: What happens in patients with hypoxia? Could fluid in the intestine increase the oxygen demand? How can we measure hypoxia in these patients to be able to give enteral nutrition?

Dr. Kudsk: Dr. Moore is the expert on hypoxia in the gut. I could provide an answer but maybe Dr. Moore should comment on that because he is the person who has been studying the gut, and I think the next presentation will be on gut failure.

Dr. Moore: I will address it in my talk but I think that you really have to ascertain that resuscitation is complete before you feed somebody, and what we know is that after shock you have a disproportion of vasoconstriction in the gut and once you resuscitate, gut perfusion does not come back to normal. We have used the gastric tonometry as a monitor in shock resuscitation and found it not to be that helpful as an endpoint for resuscitation. However, it is helpful when you start feeding patients after shock resuscitation. If PrCO$_2$ goes up the patient is not going to tolerate enteral nutrition. So that is my fast answer of how we currently could monitor gut perfusion.

Dr. McClave: I am still struggling to understand the TH1 and TH2 subset because I think they set a tone in the environment at the level of the gut and, in inflammatory bowel disease, chronic parasitic infection generates a TH2 response that downregulates the inflammatory response and you are less likely to get invasive pneumococcal disease. If you have bacterial and viral infection it is a TH1 response, it is more inflammatory, and you are more likely to get invasive pneumococcal disease. I wonder in the discussion we have had about compensatory anti-inflammatory response syndrome (CARS) if this is the difference between a TH1-predominant or a TH2-predominant environment? You just made the comment that the difference in TH1-inflammatory TH2 downregulates, though systemically it is reversed at the level of the gut. Could you clarify that? And the second point is have you interpreted that correctly?

Dr. Kudsk: We have just now started to add injury in our models. We have tried to define the system and all the permutations caused by diet. As I have looked at some of those slides with the CARS, when IL-4 and IL-10 go up, I am wondering whether that is the period of time when there is a reduction in IgA. There are bacteria present because the IgA levels are dropping. The bacteria become more virulent. There is work done by Alverdy et al. [2] on the nonfed gut and bacteria. While we see a reduction in IgA in my models, they see these bacteria becoming stressed and responding by producing adhesins which make them more attachable to the mucosa. I speculate that the increase in serum IL-4 and IL-10 is a spillover from the gut which is trying to defend against the bacteria.

Dr. McClave: You don't interpret the drop in IgA as an effect of the downregulated response by IL-4?

Dr. Kudsk: There are two things that I believe are affecting the IgA. One is the reduction in cell mass and the second is the change in cytokines. So both issues play a role prior to the bacterial infection. I haven't studied how the mucosa responds once bacteria have attached.

Dr. McClain: Some of the immunology that you are talking about really is similar to the immunology of Crohn's disease, especially when you increase the endocrine levels you increase neutrophils and myeloperoxidase activity. Do you think that maybe what you are seeing with TPN versus enteral nutrition is merely a rapid alteration in gut flora that is causing this inflammatory response in TPN, and certainly in inflammatory bolus where you see probiotics now attenuate that response? That can also explain why, when you give the TPN fluid orally, you get less of an inflammatory response because you don't change the gut bacteria.

Dr. Kudsk: There are several things happening simultaneously, downregulation of cytokines and a downregulation of the basic immunity, IgA, which keeps bacteria out of our system. It has been shown in animal models that starved animals maintain a barrier there to keep the bacteria out. If an inflammatory focus occurs, however, the whole system breaks down. But as the gut is starved while TPN is given to prevent malnutrition, the bacteria become more virulent. We plan to inject exogenous IgA to determine whether we can keep the bacteria, from becoming more virulent. That will tell me whether these bacteria are responding to a weaker host or whether they are trying to survive.

Dr. Heyland: I just want to understand your perspective on TPN a bit more. You as well as several others in other populations have demonstrated in clinical trials that there is a consistent that enteral nutrition is associated with a reduction in infectious morbidity in critical illness. You also say that TPN is more deficient than being actually a toxin or doing harm to the patient. What about the association of parenteral nutrition and hyperglycemia and its subsequently increased infectious morbidity, and what about the discussion we had yesterday related to lipids and the lipid component of the TPN, its immunosuppression, and the trials that actually would hold the lipid part of the TPN and they demonstrate a reduction of infectious morbidity? So I guess when I look at it that way I think maybe there are toxicities associated with particular kinds of TPN or at least a misuse of TPN that may explain these clinical trials. Do you want to comment on that?

Dr. Kudsk: I am glad you raised that point. Let's talk about lipid first. I haven't done studies with lipids. One of the reasons we use a TPN solution that is glucose-based is because of the controversy whether the lipid itself is an immunosuppressor. If these experiments were performed with lipid, one could argue that it is the lipid that caused the immunologic deficiency. With regard to glucose, I am surprised at how people have accepted these data on hyperglycemia, and been so willing to accept it. You know as soon as the article came out in the *New England Journal of Medicine* [3], we had more insulin drips going in our ICU than ever before, and some of these patients had blood sugars as low as 47. There is going to be a price to be paid for that. Pomposelli et al. [4] wrote that the reason for the increased infections in the VA Cooperative Study and in the Moore et al. [5] study is that the patients had high blood sugars. But what is not known is when those blood sugars were drawn. Were they drawn before the infection or during infection? All we know is the peak glucose. As patients become infected, their blood sugars go up. We went back then to our study population and looked at 95 of the 98 randomized patients in our enteral/parenteral trial [6]. We had drawn blood sugars sequentially over the first 5 days in 86 of them. I analyzed them and found that blood sugar had nothing to do with the outcome and published this about a year ago [7], but it is never brought up that the study shows that glucose did not play a significant role in our population. There was a difference of about 15 mg% over the course of the experiment between the enterally and parenterally fed patients but nowhere near the 180–190 mg/dl associated with infection. The incidence of blood sugars over 200 mg/dl was far higher in the enteral group than in the parenteral group. The people who had the highest blood sugars were not the ones who got infected. So the difference between enteral and parenteral feeding on infection cannot be explained by hyperglycemia from my data. 63% of those patients in the Van Den Berghe et al. [3] study were cardiac patients. A recent study that just came out in the *American Journal of Surgery* [8] showed no impact of diabetes on the postoperative outcome in patients having cardiac surgery. It seems to me that glucose may be working through some other mechanisms such as inotropic effects. I think it is amazing what people have accepted without question. I suspect that there will be publications that show that insulin did not have an effect on outcome.

Dr. Déchelotte: In your studies in animals did you also try to correlate your observations with IgA and IL-10 to the glutathione status in the gut or in the lung and also the production of chemokines?

Dr. Kudsk: Yes I do have those data. With intravenous TPN glutathione drops significantly.

Dr. Déchelotte: On the clinical point of view, in the clinical settings, what would you suggest to be the best way of assessing the effects of enteral nutrient supply on lung immunity? Does it make sense to determinate the aurine tricarboxylic acid concentration in BAL fluids or in the saliva for instance. What is your experience?

Dr. Kudsk: Salivary IgA can be used but it is very difficult to collect it in ICU patients. But BAL is a technique which is useful in the clinical population. I would love to get a piece of small gut from these people but that is impossible. You can get a nip of the mucosa but that is not what we are talking about, we are talking about mass along the whole gastrointestinal tract.

Dr. Schultz: Thinking about the intraepithelial lymphocytes and the context of your experiments, do you think there is any correlation between the gut and the nasal mucosa in terms of the concentrations of the γδ T cells, especially because these cells are producing α in a very high concentration?

Dr. Kudsk: The γδ cells are in the intraepithelial space much more than within the lamina propria. The person who is the expert on that is Dr. Teitelbaum at the University of Michigan. Those cells make IFN-γ, and they are important in controlling tight junctions between the epithelial cells. They also may provide another signal to the underlying gut-associated lymphoid tissue (GALT) cells, but he is working on what the intraepithelial lymphocytes do.

Dr. Nitenberg: In your experimental data you always get better results with a chow diet than with commercial diets and than with intravenous administration supplemented either with bombesin or with glutamine. Could you comment on that?

Dr. Kudsk: I think there are two things. The complex enteral diet (CED) produces similar results but is less stimulating than chow. This is one thing that chow provides that the CED does not. The CED animals are continuously infused and the animals that get chow have intermittent feeding. I looked at the gastrointestinal tract of animals that got intravenous TPN, intragastric TPN as a perfusion, and others that drank the TPN solution. Clearly intermittence of feeding plays a role [9]. Now I believe that it is an effect of the neuropeptides.

Dr. Nitenberg: Do you think it is important to have gastric feeding instead of jejunal feeding?

Dr. Kudsk: To try to put a jejunal catheter in mice would be difficult. The stomach does, however, generate a stronger hormonal response.

Dr. Chioléro: In patients difficult to feed by the enteral route, septic patients for example, would you add parenteral nutrition, practically?

Dr. Kudsk: Yes, when they are frankly septic and hyperglycemic and unstable I don't really feed them anything. If they are being fed into the small intestine and they become septic and unstable, we stop small bowel feeding at that time.

Dr. Chioléro: Yes, but if the evolution is prolonged, sepsis can last days and days, so then comes a day where you should feed these patients and when the enteral route does not work well, what would you do practically?

Dr. Kudsk: It depends upon the severity of the sepsis. If you are talking about severe sepsis with catecholamines in high levels that should resolve within a day or 2 or the patient dies, but if you are talking about very sick patients who respond to resuscitation and are better the next day, that is when we feed them intravenously and switch them to enteral feeding as soon as possible.

Dr. Bozzetti: What is the minimal dose that you expect to be beneficial in clinical practice, the minimal dose of enteral feeding?

Dr. Kudsk: There are very little data on that. We only have a study by Alexander [10] in which he gave animals 100% TPN, 75% TPN and 25% enteral, 50–50, 25–75, and 100% enteral. In that particular experiment when he went from 25% enteral to 50% enteral was when the big reduction in translocation occurred. That was using a burn model.

Dr. McClave: A lot of the stimulation for GALT are ubiquitous organism and so I would expect those same organisms to be in the nasal cavity and colonizing an endotracheal tube and stimulating mucosa-associated lymphoid tissue (MALT) in the lungs. So I would expect these same systems, the nasopharyngeal-associated lymphoid tissue (NALT) and the MALT, in the lungs to have exposure, process the lymphocytes and have them home back to those areas, and yet you have shown in your experiments, when you don't feed the gut the IgA levels fall off as if those systems atrophy. So my question is when you look at NALT and MALT how much of their mass is due to their own processing and homing mechanisms versus immune tissue being processed at the level of gut and coming up these sites? Is that something you can answer?

Dr. Kudsk: We did the second experiment to generate immunity because patients who get put in the ICU and have to generate resistance and defenses against new bacteria are generally resistant to gram-negative bacteria. As they get challenged with bacterial overgrowth, they need to respond to them. I think that the defect occurs because this whole system is being downregulated and also there is an impairment to a new challenge.

Dr. McClave: Let me clarify it. How much of these distant site MALT in the lungs, not in the nasal cavities, are dependent on their own antigen processing versus antigen processing in immune tissue, come from the gut to these distant sites?

Dr. Kudsk: An experiment we have never done is to divide the esophagus of these animals and immunize via the nasal passages so the antigen can't go into the stomach and see if protection develops in the gut. Then immunize another group of mice into the stomach to see how much protection there is in the airway. In human studies, a type-specific *Escherichia coli* was given to the mothers towards the later part of the pregnancies [11]. Whereas the colostrum had no specific IgA before immunization, after the subjects had been immunized then suddenly the colostrum provided IgA against that particular *E. coli*. So clearly a distribution does occur in humans. How much of the antigen is processed within the nasal passages, I don't think anybody knows.

Dr. Baracos: I am sitting back here cogitating on amino acid requirements for gut-associated immunity and starting to understand some of the things that were said by Dr. Cynober. There is group of people who spend their time and energy studying first the path metabolism of amino acids in the gut. So they are looking at what disperses from the lumen and what appears on import blood, and they spend their time fantasizing about what the amino acids might have been utilized for in the first path. I wonder if you know what the respective culture of that profile of amino acids might be in the gut-associated immune cells as opposed to the enterocytes? Then, if I understood Dr. Cynober correctly, was he suggesting that if you knew what that culture in your amino acid solution was to optimize gut-associated immunity if delivered parenterally, would it be based on that first path culture?

Dr. Kudsk: I haven't studied that very much but I think back to an article in 1969 by Hirschfield and Kern [12]. They looked at animals that were given amino acids both in the well-fed state and animals that had been fasted, and then during recovery. What they found was that in the animals that had a fed gut, the amino acids basically passed across the mucosa. When the animals had been fasted and had gastrointestinal tract atrophy, then almost none of the amino acids passed through into the vascular system until the mucosa had regained its thickness, or nearly regained it. Then it allowed the amino acids to go into the systemic circulation.

Dr. Allison: If you put some non-absorbed thing into the gut just like bulk, would that have the same effect? I mean have you got to put substrates that are metabolized bulk substrates in?

Dr. Kudsk: Spaeth et al. [13] did that and studied bacterial translocation. They gave animals just bulk and found that bacterial translocation was reduced by it. I believe that as the bulk moves it stimulates neuropeptide release which stimulates normal levels of IgA and there is less bacterial translocation.

Dr. Déchelotte: I have an additional comment on the point made by Dr. Baracos about absorption and splanchnic extraction because there have been several studies performed in humans, in healthy humans, by Dr. Mathews and myself, demonstrating the kinetics of glutamine absorption with this quite saturable uptake process in humans. Splanchnic extraction strongly depends of course on the nutritional status and the quantity of glutamine supplied: the highest glutamine supply, the lowest splanchnic extraction.

Dr. Kudsk: Is there a difference in absorption between someone who has been fasted for 5 or 6 days and someone who is just postprandial?

Dr. Déchelotte: To this specific point I don't have any answer.

Dr. Cynober: There are classic studies which support this idea and what you mentioned before.

Dr. Rosenfeld: How much is the minimal amount to have these results in patients with enteral nutrition because sometimes it is very difficult to feed them?

Dr. Kudsk: Again I go back to the only study we have, the one with the burned guinea pigs [10] which took between 25 and 50% of the calculated nutrient goal for guinea pigs to maintain integrity with no bacterial translocation.

Dr. Peeters: Thank you very much. Maybe you will allow me to summarize. We heard quite a lot of proof for the statement we all made 25 years ago, if we want to feed a patient, feed him through the gut, and if you can't give him parenteral nutrition, it all depends on the energy you want to put in, the way you want to try to feed into the gut. Thank you very much for your presentation.

References

1. Hanna MK, Zarzaur BL, Fukatsu K, et al. Individual neuropeptides regulate gut-associated lymphoid tissue integrity, intestinal immunoglobulin A levels, and respiratory antibacterial immunity. *JPEN J Parenter Enteral Nutr* 2000; 24: 261–9.
2. Alverdy J, Holbrook C, Rocha F, et al. Gut-derived sepsis occurs when the right pathogen with the right virulence genes meets the right host: Evidence for in vivo virulence expression in *Pseudomonas aeruginosa. Ann Surg* 2000; 232: 480–9.
3. Van Den Berghe G, Wouters P, Weekers F, et al. Intensive insulin therapy in the critically ill patient. *N Engl J Med* 2001; 345: 1359–67.
4. Pomposelli JJ, Baxter JK 3rd, Babineau JJ, et al. Early postoperative glucose control predicts nosocomial infection rate in diabetic patients. *JPEN J Parenter Enteral Nutr* 1998; 22: 77–81.
5. Moore FA, Feliciano DV, Andrassy RJ, et al. Early enteral feeding, compared with parenteral, reduces postoperative septic complications. The results of a meta-analysis. *Ann Surg* 1992; 216: 172–83.
6. Kudsk KA, Croce MA, Fabian TC, et al. Enteral versus parenteral feeding. Effects of septic morbidity after blunt and penetrating abdominal trauma. *Ann Surg* 1992; 215: 503–13.
7. Kudsk KA, Laulederkind A, Hanna MK. Most infectious complications in parenterally fed trauma patients are not due to elevated blood glucose levels. *JPEN J Parenter Enteral Nutr* 2001; 25: 174–9.
8. Hamdan AD, Saltzberg SS, Sheahan M, et al. Lack of association of diabetes with increased postoperative mortality and cardiac morbidity: Results of 6565 major vascular operations. *Arch Surg* 2002; 137: 417–21.
9. Kudsk KA, Stone JM, Carpenter G, Sheldon GF. Effects of enteral vs. parenteral feeding of malnourished rats on body composition. *Curr Surg* 1981; 38: 322–3.
10. Alexander JW. Bacterial translocation during enteral and parenteral nutrition. *Proc Nutr Soc* 1998; 57: 389–93.
11. Goldblum RM, Ahlstedt S, Carlsson B, et al. antibody-forming cells in human colostrum after oral immunisation. *Nature* 1975; 257: 797–8.
12. Hirschfield JS, Kern F Jr. Protein starvation and the small intestine. 3. Incorporation of orally and intraperitoneally administered 1-leucine 4,5-3H into intestinal mucosal protein of protein-deprived rats. *J Clin Invest* 1969; 48: 1224–9.
13. Spaeth G, Specian RD, Berg RD, Deitch EA. Bulk prevents bacterial translocation induced by the oral administration of total parenteral nutrition solution. *JPEN J Parenter Enteral Nutr* 1990; 14: 442–7.

Cynober L, Moore FA (eds): Nutrition and Critical Care.
Nestlé Nutrition Workshop Series Clinical & Performance Program, Vol 8, pp 149–170
Nestec Ltd., Vevey/S. Karger AG, Basel, © 2003.

Gut Dysfunction and Intolerance to Enteral Nutrition in Critically Ill Patients

Frederick A. Moore[a] *and Norman W. Weisbrodt*[b]

Departments of [a]Surgery and [b]Integrative Biology and Pharmacology,
University of Texas – Houston Medical School, Houston, Tex., USA

Introduction

For patients who survive the first 48 h of intensive care, sepsis-related multiple organ failure (MOF) is the leading cause for prolonged intensive care unit (ICU) stays and deaths. Several lines of clinical evidence convincingly link gut injury and subsequent dysfunction to MOF [1]. First, patients who experience persistent gut hypoperfusion (documented by gastric tonometry) after resuscitation are at high risk for abdominal compartment syndrome (ACS), MOF, and death [2]. Second, epidemiologic studies have consistently shown that the normally sterile proximal gut becomes heavily colonized with a variety of organisms. These same organisms have been identified to be pathogens that cause late nosocomial infections. Thus, the gut has been called the 'undrained abscess' of MOF [3]. Third, gut-specific therapies (selective gut decontamination, early enteral nutrition (EN), and most recently immune-enhancing enteral diets) have been shown to reduce these nosocomial infections [4–7]. Of these gut-specific therapies, early EN is most widely employed. However, the most severely ill patients who should benefit most from early EN are frequently intolerant to it and are at increased risk for EN-related complications [8–11]. The purpose of this chapter will be to first provide a brief overview of why critically ill patients (using trauma patients as a model)

Supported by grants, NIGMS P50 GM38529 and NIGMS U54 GM62119, from the National Institutes of Health.

develop gut dysfunction and how gut dysfunction contributes to adverse outcomes. The discussion will then focus on the pathogenesis and clinical monitoring of specific gut dysfunctions that contribute to intolerance to EN. Based on this information, potential therapeutic strategies to prevent and/or treat gut dysfunction and to enhance tolerance to EN will be discussed.

How Gut Dysfunction Contributes to Adverse Patient Outcome

Multiple Organ Failure

A recent paradigm of post-injury MOF pathogenesis is depicted in figure 1 [12]. MOF occurs as a result of a dysfunctional inflammatory response and it occurs in two different patterns (i.e. early vs. late). After a traumatic insult, patients are resuscitated into a state of systemic hyperinflammation, now referred to as the systemic inflammatory response syndrome (SIRS). The intensity of SIRS is dependent upon (1) inherent host factors, (2) the degree of shock, and (3) the amount of tissue injured. Of the three, shock is the predominant factor [13]. Mild to moderate SIRS is most likely beneficial while severe SIRS can result in early MOF. As time proceeds, negative feedback systems downregulate certain aspects of acute SIRS to restore homeostasis and limit potential autodestructive inflammation. This latter response has recently been dubbed the compensatory anti-inflammatory response syndrome and results in delayed immunosuppression [14]. Mild to moderate delayed immunosuppression is clinically insignificant, but severe immunosuppression is associated with late infections. These late infections can worsen early MOF or precipitate late MOF.

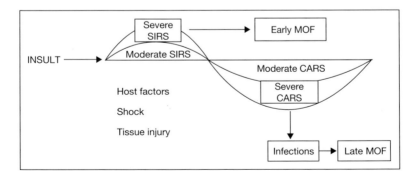

Fig. 1. Postinjury MOF occurs as a result of a dysfunctional inflammatory response. SIRS = Systemic inflammatory response syndrome; ICU = intensive care unit; MOF = multiple organ failure; CARS = counter anti-inflammatory response syndrome; TPN = total parenteral nutrition.

The gut is believed to be both an instigator and victim of this dysfunctional inflammatory response (fig. 2) [1]. Shock is associated with obligatory gut ischemia [15]. With resuscitation, reperfusion results in a local inflammatory response that can injure the gut setting the stage for ACS (see below) [16]. Additionally, the reperfused gut releases mediators that amplify SIRS [17–19]. Moreover, for patients undergoing laparotomy, bowel manipulation and anesthetics cause further gut dysfunction [19]. Finally, standard ICU therapies (morphine, H$_2$ antagonists, catecholamines, and broad-spectrum antibiotics) and intentional disuse (use of TPN rather than EN) promote additional gut dysfunction [20]. The end result is progressive dysfunction (table 1) characterized by gastroesophageal reflux, gastroparesis, duodenogastric reflux,

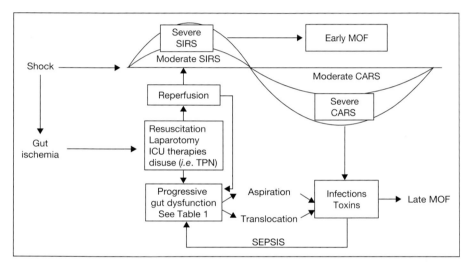

Fig. 2. The gut is the instigator and victim of a dysfunctional inflammatory response. SIRS = Systemic inflammatory response syndrome; MOF = multiple organ failure; CARS = counter anti-inflammatory response syndrome.

Table 1. Progressive gut dysfunction in critically ill patients

Gastroesophageal reflux/aspiration
Gastroparesis
Duodenogastric reflux
Gastric alkalinization
Decreased mucosal perfusion
Impaired intestinal transit
Increased colonization
Increased permeability
Decreased mucosal immunity

Table 2. Gut dysfunctions that contribute to intolerance of enteral nutrition in critically ill patients

Dysfunction	Pathogenesis	Clinical monitors

Gastroesophageal reflux	NG tube
	Morphine
	Sepsis mediators
	High ICP
		Vomiting/
		  regurgutation
		? Glucose in sputum
		? Blue food coloring
		  in sputum

Gastroparesis	Morphine Dopamine Sepsis mediators High ICP	NG tube output Gastric residual volumes ? Saline load test
Decreased mucosal perfusion	Sympathetic nerves Angiotensin II	Gastric tonometry
Impaired intestinal transit	Neural reflex Decreased hormone Inflammatory mediators	? Bowel sounds Distention ? Contrast studies Diarrhea
Decreased gut absorptive capacity	Calcium overload ATP depletion Decreased enzyme activity Decreased transporter activity Decreased surface area Hypoalbuminemia	Diarrhea

gastric alkalinization, decreased mucosal perfusion, and impaired intestinal transit. As time proceeds, the normally sterile upper gut becomes heavily colonized, mucosal permeability increases and local mucosal immunity decreases [21–23]. Intraluminal contents (e.g. bacteria and their toxic products) then disseminate by aspiration or translocation to cause systemic sepsis which then promotes further gut dysfunction [24, 25].

Abdominal Compartment Syndrome

Intra-abdominal pressure (IAP) is monitored by urinary bladder pressure (UBP) measurements and when UBP exceeds 25 cm H_2O, extra-abdominal organ functions may become impaired. By definition, this is ACS. There are two types of ACS: primary and secondary [2]. Primary ACS occurs in patients with abdominal injuries that typically have undergone 'damage control' laparotomy (where obvious bleeding is rapidly controlled and the abdomen is packed) and have entered the 'bloody viscus cycle' of coagulopathy, acidosis, and hypothermia which promotes ongoing bleeding. Accumulation of blood, worsening bowel edema from resuscitation, and the presence of intra-abdominal packs all contribute to increasing IAP that causes ACS. Secondary ACS occurs when an extra-abdominal injury (e.g. pelvic fracture or mangled extremity) requires massive resuscitation which causes bowel edema which increases IAP to cause ACS. Markedly elevated IAP also decreases gut perfusion which may adversely affect a variety of gut functions. ACS is a harbinger of MOF and failure to promptly recognize and treat it contributes to bad outcomes.

Nonocclusive Small Bowel Necrosis

Nonocclusive small bowel necrosis (NOBN) is a relatively rare, but frequently fatal entity that is associated with the use of EN in critically ill patients [11]. Patients typically present with complaints of cramping abdominal pain, progressive abdominal distention associated with SIRS. Computed tomography will reveal a thickened dilated bowel with pneumatosis intestinalis. For those who progress and require exploratory celiotomy, extensive patchy necrosis of the small bowel is found. Pathologic analysis of the resected specimens yields a spectrum of findings from acute inflammation with mucosal ulceration to transmural necrosis and multiple perforations. The consistent association with EN indicates that inappropriate administration of nutrients into a dysfunctional gut plays a pathogenic role. There are two popular hypotheses. First, metabolically compromised enterocytes become adenosine triphosphate (ATP) depleted as a result of increased energy demands induced by the absorption of intraluminal nutrients [26]. The second hypothesis is that when nutrients are delivered into the dysmotile small bowel, fluid shifts into the lumen as a result of the presence of hyperosmolar enteral formula. Additionally, CO_2 may be produced as a result of fermentation of carbohydrates by colonized bacteria. Increased intraluminal fluid and gas cause small bowel distention which, when massive, causes hypoperfusion [11].

How Gut Dysfunctions Contribute to Intolerance to Enteral Nutrition

The gut is a complex organ that performs a variety of functions, some of which are vital for ultimate survival of critically ill patients (e.g. barrier function, immune competence, and metabolic regulation). Unfortunately, gut dysfunction in critically ill patients is poorly characterized and routine monitoring of gut function is crude. Currently, the best parameter of gut function is tolerance to EN. For several reasons, this is an attractive parameter to monitor and potentially modulate. First, tolerance to EN requires integrative gut functioning (e.g. secretion, digestion, motility, and absorption). Second, locally administered nutrients may improve perfusion and optimize the recovery of other vital gut functions (e.g. motility, barrier function, mucosal immunity) [27, 28]. Third, tolerance correlates with patient outcome and improving tolerance will likely improve patient outcome. Fourth, refined therapeutic interventions to improve EN tolerance will lessen the need to use TPN and decrease EN-associated complications.

Of the gut dysfunctions outlined in table 1, gastroesophageal reflux (GER), gastroparesis, decreased mucosal perfusion, impaired intestinal transit, and impaired gut absorptive capacity (GAC) are likely contributors to intolerance to EN. A brief overview of the pathogenesis of each of these dysfunctions and how they are monitored clinically will be reviewed to provide the rationale for proposed therapeutic strategies to improve tolerance to EN.

Gastroesophageal Reflux

GER is an important contributing factor to aspiration of EN which is a common cause of pneumonia in ICU patients. Reflux will occur whenever the pressure difference between the stomach and esophagus is great enough to overcome the resistance offered by the LES. Increases in gastric pressure can be due to distention with fluids and failure of the stomach to relax to accommodate fluid. Decreases in resistance at the lower esophageal sphincter (LES) can be due to relaxation of LES muscle in response to many stimuli including mediators released during injury and resuscitation [29]. Additional contributing factors include: (a) forced supine position; (b) the presence of a nasoenteric tube; (c) hyperglycemia, and (d) morphine.

Commonly used clinical monitors include laboratory testing for the presence of glucose in tracheal secretions or by observing blue food dye (BFD) which has been added to the enteral formula in tracheal aspirates [30]. Detection of glucose lacks specificity. False-positive results can occur with high serum glucose levels or the presence of blood in tracheal secretions. The use of BFD is poorly standardized and lacks sensitivity. More importantly, however, several reports document absorption of BFD in critically ill patients and is associated with death. This is presumably due to a toxic effect that BFD has on mitochondrial function. A recent consensus conference recommended that both of these techniques be abandoned [31]. Unfortunately, there are no simple monitors of GER other than observing for vomiting or regurgitation which are not very sensitive. The head of the bed should be elevated 30–45° to decrease the risk that, when GER occurs, it is less likely to result in pulmonary aspiration. Gastric residual volumes (GRVs; see below) should be monitored with the presumption that a distended stomach will lead to a higher volume GER.

Gastroparesis

Recent studies have confirmed that gastroparesis is common in ICU patients [32]. Gastroparesis predisposes for increased duodenogastric reflux (a potential contributing factor for gastric alkalinization) and GER (a contributing factor for aspiration). The mechanisms responsible for gastroparesis in critical illness have not been well studied. Potential factors include: (a) medications (e.g. morphine, dopamine); (b) sepsis mediators (e.g. nitric oxide); (c) hyperglycemia, and (d) increased intracranial pressure.

The common clinical monitors for gastroparesis are intermittent measurement of GRVs when feeding into the stomach or measurement of continuous suction nasogastric tube output when feeding postpylorically. The practice of using GRVs is poorly standardized and is a major obstacle to advancing the rate of EN [33]. GRVs appear to correlate poorly with gastric. GRVs of $<200\,cm^3$ generally are well tolerated. GRVs of $200–500\,cm^3$ should prompt careful clinical assessment and the initiation of a prokinetic agent. With GRVs of $>500\,cm^3$, EN should be stopped. After clinical assessment excludes small bowel ileus or obstruction, placement of a post-ligament of Treitz feeding tube should be considered.

Impaired Mucosal Perfusion

Shock results in disproportionate splanchnic vasoconstriction. The gut mucosa appears to be especially vulnerable to injury during hypoperfusion. The arterioles and venules in the small bowel mucosal villi form 'hairpin loops' [34]. This anatomic arrangement improves absorptive function, but it also permits a countercurrent exchange of oxygen from the arterioles to the venules in the proximal villus. Under hypoperfused conditions, a proximal 'steal' of oxygen is believed to reduce the pO_2 at the tip of the villi to 0. The gut mucosa is further injured during reperfusion by reactive oxygen metabolites and recruitment of activated neutrophils. This mucosal injury, however, appears to repair itself rather quickly. Mucosal blood flow, however, does not always return to baseline with resuscitation and this is in part due to defective vasorelaxation [35]. The gut mucosa is also vulnerable to recurrent episodes of hypoperfusion from ACS, sepsis, and the use of vasoactive drugs. Whether recurrent hypoperfusion results in additional ischemia/reperfusion injury is not known, but it is reasonable to assume that hypoperfusion would decrease gut nutrient absorption and render the patient more susceptible to NOBN.

Monitoring gastric mucosal perfusion in the clinical setting can be done by gastric tonometry [15]. With hypoperfusion, intramucosal CO_2 increases due to insufficient clearance of CO_2 produced by aerobic metabolism or due to buffering of extra hydrogen ions produced in anaerobic metabolism. As intramucosal CO_2 accumulates, it diffuses into the lumen of the stomach. The tonometer measures the CO_2 that equilibrates in a saline-filled balloon (a newer monitor uses an air-filled balloon) that sits in the stomach. This is the regional CO_2 tension ($PrCO_2$) and is assumed to equal the intramucosal CO_2 tension. Using this measured $PrCO_2$ and assuming that arterial bicarbonate equals intramucosal bicarbonate, the intramucosal pH (pHi) is calculated by using the Henderson-Hasselbalch equation. Numerous studies have documented that a persistently low pHi (or high $PrCO_2$ level) despite effective systemic resuscitation predicts adverse outcomes. Unfortunately, alternative resuscitation strategies have not been able to increase pHi to improve outcome and thus this monitoring tool is in search of a novel application. We have found the new Tonocap which is a combined capnograph and semi-continuous air tonometer to be useful in identifying patients early in resuscitation who are at high risk of developing ACS. After resuscitation, we have also found it to be valuable in identifying patients who will not tolerate EN. If $PrCO_2$ is high (>90 mm Hg) we do not start EN. If $PrCO_2$ is low, but rises with initiation of EN, we proceed cautiously in the advancement of rate of feeding.

Impaired Intestinal Transit

Laboratory models of shock, bowel manipulation and sepsis demonstrate that small bowel transit is impaired [19, 24, 36]. In all of these models, cytokines and other mediators are produced by cells in the intestine that impair enteric nerve and/or intestinal smooth muscle function [24, 37]. This impairment in turn is expressed as a decrease in the number and/or force of contractions, or as an abnormal pattern of contractions. Although the results in animal models are convincing, surprisingly, clinical studies indicate that small bowel motility and transit are more often than not well preserved after major elective and emergency laparotomies [10]. This observation coupled with the observation that small bowel absorption of simple nutrients is relatively intact provided the rationale for early jejunal feeding.

Clinical studies have documented that over 85% of critically ill patients tolerate early jejunal feeding [8, 9]. In a recent study, severely injured patients had jejunal manometers and feeding tubes placed at secondary laparotomy [10]. Surprisingly, 50% had fasting patterns of motility that included components of the normal migrating motor complexes (MMCs). These patients tolerated advancements of EN without problems. The other 50% who did not have fasting MMCs did not tolerate early advancement of EN. Of note, none of the patients converted to a normal fed pattern of motility once they reached full-dose enteral feeding. This could be due to infusion of caloric loads insufficient to bring about conversion. On the other hand, the failure to develop fed activity, a pattern of motility promoting mixing and absorption, might explain why diarrhea is a common problem in this patient group.

Although manometry can be used to monitor motility, it is not practical. Unfortunately, simpler indicators of motility such as the presence of bowel sounds or the passing of flatus are unreliable. Other, minimally invasive methods to monitor transit are needed. Contrast studies through the feeding tubes are relatively simple, but not validated.

Impaired Gut Absorptive Capacity

Small bowel absorption of glucose and amino acids is depressed after trauma and sepsis [38]. Multiple factors have been identified including: (a) cytosolic calcium overload; (b) ATP depletion; (c) diminished brush border enzyme activity; (d) decreased carrier activity; (e) decreased absorptive epithelial surface area, and (f) hypoalbuminemia. In a recent animal study [26], intestinal ischemia/reperfusion caused significant mucosal injury and significant depletion of mucosal ATP. When this was combined with exposure of the bowel to alanine, the damage and ATP depletion were more severe and the absorption of glucose was impaired. In contrast, exposure of the bowel to glucose or glutamine preserved the ATP level, protected against mucosal injury and improved GAC.

The clinical significance of these observations remains unclear since most patients tolerate EN when delivered into the small bowel. However, decreased GAC may be a cause for diarrhea and may explain why patients commonly experience diarrhea with reinstitution of EN after prolonged bowel rest. Unfortunately, there are no clinical monitors for GAC.

Diarrhea may be indicative of depressed GAC, but there are other causes for diarrhea in the critically ill including: impaired transit (described above); bacterial overgrowth (e.g. reduced short-chain fatty acid (SCFA) production or the presence of *Clostridium difficile*); contaminated enteral formulas; abnormal colonic responses to EN (e.g. ascending colon secretion rather than absorption, or impaired distal colon motor activity), and administration of drugs which contain sorbitol (e.g. medical elixirs) or magnesium (e.g. antacids).

Strategies to Improve Tolerance of Enteral Nutrition

Gut-Specific Resuscitation

If shock-induced gut hypoperfusion is assumed to be a prime inciting event for gut dysfunction, then resuscitation protocols need to be devised to optimize early gut perfusion and prevent reperfusion injury. Traditional resuscitation is aimed at optimizing systemic perfusion and the standard of care is to first administer 50 ml/kg of isotonic crystalloids (3 liters in the normal adult), then to add packed red blood cells (PRBCs) to the regimen at a ratio of 3:1 crystalloid:blood. While this approach is effective in most patients, it is associated with problematic bowel edema in patients at high risk for MOF. Alternative resuscitation strategies to reduce reperfusion injury and reduce bowel edema may include the earlier use of PRBCs or new blood substitutes and to use hypertonic saline or colloids instead of isotonic crystalloids.

How bowel edema effects bowel function needs to be better clarified. However, it is reasonable to assume that a grossly edematous bowel will have abnormal motility and not optimally absorb nutrients. With more severe bowel wall edema, patients develop IAP which can worsen bowel perfusion and set up a vicious cycle that leads to ACS. Routine UBP monitoring is recommended with massive resuscitations. We and others have also found that gastric tonometry is valuable in early identification of ACS.

157

Enteral Feeding Protocols

Once resuscitation is judged to be complete, enteral access should be obtained. Controversy exists over the optimal level of feeding (i.e. stomach vs. duodenum vs. jejunum). While comparative trials do not exist, clinical experience shows that feeding past the ligament of Treitz (via surgically placed jejunostomy or endoscopically placed nasojejunal tubes) is highly successful [8, 9]. While we recommend jejunal feeding in high-risk patients, access past the ligament of Treitz is not readily available in most ICUs. Recent trials that have compared gastric to duodenal feeding are underpowered, but collectively they show that duodenal feeding more rapidly achieves nutritional goals and reduces the risk for aspiration [39–41]. Regardless of the level of feeding, all patients should have the head of the bed elevated (reverse Trendelenburg preferred) to 30–45° to reduce the risk of aspiration. Feeding should be started at a low rate (e.g. $15\,cm^3/h$) of continuous infusion and advanced at set intervals (e.g. every 8–12 h) to a modest goal (60 ml/h) while monitoring and treating signs and symptoms of intolerance (tables 3, 4). When feeding into the stomach, fear of aspiration is a major concern and increased GRV is the primary reason that limits advancement of the rate of feedings. On the other hand, diarrhea and abdominal distention are the major problems encountered in postpyloric feeding. Diarrhea can generally be successfully managed (table 4), but distention is not as amenable to intervention and may be the harbinger of NOBN.

Of note, the goals of early EN have changed. Traditionally, EN was rapidly advanced to high rates ($125–150\,cm^3/h$) to place the patient in positive caloric and nitrogen balance as soon as possible so as to prevent acute protein malnutrition. This rapid advancement is associated with high rates of intolerance and failure of EN. However, it appears that early EN exerts beneficial effects at lower rates of infusion (i.e. $60\,cm^3/h$) presumably by promoting vital gut functions (motility, mucosal immunities and barrier function) and enhancing systemic immunity. Advancement beyond $60\,cm^3/h$ to place the patient in positive caloric and nitrogen balance should be done slowly over the first week of ICU treatment. If patients cannot achieve 60% of this targeted goal by ICU day 7, concurrent TPN should be started.

Clinical studies have demonstrated that clinical signs of NOBN are not reliable [11]. This rare but devastating complication can occur when the clinical status of the patient deteriorates. For patients who are at perceived high risk for NOBN (table 4), EN should be temporally stopped and if the condition persists low-dose ($15\,cm^3/h$) elemental formulas with high glucose and glutamine levels are initiated.

Modified Enteral Formulas

The earliest enteral diets used in critically ill patients were formulated (i.e. elemental amino acids, low fat) to enhance tolerances. It has subsequently been observed that critically ill patients can tolerate more complex formulas

Table 3. Monitoring and management of intolerance to enteral nutrition

Indicator	Severity	Definition	Treatment
Vomiting	(witnessed)	Gastric contents in oropharynx	Place NG suction catheter, check oropharynx function Check existing NG function Decrease TF infusion rate by 50%
High NG tube output (for post-pyloric feeding)	(measured)	>1,200 cm^3/12 h	Check existing X-ray for post-pyloric placement of feeding tube If >48 h since last X-ray, order KUB If not tube post-pyloric, hold TF order new feeding tube placement Check NG aspirate for glucose If glucose present and feeding tube post-pyloric, hold TF and reassess in 12 h Retest NG aspirate for glucose 12 h
High gastric residual volumes (for gastric feeding)	Mild	75–200 cm^3	Tighten glycemic control Minimize narcotics
	Moderate	200–500 cm^3	As above Prokinetics Clinical assessment
	Severe	>500 cm^3	Stop gastric feeding Clinical assessment Post ligament of Treitz tube
PrCO$_2$ by tonometry If patient is in permissive hypercapnia (PaCO$_2$ >50 mm Hg) use PrCO$_2$–PaCO$_2$ gap Otherwise use PrCO$_2$ reading	Moderate	70 mm Hg <PrCO$_2$ <90 mm Hg >8 h or PrCO$_2$–PaCO$_2$ gap = 30–50 mm Hg	Change to elemental diet at present rate and advance as per protocol If already on elemental diet, continue to advance as per protocol
	Severe	PrCO$_2$ >90 mm Hg for >8 h or PrCO$_2$–PaCO$_2$ gap >50 mm Hg	Stop TF infusion Re-evaluate in 6 h If PrCO$_2$ is moderate, start elemental formula at 15 ml/h and advance per protocol If PrCO$_2$ is still severe, start elemental formula at 15 ml/h and do not advance rate until PrCO$_2$ is moderate

Table 4. Monitoring and management of intolerance to enteral nutrition

Indicator	Severity	Definition	Treatment
Abdominal distention and/or cramping or tenderness (if detectable)	Mild	Hx and/or PE	Maintain TF infusion rate Re-examine in 6 h
	Moderate	Hx and/or PE	Stop TF infusion Order AP supine KUB X-ray – assess for small bowel obstruction if SBO, notify primary team Place gastric tonometer NG catheter – replace existing NG catheter if not gastric tonometer Re-examine in 6 h If moderate distension for ≥24 h, switch to elemental for 72 h
	Severe	Hx and/or PE	Stop TF infusion Set i.v. fluid infusion rate = 250 ml/h Consider CBC, lactate, ABG, Chem7, CT scan abdomen
Diarrhea	Mild	1–2 × per shift or 100–200 cm³/12 h	Maintain or increase TF infusion rate per protocol
	Moderate	3–4 × per shift or 200–300 cm³/12 h	Maintain TF infusion rate Re-examine in 6 h
	Severe	>4 × per shift or >300 cm³/12 h	Decrease TF infusion rate by 50% Give diphenoxylate/atropine (Lomotil) 10 cm³ every 6 h via feeding tube Review MAR; note antibiotic, other GI drugs Order stool studies; fecal leukocytes, toxin assays If persistent (with diphenoxylate/atropine) >48 h, switch to elemental feeding
Perceived high risk for nonocclusive bowel necrosis	Inotropes Low dose High dose		 Re-assess 6 h Stop EN if clinical course worsening
	Vasopressors Norepinephrine, phenylephrine		 Start elemental diet at 15 cm³/h and do not advance

Table 4. (continued)

Indicator	Severity	Definition	Treatment
	Epinephrine, high-dose dopamine		Reassess in 24 h
	Worsening respirator failure		Start elemental diet at 15 cm³/h and do not advance
	Prone position Paralytics		Reassess in 24 h
	Intermittent dialysis		Start elemental diet at 15 cm³/h and do not advance
	With hypotension Or need for vasopressors		Reassess in 24 h

and that the use of new immune-enhancing formulas is associated with better outcomes. Research needs to be done on determining how to modify these formulas to enhance tolerance in the most stressed patient. For example, the addition of soluble fiber to standard enteral formulas may decrease the incidence of diarrhea. Pectin and partially hydrolyzed guar are soluble fibers that are fermented in the colon to produce SCFAs [42]. SCFAs have positive trophic effects on colonocytes and promote water absorption. Other proposed mechanisms by which fibers may decrease diarrhea is by prolonging intestinal transit time, decreasing *Clostridium difficile* toxin production and by binding bile salts.

Prokinetic Agents

Because gastroparesis and ileus are commonly seen postoperatively and following resuscitation, and because they can complicate initiation of enteral feeding, agents to 'normalize' gastrointestinal (GI) motility have been sought [43, 44]. Evaluation of such prokinetic agents is difficult because it is not enough to just stimulate contractions. Contractions at adjacent sites must be coordinated in order for normal digestion, absorption, and transit to take place. Coordinated contractions are under the control of hormonal and neural, both central and peripheral, pathways and it is these pathways that are affected by the cytokines and other mediators that are upregulated following a traumatic insult [45]. Prokinetic strategies are aimed at either blocking these mediators or of overriding them by stimulating normal pathways.

Opiate Antagonist. One major cause of ileus is stimulation of opioid receptors. Stress provokes release of endogenous opioids and opioids are the most common treatment for pain in ICU patients. In animal models and humans, both endogenously released and exogenously administered opioids

161

act on receptors in both the central nervous system (CNS) and in the enteric nervous system (ENS) to alter intestinal function, especially motility [46]. Although actions at both the CNS and ENS are involved, recent studies indicate that if opioid actions at the ENS are blocked, ileus may be prevented or resolved without interfering with the desired opioid actions on the CNS and other systems. An investigational opioid receptor antagonist that has limited systemic absorption after oral administration and minimal access to the CNS has been shown to speed recovery of bowel function and shorten the duration of hospitalization after surgery [47]. This study needs to be expanded to include additional patients, especially those who have undergone resuscitation.

Erythromycin. Agents like erythromycin that act on receptors for motilin, the naturally occurring hormone responsible in part for regulating normal GI motility, have been shown to enhance gastric emptying and intestinal transit in animal models and in some clinical trials. However, their effectiveness postoperatively has been disappointing [42, 43, 48]. In addition, in animal studies, the dose of erythromycin that can initiate an MMC is close to that which can induce nausea and vomiting [49]. If the same occurs in humans, this will limit its usefulness. Other 'motilides' are under investigation, but their usefulness has not been established.

Serotonin (5-HT) Antagonists and Agonists. One of the major transmitters within the ENS is serotonin. By acting at various serotonin receptors, it can either enhance or inhibit intestinal contractions and transit. In animal and some human studies, motility has been enhanced by 5-HT_3 receptor antagonist and by 5-HT_4 agonists [50]. Although the results were never that impressive or consistent, a few agents have been used in clinical situations. Side effects, however, have resulted in their being removed from the market. Still, this is a fertile area for future research.

Antioxidants

The cycle of organ hypoperfusion during shock followed by reperfusion following resuscitation results in the formation of reactive oxygen species that are detrimental. Thus, it is logical to propose that administration of antioxidants could prove beneficial. In many animal models, administration of agents such as superoxide dismutase, ethyl pyruvate, and melatonin limit damage induced by ischemia/reperfusion [51, 52]. In a recent study, administration of α-melanocyte-stimulating hormone to rats preserved both the function and the structural integrity of the intestine following mesenteric ischemia/reperfusion [36].

Probiotics and Prebiotics

A probiotic is defined as a live microbial feed supplement which beneficially affects the host by improving its intestinal microbial balance [53]. Probiotics are most commonly lactobacilli, bifidobacteria or saccharomyces and are available in the form of powders, capsules, and enriched yoghurts.

A prebiotic is defined as a nondigestible food ingredient that beneficially affects the host by selectively stimulating the growth and/or activity of specific bacteria in the colon. Probiotics are usually nondigestible oligosaccharides. The most extensively studied are the fructoligosaccharides (FOS) such as oligofructose and inulin. FOS are fermented in the colon which promotes the proliferation of bifidobacteria with a reduction in clostridia and fusobacteria. Manipulation of the colonic microflora may reduce the incidence of EN-associated diarrhea by suppressing enteropathogens and by producing SCFA.

References

1. Hassoun HH, Mercer DW, Moody FG, Weisbrodt NW, Moore FA. Postinjury multiple organ failure: The role of the gut. *Shock* 2001; 15: 1–10.
2. Balogh Z, McKinley BA, Holcomb JB, et al. Both primary and secondary abdominal compartment syndrome (ACS) can be predicted early and are harbingers of multiple organ failure. *J Trauma* 2002, in press.
3. Marshall JC, Christou NV, Meakins JL. The gastrointestinal tract: The 'undrained abscess' of multiple organ failure. *Ann Surg* 1993; 218: 111–9.
4. Heyland DK, Cook DJ, Jaeschke R, et al. Selective decontamination of the digestive tract: An overview. *Chest* 1994; 105: 1221–9.
5. Moore EE, Jones TN. Benefits of immediate jejunal feeding after major abdominal trauma: A prospective randomized study. *J Trauma* 1986; 26: 874–83.
6. Moore FA, Feliciano DV, Andrassy R, et al. Enteral feeding reduces postoperative septic complications: A meta-analysis. *Ann Surg* 1992; 216: 62–71.
7. Moore FA. Effects of immune-enhancing diets in infectious morbidity and multiple organ failure. *JPEN J Parenter Enteral Nutr* 2001; 25: 1–8.
8. Jones TN, Moore FA, Moore EE, McCroskey BL. Gastrointestinal symptoms attributed to jejunostomy feeding after major abdominal trauma: A critical analysis. *Crit Care Med* 1989; 17: 1146–50.
9. Kozar RA, McQuiggan MM, Moore EE, et al. Postinjury enteral tolerance is reliably achieved by a standardized protocol. *J Surg Res* 2002; 104: 70–5.
10. Moore FA, Cocanour CS, McKinley BA, et al. Migrating motility complexes persist after severe traumatic shock in patients who tolerate enteral nutrition. *J Trauma* 2001; 51: 1075–82.
11. Marvin RG, McKinley BA, McQuiggan M, et al. Nonocclusive bowel necrosis occurring in critically ill trauma patients receiving enteral nutrition manifests no reliable clinical signs for early detection. *Am J Surg* 2000; 179: 7–12.
12. Moore FA, Sauaia A, Moore EE, et al. Postinjury multiple organ failure: A bimodal phenomenon. *J Trauma* 1996; 40: 502–9.
13. Sauaia A, Moore FA, Moore EE, et al. Multiple organ failure can be predicted as early as 12 hours postinjury. *J Trauma* 1998; 45: 291–303.
14. Bone RC. Sir Isaac Newton, sepsis, SIRS, and CARS. *Crit Care Med* 1996; 24: 1125–28.
15. Fiddian-Green RG. Studies in splanchnic ischemia and multiple organ failure. In: Marston A, Bulkley GB, Fiddian-Green RG, Haglund U, eds. *Splanchnic ischemia and multiple organ failure*. London: Arnold/St Louis: Mosby, 1989; 349–63.
16. Simpson R, Alon R, Kobzik L, et al. Neutrophil and non-neutrophil-mediated injury in intestinal ischemia/reperfusion. *Ann Surg* 1993; 218: 444–54.
17. Moore EE, Moore FA, Franciose RJ, et al. Postischemic gut serves as a priming bed for circulating neutrophils that provoke multiple organ failure. *J Trauma* 1994; 37: 881–7.
18. Manious MR, Ertel W, Chaudry III, et al. The gut: A cytokine-generating organ in systemic inflammation? *Shock* 1995; 4: 193.
19. Schwarz NT, Beer-Stolz D, Simmons RL, Bauer AJ. Pathogenesis of paralytic ileus. Intestinal manipulation opens a transient pathway between the intestinal lumen and the leukocytic infiltrate of the jejunal muscularis. *Ann Surg* 2002; 235: 31–40.

20. Kueppers PM, Miller TA, Chen C-Y, et al. Effect of total parenteral nutrition plus morphine on bacterial translocation in rats. *Ann Surg* 1993; 217: 286–92.
21. Li J, Kudsk KA, Gozinski B, et al. Effects of parenteral and enteral nutrition on gut-associated lymphoid tissue. *J Trauma* 1995; 39: 44–52.
22. Hieuwenheijs VB, Verheem A, van Duihvenbode-Beumer J, et al. The role of interdigestive small bowel motility in the regulation of gut microflora, bacterial overgrowth, and bacterial translocation in rats. *Ann Surg* 1998; 228: 188.
23. Faries PL, Simon RJ, Martella AT, et al. Intestinal permeability correlates with severity of injury in trauma patients. *J Trauma* 1998; 44: 1031.
24. Weisbrodt NW, Pressley TA, Li Y-F, et al. Decreased ileal muscle contractility and increased NOS II expression induced by lipopolysaccharide. *Am J Physiol* 1996; 271: G454–G60.
25. Mercer DW, Castaneda A, Denning JW, et al. Effects of endotoxin on gastric injury from luminal irritants in rats: Potential roles of nitric oxide. *Am J Physiol* 1998; 38: G449–G59.
26. Kozar RA, Schultz SG, Hassoun HT, et al. The type of sodium-coupled solute modulates small bowel mucosal injury, transport function and ATP after ischemia/reperfusion injury in rats. *Gastroenterology,* in press.
27. Houdjuk APJ, Van Leeuwen PAM, Boermeester MA, et al. Glutamine-enriched enteral diet increases splanchnic blood flow in the rat. *Am J Physiol* 1994; 267: G1035–G40.
28. Mainous MR, Block EF, Deitch EA. Nutritional support of the gut: How and why. *New Horiz* 1994; 2: 193–201.
29. Fan YP, Chakder S, Gao F, et al. Inducible and neuronal nitric oxide synthase involvement in lipopolysaccharide-induced sphincteric dysfunction. *Am J Physiol Gastrointest Liver Physiol* 2001; 280: G32–G42.
30. Maloney JP, Ryan TA. Detection of aspiration in enterally-fed patients: A requiem for bedside monitors of aspiration. *JPEN J Parenter Enteral Nutr*, in press.
31. McClave SA, Demeo MT, Delegge MH, et al. North American Summit on Aspiration in the critically ill patient: Consensus statement. *JPEN J Parenter Enteral Nutr,* in press.
32. Dive A, Miesse C, Galanti L, et al. Effect of erythromycin on gastric motility in mechanically ventilated critically ill patients: A double-blind, randomized, placebo-controlled study. *Crit Care Med* 1995; 23: 1356–62.
33. McClave SA, Snider HL. Clinical utility of gastric residual volumes as a monitor for patients on enteral tube feeding. *JPEN J Parenter Enteral Nutr,* in press.
34. Lundgren O, Haglund U. The pathophysiology of the intestinal countercurrent exchanger. *Life Sci* 1978; 23: 1411–22.
35. Reilly PM, Bulkley GB. Vasoactive mediators and splanchnic perfusion. *Crit Care Med* 1993; 21: S55–S68.
36. Hassoun HT, Moore FA, Kozar RA, et al. α-Melanocyte stimulating hormone protects against mesenteric ischemia/reperfusion injury. *Am J Physiol* 2002; 282: G1059–G68.
37. DeWinter BY, Boeckxstaens GE, DeMan JG, et al. Effect of adrenergic and nitrergic blockade on experimental ileus in rats. *Br J Pharmacol* 1997; 120: 464–8.
38. Singh G, Chaudry KI, Chudler LC, et al. Depressed gut absorptive capacity early after trauma-hemorrhagic shock: Restoration with diltiazem treatment. *Ann Surg* 1991; 214: 712–8.
39. Kortbeek JB, Haigh PI, Doig C. Duodenal versus gastric feeding in ventilated blunt trauma patients: A randomized controlled trial. *J Trauma* 1999; 46: 992–8.
40. Heyland DK, Drover JW, MacDonald S, et al. Effect of postpyloric feeding on gastroesophageal regurgitation and pulmonary microaspiration: Results of a randomized controlled trial. *Crit Care Med* 2001; 29: 1495–1501.
41. Kearns PJ, Chin D, Mueller L, et al. The incidence of ventilator-associated pneumonia and success in nutrient delivery with gastric versus small intestinal feeding: A randomized clinical trial. *Crit Care Med* 2000; 28: 1742–6.
42. Schultz AA, Ashby-Hughes B, Taylor R, et al. Effects of pectin on diarrhea in critically-ill tube-fed patients receiving antibiotics. *Am J Crit Care* 2000; 9: 403–11.
43. Chapman MJ, Fraser RJ, Kluge MT, et al. Erythromycin improves gastric emptying in critically ill patients intolerant of nasogastric feeding. *Crit Care Med* 2000; 28: 2334–7.
44. Sarna SK, Gonzales A, Ryan RP. Enteric locus of action of prokinetics: ABT-229, motilin, and erythromycin. *Am J Physiol Gastrointest Liver Physiol* 2000; 278: G744–G52.
45. Collins SM. The immunomodulation of enteric neuromuscular function: Implications for motility and inflammatory disorders. *Gastroenterology* 1996; 111: 1683–99.

46. Burks TF, Fox DA, Hirning LD, et al. Regulation of gastrointestinal function by multiple opioid receptors. *Life Sci* 1988; 43: 2177–81.
47. Taguchi A, Sharma N, Saleem RM, et al. Selective postoperative inhibition of gastrointestinal opioid receptors. *N Engl J Med* 2001; 345: 935–40.
48. Bungard TJ, Kale-Pradhan PB. Prokinetic agents for the treatment of postoperative ileus in adults: A review of the literature. *Pharmacotherapy* 1999; 19: 416–23.
49. Otterson MF, Sarna SK. Gastrointestinal motor effects of erythromycin. *Am J Physiol* 1990; 259: G355-.G63.
50. Aros SD, Camilleri M. Small-bowel motility. *Curr Opin Gastroenterol* 2001; 17: 140–6.
51. Kaez A, Demirbag M, Ustundag B, et al. The role of melatonin in prevention of intestinal ischemia-reperfusion injury in rats. *J Pediatr Surg* 2000; 35: 1444–8.
52. Sims CA, Wattanasirichaigoon S, Menconi MJ, et al. Ringer's ethyl pyruvate solution ameliorates ischemia/reperfusion-induced intestinal mucosal injury in rats. *Crit Care Med* 2001; 29: 1513–18.
53. Whelan K, Gibson GR, Judd PA, et al. The role of probiotics and prebiotics in the management of diarrhoea associated with enteral tube feeding. *J Hum Nutr Diet* 2001; 14: 423–33.

Discussion

Dr. Martindale: Do you think we should all be using a tonometer routinely in our intensive care units (ICUs)?

Dr. Moore: It isn't that practical. The tonometer is an attractive concept but we would hope that in some future studies we could provide some good data. This is our experience: we do it routinely in all our shock resuscitation patients. They have a tonometer in, it stays until we get the patients up to their full dose of enteral nutrition and then the tonometer is removed.

Dr. Peeters: I might add that some of the data that we showed on tonometry came from our hospital, and I must say that it is an enormous burden of work when you have to use those things. I don't think it is very practical.

Dr. Chioléro: I have a further question on gastric tonometry. If I correctly understood, in patients with an increased CO_2 gap, you would not start early feeding or you would be more cautious?

Dr. Moore: There are levels that make us nervous: A $PrCO_2$ of 70 would make me be cautious, but above 90 we would not feed. Most of our patients after shock resuscitation are in the 50–60 range, so we would start feeding and watch and see where the $PrCO_2$ goes to. Now I must make a comment for people who are unfamiliar with this technology. The saline tonometry was extremely labor intensive. Gas tonometry is a nasogastric tube through which you intermittently put gas down into the balloon and you aspirate it back and analyze it like end tidal CO_2. So it is not as labor intensive as the saline technology.

Dr. Ribeiro: Regarding those patients with nonocclusive bowel ischemia which developed late related to enteral nutrition, did you consider the possibility of a certain degree of intolerance from the beginning that you could have assessed?

Dr. Moore: Since we have refined this enteral feeding protocol we haven't seen any cases of this. What we have learned, and I think Dr. Kudsk mentioned it earlier, is that when somebody suddenly gets septic, the first thing you have to do is turn off the enteral feeding. The second thing is if you start advancing in care and you can't assess tolerance, then you should stop enteral feeding. So when we start getting critical hypoxemia and start flipping people over in the bed and paralyzing them, I am a little skeptical that enteral nutrition is going to change the outcome of that patient, and I certainly don't want to contribute to their demise. So we have set criteria where we cut back to 15 cm^3/h. Actually we give the patients Gatorade based upon the work that

Dr. Kozar did in the laboratory, and then we would wait a day or so and see if the patients get better. If they don't get better then we would start supplement with total parenteral nutrition (TPN).

Dr. Cynober: I understand that initial resuscitation is something crucial to protect against gut injury and I would like to know the importance of very early resuscitation. For example in a number of countries the dogma is to transport the patient as soon as possible to emergency units or ICUs, and in other countries the dogma is to make the initial resuscitation on site. Is there some objective data about the timing of initial resuscitation on gut function and metabolic alterations?

Dr. Moore: A major limitation in our resuscitation strategies is that we focus on systemic resuscitation and there has not been any emphasis to think about how you could decrease edema and inflammation in the gut. Therefore I think that earlier resuscitation would be advantageous, in fact that is what our data show. Abdominal compartment syndrome is the most extreme form of shock-induced gut dysfunction, and when these patients come to our ICU they have it. This means that we need to get a hold of these patients earlier on and begin to do more judicious resuscitation that is really directed at limiting this gut edema. We can argue about crystalloids versus colloids, and we certainly could argue for a long time about it, but it is the American standard to give crystalloids. In our basic laboratory models it is very surprising how efficacious hypertonic saline is. We can totally abrogate the impaired transit with gut ischemia reperfusion, the influx of neutrophils, protection of mucosa, and so we are quite interested in using hypertonic saline to try to figure out the mechanisms that are causing the inflammation in the gut. I assume that other resuscitation fluids could be equally good. We are interested in hemoglobin solutions. I think at some point they will become available to us. They are probably going to allow you to perfuse the gut better. So you have this defect in vaso-relaxation, the gut is vaso-constricted, the artificial hemoglobin solution should actually perfuse the gut a lot better than the resuscitation we have currently.

Dr. Berger: About gut edema, do you have any data from your patients regarding absorption capacity of that gut?

Dr. Moore: Gut absorption is a very difficult thing to quantitate and we actually had a methodology to look at gut absorption but it did not work out. In the laboratory when we looked at gut edema and its affect on absorption using the Ussing chamber. The gut edema adversely affects transit but that level of gut edema does not seem to affect the Ussing chamber numbers. The problem with the Ussing chamber is that it is really a tissue that is sort of dying as you are studying it, so sometimes it is difficult to know whether it is accurate or not, but that is the best we understand at the animal level.

Dr. Planas: Sorry, but I was unable to see in your protocol at what frequency you monitor the gastric residual volume in your patients? Second question, is it not too high to wait until 400 ml to stop enteral nutrition? And third, what do you do with the gastric residual?

Dr. Moore: I think I will refer this to Dr. McClave since he is the person who has the most experience with this.

Dr. McClave: We have just finished a study in which we put yellow colometric microspheres into the formula and infused them into the stomach, and then every 4 h we checked the residual volumes. The patients were on ventilation so we checked the tracheal and oropharyngeal secretions, and then we could put the secretions under a fluorometer and we knew exactly when the yellow bits were coming from the stomach after the oropharynx and the trachea. In the range of residual volumes of at least 400 cm^3, there was absolutely no correlation between gastric residual volumes and whether they were aspiring or regurgitating. They were regurgitating 30% of the time, aspiring about 22% of the time and there was no connection. So I think it is one of these monitors that is not a good marker of tolerance, and I think it results in more inappropriate sensation.

Dr. Zazzo: In your last study did you correlate the presented enteral tolerance with the volume of resuscitation and/or duration of shock and/or systemic acidosis or lactate level?

Dr. Moore: We did not do that because in the end the study was not large enough to make any of those correlations. Most of the patients that go into that resuscitation protocol receive in excess of 15 units of blood and for every unit of blood they are receiving at least 1 liter of crystalloid, so that is the degree of shock. Most of those people start off with a lactate level that is somewhere in the range of about 5. At the end of resuscitation we don't always normalize lactate, and that is usually a predictor of pretty bad outcome.

Dr. Allison: We think of the capillary permeability being increased with injury in shock, and this creates the appearance of edema in the skin when you resuscitate. But the starling balance across the capillary membrane is different in the skin and the gut. For example, in the liver it is very much in favor of leaking and a fast flux. I don't quite recall whether there are any data on the gut itself. In other words the gut may be even more vulnerable to edema than the systemic tissues.

Dr. Moore: It is somewhere between the skin and the liver. It is actually kind of interesting when you operate on these patients because some of them don't have gut edema and other ones really get bad edema. One of our pediatric surgeons is interested in this. His animal models have shown that it is intra-abdominal hypertension in ranges that you and I wouldn't be nervous with which should be about 15. A bladder pressure of 15 would cause venous obstruction. When you have this venous obstruction and you start resuscitating the patient more, you just get into this crystalloid loading because the reason we are doing it is because they have high intra-abdominal pressures. So we continue to volume load them, the pressure is going higher and then somewhere in the range of 25 or 30 the lymphatics turn off because of pressure, and then you get really bad edema. So I think that what we learned from our resuscitation protocol is that when those patients get those high intra-abdominal pressures we have to really rethink what we are doing, and I don't know if decompressing the abdomen of everybody is going to be appropriate. But there are things like paralyzing somebody to reduce the intra-abdominal pressure; you can go to inotropes, or colloids. While there is a US bias that we shouldn't use a lot of colloids, we would like to study this more in animals before we start doing it in people.

Dr. Carlson: The practice of open abdomen surgery or damage control surgery in the US is very different to the UK. In the UK we have used the open abdomen exclusively in the management of severe abdominal sepsis. But our experience in the UK has been rather different in that we tend leave the abdomen really open, whereas I noticed in one of your slides you had a kind of piece of plastic which looked pretty tight. I guess the question is to what extent do you think you might be able to abrogate some of these problems by literally completely leaving the abdomen open and decompressing it.

Dr. Moore: In that particular patient, when that bag was placed it was extremely loose, and I guess we and other US surgeons have evolved this from when we do damage control. The idea was that you stop the bleeding by putting the packs in and then you would tamponade the abdominal bleeding, intentionally causing a lot of pressure. That would really set you up to get an abdominal compartment syndrome because then you go back to the ICU, increased bladder pressure, start some more bleeding, and then you have intra-abdominal hypertension. So what the dogma is now is that we should place bags on everybody. Despite that, we are seeing this problem occurring in that particular patient, he really did have bladder pressures that had gone to high levels, and he had to be taken back and have a bigger

167

bag placed. I don't know how I could get an abdomen much more opened than by making an incision from here to here and put a big bag on it. I would be happy if you tell me how to do that.

Dr. Déchelotte: It makes sense not to overfeed a gut when the early phase of vaso-relaxation has not yet occurred, but on the other hand I was told this morning that it contributes to systemic inflammatory response syndrome. So what would you expect from a combination of nutrients to be given very early to this kind of patient to enhance some vaso-relaxation. There are a few papers with glutamine in ischemic reperfusion with the enteral blood flow in nonstressed animals. In your trauma models did you check whether you could enhance that?

Dr. Moore: It is very hard in the patients to prove that the gut is priming the systemic neutrophils because we would have to have a catheter in the portal vein or in the lymphatics. But what we know is that, when we look at circulating neutrophils, the priming starts within 3 h of resuscitation. It peaks at about 12 h and at about 24 h it starts coming down. After 24 h the circulating neutrophils don't work anymore, and that is because all the ones that are dangerous have already sequestered in the lung. So unless you are going to do something very early, like in the helicopter. This will be feasible in the future, right now I don't know how we would deliver that. I assume we could give some sort of intraluminal something to stop it or intravenous injection to stop the ischemia reperfusion insult to the gut.

Dr. Rosenfeld: What is your comment about active oxygen saturation when you evaluate the gut perfusion, SHO_2?

Dr. Moore: I have no experience on that. Enlighten me how that might work.

Dr. Rosenfeld: There is some work from Takala about the SHO_2 and vasoactive drugs to improve gut perfusion.

Dr. Moore: That requires the placement of some fairly sophisticated catheters. If I recall his studies he was measuring hepatic venous outflow, and to do that you have to have a special catheter that can be flooded into the liver. He did show interesting results that inotropes and vasodilators, which we would normally think would improve gut perfusion, really were harmful. So a lot of what we do in clinical medicine, we don't really understand the effects on the gut.

Dr. Rosenfeld: We don't have very good data because tonometry is controversial too. You showed excellent data right now and we are measuring intra-abdominal pressure to better resuscitate our patients and we see this as a way to monitor, but we need to monitor gut perfusion to better check if the gut is really in a good situation to enterally feed these patients.

Dr. Moore: I actually have recruited a bioengineer and his project is going to take all the available monitoring techniques that we can think of, and start trying them, because at this point they really are extremely crude. We put an nasogastric tube into somebody, we feel and we listen to their abdomen, which is a pretty crude approach to figure out what is happening to the gut. We hope that in the future we will come across with some easy way to monitor. I actually think if we could find a good way of identifying gut motility that would be a good sign of who could be fed, so that is what the manometry data shows us.

Dr. Martindale: What do you think about the optimal substrate? You mentioned you gave Gatorade at 15 cm³/h. Why aren't you using something like glutamine? I think your own data show that glutamine is beneficial.

Dr. Moore: We will have more definitive data. Gatorade is just sugar and salt, it can't hurt anybody. When we place patients on low-dose elemental diets, the Gatorade was cheaper.

Dr. McClave: An issue of the goal of enteral feeding is what volume or amount we need to get the job done. Dr. Kudsk alluded to a study by Alexander in which they actually showed that if the animals were unstressed they took 25% of kilocalories to stop translocation, but if they were injured the animals first took 50% of the kilocalories. Dr. Demayo did permeability studies in Chicago. He studied bone marrow transplant patients and ranked them by the percent of kilocalories they got and the number he came up with was 50% of kilocalories: below that permeability went way up, and above 50% permeability was contained and maintained. So my question is how do you come up with that 60 cm^3/h, that magic number, and do you think that is enough to get the job done?

Dr. Moore: I don't have any other data than what you repeated. But historically we started our enteral feeding protocol 20 years ago. We were trying to meet the patients metabolic demands within 72 h, and that meant we pushed patients to about 2,500 cm^3/day. We published studies on that and what we found was that when you start really getting to the higher volume you start having intolerance. Now when we come to 60 cm^3/h, if you believe in the immune-enhancing diet studies and you think that they are efficacious, go and see how much they are getting in, they are only getting about 1,200 cm^3, and so that is how we came up with 50–60 cm^3/h. It is probably not an unreasonable goal in the short run, and then by ICU day 7 we tried to get people up into a positive caloric and positive nitrogen goal and, if we are not at that level by day 7, then they get started on supplemental TPN, and I would say probably about 10% of our ICU patients get put on to some supplemental TPN, and we tend to go hypocaloric in large patients.

Dr. Herndon: I would like to congratulate you on your nice presentation and your emphasis on monitoring gastrointestinal function and making improvements in that area. I was surprised at how conservative you are, unusually so. We have done several clinical experiments recently in which we have given animals 60% total body surface burns and effectively completely resuscitated the animals orally. They can even be improved by using hypertonic saline resuscitation, but you can resuscitate a pig with a 60% burn with World Health Organization tablets in water, something that may be pertinent if we are faced with mass disasters. Your delay of 2–3 days before you start feeding is to me very conservative. We begin feeding within 3–4 h of the time of resuscitation and we find motility is quite adequate, and in fact it is a period in which you can avoid ileus by early feeding. Regarding Dr. Kudsk's data about bombesin, we used bombesin a long time ago and it worked well. IGF-1 can also be used as a stimulatory agent given early. There are some other drugs that can be given early that would stimulate motility. My second comment would be that this abdominal compartment syndrome seems to be an institution-specific phenomenon.

Dr. Moore: Let me answer the first question. When I am talking about minor injury patients, I don't mean burn patients. I think burn patients are different. There are certainly manometric studies that show that burn patients do not have this gastric apnea, that is without feeding, so I think they are different animals. As far as aggressive early feeding, in our original studies we started feeding in the operating room. So for the less severely injured patients it is clearly feasible to start feeding early. I don't think that. I guess my theories on ICU care are that you have to have a goal you are trying to achieve, and during resuscitation of the patients is not the time to be starting enteral feeding into the under-perfused gut. As I showed with the data from gastric tonometry, a certain portion of these patients really are hypoperfused and I think if you start feeding you will run into significant problems. As far as the institution specificity, I will be happy to show you a review article of the literature.

Dr. Herndon. Let me finish my question before you answer. I do think that, if you look at the patients who develop this kind of massive edema, delay in resuscitation is a very important issue as well as the amount of fluid that is given in the emergency room, as you showed in your own slides. We did a study on 169 patients looking at this phenomenon and those individuals who developed it. Abdominal compartment syndrome had a 2-hour delay to get intravenous infusions started. They were patients who already had very high lactic acid and lactate levels when they arrived and began resuscitation. They had high osmolarity. Also predictive, and you might look at it in the future, is the thromboxane level, it is elevated 200-fold in people who are predisposed to this particular kind of problem. Your comments that hypertonic saline and colloid-based resuscitation may decrease this phenomenon I think are well founded.

Dr. Moore: It is very interesting to see the people that develop this massive edema in the operating room because there really are these patients for whom an ultrasound was done in the emergency department, the blood pressure is 60, and you are saying we have got to get out of here, and there is no attempt to resuscitate them because we don't want to increase their pressure and just have them bleed more. You get the patient to the operating room, open up and find something that is really bleeding. You pack it and ask the anesthesiologist to start resuscitating. My colleagues just claim that this is a starling phenomenon and has nothing to do with ischemia/reperfusion. I think it really does. Anyway I agree with you that this entity, the problem when you look at the incidence of this syndrome, really is the denominator. So when people study it they either say I am looking at all the patients in the ICU then the incidence is about 0.5%, or they look at all the patients who are under damage control and the incidence is 40%. So if you take the most severely ill patients you are going to find it. If you look at our denominator we have had 196 patients over a 3-year period, that represents about 5% of our trauma admissions to the ICU, and those are extremely sick patients.

Dr. Nitenberg: For gastric residual volume I do not have the same experience because in our country Blechner and Mintake observed that there was an apparent correlation between a gastric residual volume over 100 ml and the risk of aspiration pneumonia. We are presently conducting a study to control that. We administer enteral nutrition until the gastric residual volume is 500 ml and then we administer prokinetics and, on the other hand, we administer prokinetics very early when the gastric residual volume is 100 ml, and we will see if there is any difference. My other comment and question are about the real value of an elevated bed to protect from aspiration pneumonia. I think there is no proof about that. There was a nice study presented last year at the European Congress of Intensive Care Medicine by people from the Netherlands, and they compared the risk of aspiration pneumonia with a bed at 45° and with the supine position. They found no difference in the rate of aspiration pneumonia. But it is very difficult to respect guidelines because they observed that the true inclination of the beds was in fact 28° because of the many interventions of nurses and physicians around the patient. I think there is a long way to go in respecting guidelines and to prevent that.

Cynober L, Moore FA (eds): Nutrition and Critical Care.
Nestlé Nutrition Workshop Series Clinical & Performance Program, Vol. 8, pp. 171 105,
Nestec Ltd.; Vevey/S. Karger AG, Basel, © 2003.

Nutrition of Premature and Critically Ill Neonates

Josef Neu[a] *and Ying Huang*[b,1]

[a]Department of Pediatrics, University of Florida, Gainesville, Fla., USA, and
[b]Shanghai Children's Hospital, Fudan University, Shanghai, P.R. China

Introduction

Advances in mechanical ventilation, the use of pulmonary surfactants, improved pharmacological management of expectant mothers and preterm infants and greater confidence in our overall intensive care techniques have resulted in a marked increase in the number of very immature infants who survive. The same ethical controversies of 20 years ago surrounding whether or not to resuscitate prematures of 26–28 weeks gestation are now focused on 22–24 weeks. Those involved with the care of these survivors are faced with a constellation of problems that include prevention of morbidity and fulfillment of genetic potential. Nutrition is becoming a key factor not only for the growth of these infants during their neonatal intensive care unit (NICU) stay, but also for prevention of morbidity and enhancement of their life-long well being.

The major goal of this review is to provide the reader with an overview of a few recent advances in nutrition that can be applied in the daily care of these patients. In addition, a few emerging concepts about conditionally essential amino acids, long-chain polyunsaturated fatty acids (LC-PUFAs) and probiotics are presented that are likely to become important modalities in the future care of these infants.

Morbidities Amenable to Improved Nutrition

Both short- and long-term morbidity that might be amenable to nutritional intervention are encountered in the NICU (table 1).

[1] Dr. Huang is the recipient of a Nestlé International Nutrition Scholarship.

Table 1. Morbidities amenable to nutritional intervention

Short term	Long term
Chronic lung disease	Poor neurodevelopment
Hospital-acquired sepsis	'Programmed' for metabolic syndrome in adulthood (syndrome X: obesity, hypertension, type-II diabetes, coronary artery disease)
Intestinal problems (necrotizing enterocolitis and perforations)	
High cost of care	

Some of the major short-term morbidity faced by very low birth weight (VLBW) infants in the NICU include: chronic lung disease; hospital-acquired sepsis; necrotizing enterocolitis (NEC), and a high cost of care. One major long-term morbidity is poor neurodevelopmental outcome. Furthermore, the concept that nutritional deprivation during critical periods of development can 'program' the individual toward a greater disposition to adult diseases has emerged [1].

Although the focus of neonatal nutrition has previously been on the period after critical illness has subsided, it has become increasingly evident that nutrition during the first few weeks of life while the infant is struggling for survival is crucial. Evaluations of growth reveal that many VLBW infants do not attain the same growth, had they remained in utero during the time they are in the NICU [2] (fig. 1). From this figure, it is evident that infants born prematurely are being discharged from the NICU 'small for gestational age' when compared to fetuses growing in utero.

Although not yet fully substantiated, postnatal growth retardation appears to be analogous to infants being intrauterine growth-retarded (IUGR), which has been associated with the development of 'metabolic syndrome' or 'syndrome X' during adult life. This syndrome includes obesity, type-II diabetes and hypertension, and is thought to be due at least partially to the development of a 'thrifty' phenotype [3] secondary to nutritional deprivation during early development. Part of this failure to reach intrauterine growth potential stems from the fear of causing NEC by too rapid advancement of enteral feedings in an individual with an immature intestine. There are also major concerns of causing metabolic imbalances with parenteral nutrition [4].

In this review, we will first discuss the macronutrient needs of the low birth weight infant and methods used to meet these needs. The emphasis will be on continuation of growth and nutrition similar to that the infant would receive and attain in utero. We will then discuss a few nutritional supplements that are emerging as potential agents in the prevention of both short- and

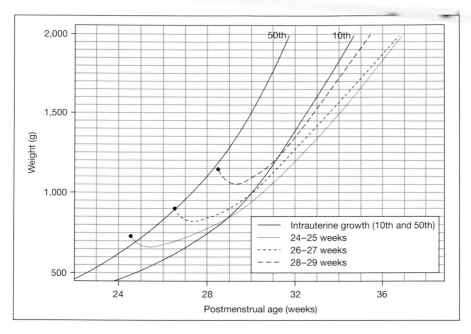

Fig. 1. Growth of fetus in utero versus growth of infants born prematurely and nourished in the NICU. From Ehrenkranz et al. [2].

long-term morbidity with an emphasis on how they relate to the gastrointestinal barrier and immune system.

Nutritional Needs of the VLBW Preterm Infant

Energy Requirements

The fetus gains approximately 5 g/day at 16 weeks of gestation, 10 g/day at 21 weeks, and 20 g/day at 29 weeks [5]. Between 24 and 40 weeks gestation, water content declines from approximately 87 to 71%, protein rises from 8.8 to 12%, and fat from 1 to 13%. The American Academy of Pediatrics has recommended that the caloric and average intake of the growing preterm infant to be approximately 120–130 kcal/kg/day [6].

Specific Nutrients

Glucose and Carbohydrates

Both hyper- and hypoglycemia are common problems in VLBW infants. Glucose utilization and production rates in VLBW average from 6 to 10 mg/kg/min [7]. The cause of hyperglycemia is not known, but may include

173

stress, relative insulin resistance and a decreased utilization of glucose secondary to lipid infusion. What constitutes 'hypoglycemia' in the preterm infants is somewhat controversial. Fetal plasma glucose levels over the second half of gestation are usually greater than 2.8–3.1 mm/l [8]. These levels are barely greater than those below which repeated measurements of low glucose concentrations are associated with increased risk of mental and motor developmental delay [9]. Thus, the 2.8- to 3.1-mm/l glucose concentration range should be the lower limit for VLBW preterm infants. Because of its critical role in brain metabolism, glucose infusions should start immediately in critically ill prematures. The role of infusing insulin in order to increase energy intake for faster growth remains controversial.

Amino Acids and Protein

Growth cannot be attained without protein or amino acids. The growth rate of lean body mass of the normally growing human fetus is about 3.6–4.8 g/kg/day [10]. This is greater than the amount of amino acid or protein intake that these infants usually are fed. With current human milk or formula-feeding regimens, it is practically impossible to achieve intakes that are necessary to achieve and maintain the desired rates of protein intake [10]. This becomes especially critical in sick VLBW infants. If they receive glucose alone, they lose in excess of 1.2 g/kg/day of endogenous protein [11]. Provision of amino acids, even if total energy intake is low, spares endogenous protein stores by enhancing the rate of protein synthesis. Providing 30 kcal/kg/day with 1.1–1.5 g intravenous amino acid changes the balance of protein from substantially negative to zero or slightly positive [12]. Higher intakes of both protein and energy result in net protein anabolism [13]. Unfortunately, many VLBW infants do not receive even such modest intravenous amino acid intakes during their first several days of life, nor do they receive enough enteral feedings to meet these requirements, thus assuring the development of a catabolic state.

The above information suggests that ideally, we should not interrupt the flow of nutrition that the fetus has been obtaining from its mother and not hesitate to provide nutrition to the infant immediately after birth. Because of gastrointestinal immaturity, it is neither possible nor prudent to attempt full nutrition by the enteral route immediately after birth. However, there are very few, if any convincing reasons to withhold intravenous glucose, amino acids, lipids, vitamins and trace elements beyond the immediate stabilization period after birth (which should not be more than 6–12 h). There is a tendency to begin parenteral amino acid intake at only 0.5 g/kg/day or less, gradually achieving an intake of 2.5–3.0 g/kg/day over a period of 7–10 days to avoid protein 'intolerance and toxicity'. This practice should become obsolete because of recent studies demonstrating that intakes up to 2.9 g/kg/day revealed little evidence of protein toxicity as measured by hyperammonemia, azotemia, or metabolic acidosis [14].

Lipids

Lipid requirements are limited to the essential fatty acids (linoleic and linolenic acid). Although lipid comprises about 50% of the nonprotein energy content of both human milk and formulas, both of which contain these fatty acids, the frequent practice of limiting enteral intake precludes the supply of these essential fatty acids, unless they are provided intravenously. Parenteral lipid emulsions provide these essential fatty acids but their use is often delayed or limited by concerns of adverse effects. These putative effects include impaired oxygenation, impaired lung function, impaired immune function, decreased platelets and increased free bilirubin levels. Despite in vitro studies which suggested effects of lipid emulsion on immune function, there is no conclusive evidence for in vivo effects. In vitro studies have shown that unesterified fatty acids can displace bound bilirubin from albumin, thus increasing free bilirubin. However, clinical studies have shown that infusion of lipid at rates up to 3 g/kg/day do not increase plasma concentrations of free fatty acids or free bilirubin [15]. Provision of lipid infusions at rates of less than 0.2 g/kg/h does not result in deterioration of oxygenation or lung function [16]. Despite thrombocytopenia being frequently listed as a side effect of intravenous lipids, provision of up to 3.3 g/kg/day has been shown to have no effect on platelet concentrations even if given for up to 4 weeks [17]. Controversy remains about whether intravenous lipids are associated with an increased incidence of sepsis. At this time there is no convincing evidence that lipids should be withheld because of an increased risk of sepsis.

Failure to provide essential fatty acids in the extremely low birth weight infant results in biochemical signs of deficiency within 72 h [18]. This can be prevented by the administration of as little as 0.5 g/kg/day of lipid emulsions. Although these emulsions contain high concentrations of linoleic and linolenic acid, they do not contain the LC-PUFAs, arachidonic (AA) or docosahexanenoic acid (DHA). These are thought to be critical nutrients for the developing central nervous system. The qualitative composition of lipids in these intravenous emulsions is quite different when compared to normal tissue and plasma lipids and human milk. The high content of linoleic and linolenic acid, but low content of saturated and monounsaturated fatty acids along with the absence of LC-PUFAs raises questions about the propriety of the present solutions for the VLBW infant. Furthermore, the concentration of n-3 fatty acid in these lipid formulations is relatively low. Whether an increased intake of these would provide an anti-inflammatory effect in these infants is not currently known.

Considerations for Enteral Feeding of the Sick Premature Infant

Gastrointestinal Development

One of the major reasons why neonatologists do not use the gastrointestinal tract of the premature infant for long periods of time after

Table 2. Summary of nutritional approach to VLBW infants

Enteral intake
    Begin as soon as possible (day 1 of life, e.g.) – minimal enteral nutrition during TPN
    Breast milk – preferably from infant's own mother, or premature formula
    Advance enteral intake as TPN is being decreased
Parenteral intake
    Begin glucose infusion immediately after birth at 4–8 mg/kg/min
    Begin amino acid infusion at 2.5–3.0 g/kg/day on day 1 of life
    Begin intravenous lipids at <0.2 g/kg/h infusion but >0.5 g/kg/day within the first
    1–2 days of life

birth is that the gastrointestinal tract of these infants is poorly developed. What are these immaturities? These consist of suck-swallow incoordination, poor gastric emptying and intestinal motility, and immaturity of luminal digestion and mucosal absorption. How quickly should enteral feedings be advanced? Because of the individual characteristics of each patient, one feeding protocol or guideline cannot be used for all infants. Clinical judgement based on available scientific data and experience presently appear to be the best criteria upon which we should base our feeding practices. However, there are data showing that advancement of enteral feedings faster than 20 ml/kg/day is associated with an increased incidence of NEC [19]. From the available studies, minimal enteral feedings should be instituted within the first days of life. What constitutes 'minimal enteral nutrition' is not clearly defined. Review of the literature supports a definition of minimal enteral nutrition as being less than 20 ml/kg/day, an amount insufficient for the demands of the rapidly growing infant, but enough to promote intestinal trophic hormone release, improve motility and prevent atrophy induced by total parenteral nutrition (TPN) and lack of enteral nutrients. There is no clear evidence that the concomitant use of umbilical catheters, continuous positive airway pressure, mechanical ventilation, indomethacin or the presence of apneic and bradycardic episodes preclude the use of minimal enteral nutrition because of an increased risk of NEC.

Feeding milk from the infant's own mother is the preferred enteral intake. This has been associated with less NEC, sepsis and better tolerance to advancement of enteral feedings [20].

Table 2 summarizes these recommendations for nutritional support.

Nutritional Supplements

The intestine is a primary origin of the systemic inflammatory response syndrome. It is therefore reasonable that nutritional agents might stabilize the intestinal mucosal barrier, alter the balance of pro- and anti-inflammatory cytokines, and prevent excessive activation of nuclear factor κB (NFκB), a transcription factor that is thought to play a major role in the production of proinflammatory mediators.

Some nutrients, such as glutamine, arginine, n-3 fatty acids, and probiotics, have been shown to influence intestinal barrier function and the immune system.

Amino Acids (Arginine and Glutamine)

Even when high quantities of amino acid or protein are provided, an inadequate intake of certain 'conditionally essential' amino acids may exist. Examples of these include glutamine, arginine, glycine, histidine, taurine and tyrosine. If these are not provided, essential amino acids are diverted away from protein synthesis. One such amino acid that has recently received increasing attention is glutamine. Supplementation in adults has resulted in improved survival; decreased hospital-acquired sepsis in bone marrow transplant and trauma patients, along with improved nitrogen balance and decreased costs of hospitalization [21]. One study of parenteral glutamine supplementation has shown decreased requirement for mechanical ventilation in neonates with a birth weight of less than 800 g [22]. Another study of enteral glutamine supplementation has suggested decreased hospital-acquired sepsis, decreased catabolism and/or improved amino acid utilization, improved tolerance to enteral feedings, decreased cost of hospitalization and appeared safe at the doses used [23].

The rationale for supplementing glutamine is based on its ubiquitous metabolic role in energy metabolism (especially in the intestine and lymphocytes), nucleotide synthesis, glucosamine synthesis, and as an antioxidant precursor. Studies in animals have demonstrated both intravenous and enteral glutamine to be protective against various forms of experimentally induced enterocolitis and it has been found to be a 'conditionally essential' amino acid during times of stress. VLBW infants are catabolic and highly stressed during their first weeks of hospitalization. Despite this, glutamine is not added to their TPN and they do not receive glutamine unless they are enterally fed (they frequently are not, as previously mentioned). This constitutes a major interruption in the flow of glutamine these infants would be receiving had they remained in utero [24]. In the study of infants, analysis of T cells found a blunting of HLA-DR+ and CD16+ T lymphocytes, which was consistent with decreased stimulation of the immune response secondary to decreased translocation of bacteria or their antigens across mucosal surfaces.

In a study of a rat model of endotoxemia, Wischmeyer et al. [25] found glutamine reduced proinflammatory cytokine release, organ damage, and mortality. In another study, 9 fasted volunteers received either glutamine or saline orally over 6 h. Duodenal biopsies were taken and cultured for 24 h with or without glutamine. This study demonstrated that glutamine pretreatment in vivo and in vitro significantly decreased production of proinflammatory cytokines (IL-6 and IL-8) by the human intestinal mucosa [26]. In a mouse model glutamine-enriched TPN preserved the expression of IL-4 and IL-10 mRNA (anti-inflammatory cytokines) in lipopolysaccharide-stimulated intestinal lamina propria [27]. Preliminary studies in Caco-2 cells by our group demonstrated that glutamine decreases IL-8 production after lipopolysaccharide stimulation (unpublished results). Investigations underway in our laboratory are designed to determine whether this downregulation is mediated via NFκB. These studies support the hypothesis that some of glutamine's beneficial effects may be a result of improved gut integrity or immune function and that glutamine could be used to regulate the intestine-mediated inflammatory response.

Arginine

Another amino acid that some consider as either essential or conditionally essential in the neonate is arginine. This amino acid plays a critical role in immune function, as a stimulant to the production of growth hormone and as a precursor to energy carriers such as creatine. As a precursor for the synthesis of nitric oxide (NO), creatine, polyamines, urea, ornithine, proline, glutamate, and other molecules with enormous biologic importance, and as a stimulant to the production of growth hormone, L-arginine plays versatile key roles in nutrition and metabolism [28].

The plasma and intracellular concentration of arginine may be critical not only for tissue growth but also for normal physiological function. It has been shown that premature infants who subsequently developed NEC have a significant lower plasma concentration of arginine [29]. This may be due to an increased metabolic demand for arginine or limited endogenous synthesis. NO plays an important role in the gastrointestinal system. In the face of inflammation or injury, NO is a mediator critical to regulation of blood flow in the intestine. Study in a neonatal piglet model of NEC suggested a potential therapeutic use of arginine, which is the substrate of NO synthase [30]. The effect may be synergistic to protein and polyamine synthesis, which also would help maintain intestinal mucosal integrity. One study in VLBW infants demonstrated a lower incidence of NEC in arginine-supplemented infants [31]. Current TPN solutions remain suboptimal for arginine for preterm infants.

Probiotics

Probiotics are defined as live microbial food supplements that beneficially affect the host animal by improving its intestinal microbial balance. Their attachment to the intestinal epithelium can strengthen the host's mucosal defenses through enhancement of secretory antibody responses, through a tightening of the mucosal physical barrier to microorganism translocation, and by a balance in T-helper cell response [32].

A better understanding of probiotic-epithelial crosstalk can be used to devise new strategies to prevent and treat bacterial infections of the gut. From the fact that largely bifidobacterial flora have been observed in breast-fed infants who show a greater resistance to various infectious diseases than do bottle-fed infants, the desire arose to generate a predominantly bifidobacterial flora in bottle-fed infants. Administration of *Bifidobacterium bifidum* to bottle-fed infants results in an increase in fecal counts of bifidobacteria and a decrease in fecal pH, which plays a role in protecting premature infants and other newborns from intestinal disease. One study documented a reduction in NEC in premature newborns given a daily enteral supplement of *Lactobacillus acidophilus* and *Bifidobacterium infantis* compared with a historical control group [33]. Additional prospective studies are needed.

Long-Chain and n-3 Polyunsaturated Fatty Acids

Dietary fatty acids such as linoleic acid (LA; 18:2 n-6) and α-linolenic acid (ALA; 18:3 n-3) of the n-6 and n-3 series of PUFAs, respectively, are considered 'essential' because they must be derived from the diet. Once ingested, the essential fatty acids are converted to longer-chain, more highly unsaturated fatty acids, including AA from LA and eicosapentaenoic acid (EPA) and DHA from ALA. Modulation of immune and inflammatory responses has been reported with increased intakes of PUFAs of the n-3 series [34]. The outcome is dependent on the type of PUFA, the target tissue, as well as the immune status of the host before exposure. Specific cellular mechanisms for these events may include modulation of transcription factor expression, e.g. NFκB; alteration of signal transduction protein (protein kinase C) activity; inhibition of cellular transport proteins (Mg^{2+}-ATPase); inhibition of apoptosis; stimulation of the antioxidant system, and modulation of cytokine and prostaglandin metabolite receptor activation. Recently, Caplan et al. [35] indicated that dietary PUFA supplementation (AA/DHA ratio of 1.5:1) significantly reduced the incidence of NEC in the neonatal rat model by downregulating platelet-activating factor (PAF) production, PAF receptor synthesis, and endotoxin translocation into the systemic circulation.

Intake of LC-PUFAs may be related to structural and functional development of sensory, perceptual, cognitive and motor neural systems. DHA is selectively incorporated, retained, and highly concentrated in the phospholipid bilayer of biologically active brain and retinal neural membranes. LC-PUFA supplementation of neonatal formula has been studied extensively for the outcomes of central nervous system development and visual acuity. Additional research is warranted to delineate the specific cellular effects of PUFA on intestinal integrity, to clarify the specific components of PUFA responsible for improved intestinal health in animals and to confirm the beneficial role of these dietary supplements for premature infants.

Conclusion

In this brief overview, the main message is that during critical illness in newborn infants, emphasis should be placed on the provision of optimal nutrition. This is necessary for alleviation of not only short-term morbidity, but for optimization of health throughout the individual's lifetime.

References

1. Godfrey KM, Barker DJ. Fetal programming and adult health. *Public Health Nutr* 2001; 4: 611–24.
2. Ehrenkranz RA, Younes N, Lemons JA, Fanaroff AA. Longitudinal growth of hospitalized very low birth weight infants. *Pediatrics* 1999; 104: 280–9.
3. Hales CN, Barker DJ. The thrifty phenotype hypothesis. *Br Med Bull* 2001; 60: 5–20.
4. Hay WWJ, Lucas A, Heird WC, Ziegler E. Workshop summary: Nutrition of the extremely low birth weight infant. *Pediatrics* 1999; 104: 1360–8.
5. Sparks JW, Cetin I. Intrauterine growth. In Hay W, ed. *Neonatal Nutrition and Metabolism*. New York: Mosby, 1991; 3–41.
6. American Academy of Pediatrics Committee on Nutrition. Nutritional needs for low birthweight infants. *Pediatrics* 1985; 75: 976–86.
7. Sunehag A, Ewarld U, Larsson A, Gustafson J. Glucose production rate in extremely immature neonates (<28 weeks) studied by use of deuterated glucose. *Pediatr Res* 1993; 33: 97–100.
8. Srinivasan G, Pildes RS, Cattamanchi G, Voora S, Lilien LD. Plasma glucose values in normal neonates: A new look. *J Pediatr* 1986; 109: 114–7.
9. Lucas A, Morley R, Cole TJ. Adverse neurodevelopmental outcome of moderate neonatal hypoglycemia. *Br Med J* 1986; 297: 1304–8.
10. Ziegler EE. Protein nutrition in premature feeding. *Nutrition* 1994; 10: 69–71.
11. Mitton SG, Calder AG, Garlick PJ. Protein turnover in sick, premature neonates during the first few days of life. *Pediatr Res* 1991; 30: 418–22.
12. Rivera A, Bell EF, Bier DM. Effect of intravenous amino acids on protein metabolism of preterm infants during the first three days of life. *Pediatr Res* 1993; 33: 106–11.
13. Denne SC, Karn CA, Ahlrichs JA, Dorotheo A, et al. Proteolysis and phenylalanine hydroxylation in response to parenteral nutrition in extremely premature and normal newborns. *J Clin Invest* 1996; 97: 746–54.
14. Thureen PJ, Anderson AH, Baron KA, Melara DL, Hay WW Jr, Fennessy PV. Protein balance in the first week of life in ventilated neonates receiving parenteral nutrition. *Am J Clin Nutr* 1998; 68: 1128–35.
15. Rubin M, Naor N, Sirota L, Moser A, Pakula R, Harell D, Sulkes J, Davidson S, Lichtenberg D. Are bilirubin and plasma lipid profiles of premature infants dependent on the lipid emulsion infused? *JPEN J Parenter Enteral Nutr* 1995; 21: 25–30.
16. Brans YW, Ritter DA, Kenny JD, Andrew DS, Dutton EB, Carrillo DW. Influence of intravenous fat emulsion on serum bilirubin in very low birthweight neonates. *Arch Dis Child* 1987; 62: 156–60.
17. Putet G. Lipid metabolism of the micropremie. *Clin Perinatol* 2000; 27: 57–69.
18. Gutcher GR, Farrell PM. Intravenous infusion of lipid for the prevention of essential fatty acid deficiency in premature infants. *Am J Clin Nutr* 1991; 54: 1024–8.
19. Anderson DM, Kliegman RM. The relationship of neonatal alimentation practices to the occurrence of endemic necrotizing enterocolitis. *Am J Perinatol* 1991; 8: 62–7.
20. Lucas A, Cole TJ. Breast milk and neonatal necrotising enterocolitis. *Lancet* 1990; 336: 1519–23.
21. Neu J, DeMarco V, Li N. Glutamine: Clinical applications and mechanisms of action. *Curr Opin Clin Nutr Metab Care* 2002; 5: 69–75.
22. Lacey J, Crouch S, Benfell K. Glutamine supplemented parenteral nutrition is associated with improved outcome in preterm infants. *JPEN J Parenter Enteral Nutr* 1996; 20: 74–80.

23. Neu J, Roig JC, Meetze WH, Veerman M, Carter C, Millsaps M, Bowling D, Dallas MJ, Sleasman J, Knight T, Auestad N. Enteral glutamine supplementation for very low birth weight infants decreases morbidity. *J Pediatr* 1997; 131: 691–9.

24. Lemons JA, Adcock EW 3rd, Jones MD Jr, Naughton MA, Meschia G, Battaglia FC. Umbilical uptake of amino acids in the unstressed fetal lamb. *J Clin Invest* 1976; 58: 1428–34.

25. Wischmeyer PE, Kahana M, Wolfson R, Ren H, et al. Glutamine reduces cytokine release, organ damage, and mortality in a rat model of endotoxemia. *Shock* 2001; 16: 393–402.

26. Coeffier M, Miralles-Barrachina O, Le Pessot, F, Lalaude O, Daveau M, Lavoinne A, Lerebours E, Dechelotte P. Influence of glutamine on cytokine production by human gut in vitro. *Cytokine* 2001; 13: 148–54.

27. Fukatsu K, Kudsk KA, Zarzaur BL, Wu Y, Hanna MK, DeWitt RC. TPN decreases IL-4 and IL-10 mRNA expression in lipopolysaccharide stimulated intestinal lamina propria cells but glutamine supplementation preserves the expression. *Shock* 2001; 15: 318–22.

28. Wu G, Meininger CJ, Knabe DA, Bazer FW, Rhoads JM. Arginine nutrition in development, health and disease. *Curr Opin Clin Nutr Metab Care* 2000; 3: 59–66.

29. Becker RM, Wu G, Galanko JA, Chen W, Maynor AR, Bose CL, Rhoads JM. Reduced serum amino acid concentrations in infants with necrotizing enterocolitis. *J Pedatr* 2000; 137: 785–93.

30. Wu G, Knabe DA. Arginine synthesis in enterocytes of neonatal pigs. *Am J Physiol* 1995; 269: R621–R9.

31. Amin HJ, Zamora SA, McMillan DD, Fick GH, Butzner JD, Parsons HG, Scott RB. Arginine supplementation prevents necrotizing enterocolitis in the premature infant. *J Pediatr* 2002; 140: 389–91.

32. Walker WA. Role of nutrients and bacterial colonization in the development of intestinal host defense. *J Pediatr Gastroenterol Nutr* 2000; 30: S2–S7.

33. Hoyos AB. Reduced incidence of necrotizing enterocolitis associated with enteral administration of *Lactobacillus acidophilus* and *Bifidobacterium infantis* to neonates in an intensive care unit. *Int J Infect Dis* 1999; 3: 197–202.

34. Calder PC. Omega 3 polyunsaturated fatty acids, inflammation and immunity. *World Rev Nutr Diet* 2001; 88: 109–16.

35. Caplan MS, Russell T, Xiao Y, Amer M, Kaup S, Jilling T. Effect of polyunsaturated fatty acid (PUFA) supplementation on intestinal inflammation and necrotizing enterocolitis (NEC) in a neonatal rat model. *Pediatr Res* 2001; 49: 647–52.

Discussion

Dr. Kudsk: What is the normal amino acid composition of mother's milk?

Dr. Neu: The protein matrix is actually a little bit less than what you find in most of the commercial formulas, and so mother's milk actually provides less total protein than do some of the commercial formulas. Now one of the things that the commercial companies have done is they have actually made fortifiers for mother's milk so that once these babies are on full enteral nutrition they actually have more protein added.

Dr. Endres: If you investigate breast milk longitudinally, you can show that the composition of amino acids is changing in the first week. For example in the colostrum there are very high amounts of taurine which decrease thereafter. This could be interpreted teleologically that the young infant is not able to produce taurine from cystine or methionine. Many amino acid solutions in pediatrics as well as infant formulae are designed on the standard of breast milk. But there are of course a lot of other issues as mentioned by Dr. Neu, e.g. if premature babies receive pumped breast milk, it should be supplemented by a fortifier so that it has a caloric density of about 85% instead of only <70 kcal/100 ml, and this should be continued after hospital discharge.

Dr. Neu: This is something that people could take hours to try to answer. I think that probably to try to answer this as concisely as possible, it is not only a nutritional fluid, it also has a lot of very bioactive components, lactoferrin, cellular components, IgA, very long chain fatty acids (e.g. docosapentaenoic acid, DHA) that we haven't been able to fully duplicate commercially yet.

Dr. Cynober: You mentioned that glutamine is the first amino acid taken up by the fetus and you mentioned that glutamate is the first amino acid released by the fetus. If I try to make a balance, the net balance is one ammonia molecule production without any energy production, without any substrate of interest production. What is the rationale about this rather surprising thing?

Dr. Neu: This is called the glutamine/glutamate shuttle, and this was a sort of schema that was developed by the people at the University of Colorado starting at the mid 1970s [1]. They found that glutamine is the major amino acid going into the placenta, it is actually enriched somewhat by the placenta. Then it goes to the mother, it goes to the fetal liver, and then more than 50% of it is converted to glutamate. The glutamine is used for various purposes in the fetus. The glutamate goes back to the placenta and enters the tricarboxylic acid cycle, and it is thought that it is actually important in the pyruvate malate conversion reaction to help maintain progesterone production. There are some studies [2] that suggest that this is a very important component of that glutamate coming back to the placenta. The fetus also is not able to make glucose through gluconeogenesis and it is thought that glutamate is the most important gluconeogenic substrate for the fetus. So there is a very interesting interrelationship with that particular glutamine/glutamate shuttle in the fetus and the mother and the placenta.

Dr. Moore: We had an interesting discussion yesterday of comparing necrotizing enterocolitis (NEC) with this nonocclusive bowel necrosis. What you are describing in these children is exactly the fear that we have in these sick adults. How do you assess bowel function or tolerance while you are advancing enteral feeding?

Dr. Neu: That is still very crude and yesterday we discussed that there are methods that we have right now to look primarily at how much gastric residual remains in the stomach 2 or 3 h after feeding, and there are certain loose criteria that we use to see if we should continue to advance feedings. One criterion is looking at abdominal distension. If there is abdominal distension, sometimes it may be too late. Our colleague Dr. Berseth [3] has done some studies looking at motility and migrating motor complexes, and she has found that this can be correlated to gut motility and capability for advancement of feedings. The only problem is that this is a technique which is, at least at this point, not very useful practically for routine use.

Dr. Martindale: My understanding is that the fetus swallows a significant amount of amniotic fluid in the last trimester and the highest amino acid in the amniotic fluid, I understand, is also glutamine. What is the reluctance of neonatologists to drip in small amounts of glutamine? I mean if the child normally would have been swallowing very large amounts of glutamine in utero, I am still not clear. It doesn't make sense to me why they want to prevent that.

Dr. Neu: This is also a question that has to do with a sort of neonatological culture and I think that we are at a point right now where we are very afraid of trying new things. Sometimes when I mention glutamine to my neonatology colleagues they ask why are you giving this drug? This is not a pharmacologic agent, this is not a drug, this is primarily a food replacement that the infant is not getting in the ICU which he/she would be getting had the infant remained in utero or was able to ingest a normal diet. This is where our discussions have been in the last couple of days, if this is something that we are trying to replace which really should be there but is not there. The Pediatrix enteral glutamine supplementation trials actually involve putting glutamine into water so that we are able to provide about 0.3 g/kg/day of glutamine to these babies enterally. That is really the approach that I would like to take if we are going to use glutamine in the future: to use it by the enteral route as a primary route. You are absolutely right about the amniotic fluid. In the last trimester of pregnancy the fetus swallows approximately 450 ml/day of amniotic fluid. You have a flux of amniotic fluid, a tremendous flux going through their gastrointestinal tract, and that would translate to about 10 liters going through the adult gastrointestinal tract a day. Nobody has even tried infusion of just amniotic fluid in those kinds of volumes because we are just scared to death of hypomotility problems in the neonate.

Dr. Zazzo: What about trace elements in neonates, the pool may be very small, and the question is, did any study you presented contain trace elements and vitamins in a large enough amount, and is this an explanation for a lack of results in the infection rate for instance?

Dr. Neu: They did supply trace elements in the total parenteral nutrition solution that they gave to these babies. It is routine practice now to give vitamins and trace elements, but we still don't know the exact requirement. But remember, both groups received the same amount of trace elements, the control and the glutamine-supplemented group received the same amount of trace elements. I see one potential flaw in that study. This is something that I am very concerned about, and we had a controversy about this the other day, about making isonitrogenous controls. The flaw is that they tried to make isonitrogenous control studies and the way they did this was that they added 20% glutamine in the glutamine-supplemented group but they took out 20% of the other amino acids including essentials. So the glutamine-supplemented group had more glutamine, but had less total amino acids including essential amino acids. So this may be a very important point in that particular study.

Dr. Herndon: There is a basic assumption, and this seems to be a neonatologist culture, that NEC comes from feeding or overfeeding, whereas the reverse may be true, that it comes from underfeeding. Can it only be studied in humans? Are there no models? Is there any experimental evidence that early feeding in neonates contributes to NEC?

Dr. Neu: There is feeding with the big F and there is feeding with the little F. The feeding with the big F is the one where we try to get to full enteral nutrition in the 1st week of life, 120 cal/kg/day in the 1st week of life. That was tried by many neonatologists back in the 1970s, and it almost invariably lead to major detrimental consequences.

Dr. Herndon: Was NEC one of those?

Dr. Neu: That is the major detrimental consequence that I am talking about. There have been several studies looking at the advancement of feeding [4, 5] and usually an advancement of $>20 \, cm^3/kg/day$ of formula has been associated with a higher incidence of NEC. But studies [5] that have been done with the minimal enteral nutrition, the little F, where you provide them with a very slow onset of enteral feeding over the 1st week of life, those studies actually suggested a lower incidence of NEC, not statistically significant but the analysis that was done suggested that there was actually less NEC. It certainly appears to be safe and has all those other positive consequences that I showed on that slide.

Dr. Calder: You mentioned the very high rate of protein accretion during the third trimester but also during that period there is a very high rate of accretion of specific fatty acids, arachidonic acid and DHA. I wonder if people have considered those specific fatty acids, and then thinking about that I remembered the study Carlson et al. [6] did of egg yolk phospholipids which showed a decreased incidence of NEC, particularly I think in preterm boys rather than girls. So there might be some functional effect in addition to the traditional structural role of those fatty acids.

Dr. Neu: Yes, I fully agree with you and that is certainly an area that we have to look at more closely, the lipid area in neonatology. I think we neonatologists have been so focused on the survival aspects that some of these things have just kind of gone by the wayside. Now we need to start looking at things like that, and the Carlson study I think was very provocative but certainly more work needs to be done in that area.

Dr. Allison: The NEC story is an interesting one. On other side of the equation is the circulation in the microvillus which is a very counter-current system, and of course feeding makes demand upon this. Is there anything you can do to improve the other part to increase the tolerance? My daughter did an observational study where she showed that all 9 cases of 180 babies admitted to her unit over a year or 18 months all followed immediately from red cell transfusion. So obviously this changes the viscosity very abruptly and this can make a critical change in the microcirculation. So is there any way to increase the tolerance by paying attention to that microcirculation to improve that?

Dr. Neu: One of the interesting aspects of the arginine supplementation trial is that in the discussion section of that article [7] in the *Journal of Pediatrics* just 3–4 months ago, they were talking about the effect of nitric oxide on the arginine supplementation. I think that is certainly one area that is very interesting. Arginine supplementation might be a way to go about that.

Dr. Moldawer: You commented on large prospective clinical trials, one with intravenous glutamine and one with enteral glutamine, and you talked briefly about some of the reasons why the enteral study was not positive. I was just curious where your thoughts were going in terms of future large clinical trials with enteral/parenteral studies. Are we going to see additional studies now? The fact that you can get beneficial effects on secondary outcomes is always optimistic, but the primary objectives tend to be looked upon a little less favorably. I was wondering if there is an effort now to redirect those studies or are we going to see more large scale?

Dr. Neu: I think it is too early to tell. What I am afraid of is that the negative result in this very large National Institutes of Health multicenter trial may have killed the enthusiasm for studying glutamine further, at least at the National Institutes of Health level.

Dr. Moldawer: That is where I was going. It is very difficult these days to get enthusiasm based on one poorly designed negative study with inappropriate entry criteria and inappropriate outcome variables, to then go ahead and design the appropriate study based on those results.

Dr. Neu: If the secondary outcome results with the enteral trial hold up, there is tremendous concern amongst neonatologists about intraventricular hemorrhage and periventricular leukomalacia. If we can demonstrate a therapy that decreases this, and if this really holds, along with further information on mechanisms for this, then I think that the enthusiasm for looking at glutamine will be reinvigorated.

Dr. Allison: You spoke about the lipids, but what about the lipid profile because of the demand of the growing brain for phospholipid and so on? Have you developed the lipid profile of your preparations far enough, or which direction are you going with that?

Dr. Neu: The answer to your first question is no, in my opinion the work on lipid profiles has not yet been fully elucidated. There are studies on the central nervous systems of human milk-fed babies and formula-fed babies looking at the brain and red cell composition [8]. I think that we have some handle on that but I don't think that those are necessary ideal studies. The gold standard we use in terms of lipid composition for feeding is human milk, but that may necessarily not be the gold standard for a baby that is born very prematurely. So there are still a lot of questions in that area and, as I mentioned, some of formula companies have put millions of dollars into the studies of long chain fatty acids, adding the long chain of fatty acid DHA to formulas, and also some arachidonic acid. Studies were done looking at the various combinations of these, and at least in Europe I think most of the formula companies include these long chain fatty acids and in the US the Food and Drug Administration has just given approval to a couple of the companies to add DHA. But we have not yet looked at the anti-inflammatory effects and more studies are needed in that particular area, and the question is should more eicosapentaenoic acid (EPA) be added and can we be getting anti-inflammation by adding EPA to the formulas?

Dr. McClain: You showed that glutamine was downregulating proinflammatory cytokines. Is there any thought that its important role in utero might be to keep a tolerance state there, which is vital for normal in utero growth?

Dr. Neu: That could be one mechanism. I think we can certainly speculate on that. There are very interesting results in both the neonatal and obstetrics literature. There is now a growing body of information that inflammation of the placenta in the mother associated with elevated amniotic fluid proinflammatory cytokine concentrations, and plasma cytokine concentrations in the fetus are associated with the development of intracranial hemorrhage and periventricular leukomalacia. This is why I think that if glutamine is downregulating the inflammatory response, it could potentially be the reason why we are seeing less intracranial hemorrhages and periventricular leukomalacia in these babies. If the glutamine administration is started shortly after these babies are born, and you downregulate that response, could this be where some of that benefit comes in?

Dr. McClain: Actually the Centers for Disease Control and Prevention in the United States is very interested in the proinflammatory cytokines, and so not only those complications but also premature delivery and overall poor outcome are associated. They are looking at this in an inner city minority population as a risk factor for all those complications.

References

1. Lemons JA, Adcock EW 3rd, Jones MD Jr, et al. Umbilical uptake of amino acids in the unstressed fetal lamb. *J Clin Invest* 1976; 58: 1428–34.
2. Battaglia F, Regnault T. Placental transport and metabolism of amino acids. *Placenta* 2001; 22: 145–61.
3. Berseth CL. Effect of early feeding on maturation of the preterm infant's small intestine. *J Pediatr* 1992; 120: 947–53.
4. Anderson DM, Kliegman RM. The relationship of neonatal alimentation practices to the occurrence of endemic necrotizing enterocolitis. *Am J Perinatol* 1991; 8; 62–7.
5. Neu J. Necrotizing enterocolitis: The search for a unifying pathogenic theory leading to prevention. *Pediatr Clin North Am* 1996; 43: 409–32.
6. Carlson SE, Montalto MB, Ponder DL, et al. Lower incidence of necrotizing enterocolitis in infants fed a preterm formula with egg phospholipids. *Pediatr Res* 1998; 44: 491–8.
7. Amin HJ, McMillan DD, Fick GH, et al. Arginine supplementation prevents necrotizing enterocolitis in the premature infant. *J Pediatr* 2002; 140: 389–91.
8. Uauy R, Hoffman DR, Peirano P, et al. Essential fatty acids in visual and brain development. *Lipids* 2001; 36: 885–95.

Cynober L, Moore FA (eds): Nutrition and Critical Care.
Nestlé Nutrition Workshop Series Clinical & Performance Program, Vol 8, pp 187–206,
Nestec Ltd.; Vevey/S. Karger AG, Basel, © 2003.

Nutritional Support of Obese Critically Ill Patients

René L. Chioléro[a], *Luc Tappy*[b] *and Mette M. Berger*[a]

[a]Surgical Intensive Care Unit, Department of Surgery and
[b]Department of Physiology, University Hospital – CHUV, Lausanne, Switzerland

Obesity: A Common Disease

Obesity is a common medical condition affecting more than 1 in 10 adults in Western European countries [1]. Its prevalence varies considerably in different countries. In Europe, it amounts to about 10–15% of the middle-aged population. It is highest in Eastern European countries, in North America, high in Africa and Eastern Asian countries, where it is strongly associated with poverty, but lower in Japan and China. There has been a progressive rise in the overall prevalence of obesity during the last decade, both in adults and children. The medical and economical consequences are enormous.

The medical spectrum of obesity is wide, ranging from simple overweight without associated medical risk, to morbid obesity with severe associated comorbidities [1]. Various diagnostic criteria have been used; the most useful and simplest relies on the body mass index (BMI) scale. According to the International Obesity Task Force of the Word Health Organization, the severity of obesity is classified into 3 main categories: (1) overweight: BMI 25–30; (2) obesity: BMI 30–40, and (3) morbid obesity: BMI over 40 kg/m². In addition to the absolute amount of body fat, as reflected by the BMI, body fat distribution is important: centralization of body fat to the abdominal visceral stores is associated with the development of systemic and metabolic complications [2]. Body fat distribution can easily be assessed in clinical practice using simple anthropometric measurements, such as waist circumference: a circumference over 102 cm in European men and 88 cm in women is an independent risk factor for a cluster of medical and metabolic complications, such as insulin resistance, glucose intolerance or noninsulin-dependent diabetes, arterial hypertension, cardiovascular diseases, stroke, high very low-density lipoprotein, low high-density lipoprotein, micro-albuminuria, hyperuricemia [2, 3]. Previously designated as the X syndrome or the insulin-resistance syndrome, it is now called the dysmetabolic syndrome. This syndrome is important in clinical nutrition, since it may influence both the nutritional requirements and the tolerance to artificial feeding, as well as the metabolic response to stress. Grossly obese patients also have an increased incidence of respiratory diseases, particularly the sleep apnea syndrome and the restrictive lung disease, venous disease, musculoskeletal degenerative disorders, liver disease (fatty liver) and metabolic disorders consecutive to bariatric surgery.

Critically Ill Obese: The Clinical Picture

There is a rise in the number of obese patients requiring intensive care unit (ICU) management parallel to the currently increasing prevalence of obesity. Despite this epidemiological reality and the well-known technical difficulties related to vascular and airway management in grossly obese patients, it is surprising to note the relative paucity of medical literature devoted to this topic. Performing a Medline search using obesity and critically ill as key words furnishes only 35 English references, while the combination 'obesity and critically ill and nutrition' limits the list to 11 references.

Although gross obesity seems to markedly affect the survival in severe blunt trauma, this seems not to be the case in patients requiring planned surgery. In a retrospective study performed in 184 patients with severe blunt trauma, mortality was markedly increased in obese patients (BMI >31, n = 19, mortality 42%), compared to overweight (BMI 27–31, n = 25, mortality 8%) and nonobese patients (n = 140, mortality 5%), despite similar severity of injury [4]. Complications were also more frequent in the severely obese group. Multiple regression analysis showed that BMI was an independent predictor of outcome. In a prospective study performed in 24,157 consecutive patients requiring general anesthesia, gross obesity (body weight, BW, >120 kg in males, >100 kg in females) was found to be a strong risk factor for postoperative critical respiratory events (relative risk 2.2) [5]. A retrospective study including 849 patients receiving various types of surgery showed that obesity was associated with higher rates of nosocomial infections, but mortality was not affected [6]. In a retrospective study performed in 5,168 cardiac surgery patients, the incidence of deep sternal wound infections was increased in obese patients, but mortality was not influenced by the presence of obesity [7]. This contrasted with malnutrition (BMI <20, serum albumin <25 g/l), in which these variables were each independently associated with increased mortality. Altogether, these data

Table 1. Demographic data of obese and nonobese patients admitted to the surgical ICU in 2000 and 2001

	Obese (BMI ≥ 30) (n = 131; 5.4%)	Other patients (n = 2,416)
Age, years		
16–59	53 (40.5%)	44.5%
60–69	42 (32.1%)	24.5%
70–79	32 (24.4%)	26.0%
≥80	4 (3%)	5.0%
BMI, kg/m²	34.8 + 4.5	–
30–39	117 (89%)	
>40	14 (11%)	
Length of ICU stay, days	7.3	4.5
ICU mortality	5 (3.8%)	192 (7.5%)

There was a trend to a lower mortality in obese patients (p = 0.08).

suggest that obesity is associated with increased morbidity after major surgery, particularly septic complications, but has no major impact on mortality. In case of more severe stress, like multiple injuries, the presence of obesity seems to markedly affect the outcome.

Table 1 summarizes our data on 131 consecutive obese patients admitted over a 2-year period to our surgical ICU. The latter represented only 5.4% of total admissions. Surprisingly mortality tended to be lower in the obese (3.8 vs. 7.5%, p < 0.08), while the ICU stay tended to be longer. Among obese patients, the longest ICU stays were related to abdominal complications of bariatric surgery. The latter patients required prolonged nutritional support (fig. 1, 2): both patients had suffered acute weight loss over a short period of time before their admission in the ICU, and were actually acutely malnourished, requiring artificial nutrition support.

Metabolic Response to Critical Illness

Extensive endocrine, metabolic and immunological changes occur in ICU patients, particularly those suffering from multiple injury, major burns, severe sepsis or severe inflammation. Resting metabolic rate increases, as well as fasting and postprandial glycemia related to insulin resistance [8]. Protein breakdown exceeds protein synthesis in both the fasting and fed state, at the cost of the muscle mass. The response to nutrition is altered: protein balance stays negative despite full nutritional support in highly stressed patients, while gluconeogenesis is not suppressed by carbohydrate administration (see Baracos, pp 1–9).

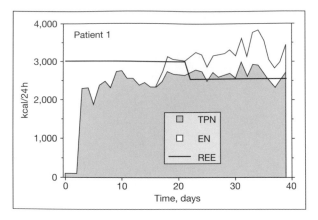

Fig. 1. Nutritional support of a 60-year-old severely obese patient (height 168 cm, admission weight 133 kg) during the first 40 days after ICU admission. The patient suffered multiple intestinal fistulae after bariatric surgery, complicated by acute respiratory and renal failure. Nutritional assessment on admission showed severe acute malnutrition, resulting from a rapid 20-kg weight loss during the 4 weeks preceding admission (BMI 54.2 → 47.1 kg/m^2). Nutritional support was first exclusively provided by the parenteral route (TPN) followed by progressive reintroduction of enteral nutrition (EN). Resting energy expenditure (REE) was determined by indirect calorimetry on days 3 and 21, amounting to 3,000 and to 2,600 kcal/day, respectively. Comparison of energy delivery (shaded area) and REE (solid line) shows that moderate hypocaloric feeding (80% REE) was delivered during the first 18 days, followed by isocaloric feeding. Note that all routes of artificial feeding were used in this patient.

The metabolic response to stress in obese critically ill patients is complex, since it occurs in a population with preexistent metabolic and endocrine abnormalities. A study performed in severely traumatized obese and nonobese patients (injury severity score >18) during the early flow phase (2–4 days after ICU admission) suggests that the metabolic response to injury is influenced by obesity [9, 10]. Compared with lean controls, the obese patients (BMI >30, range 30.8–41.8) had a similar degree of hypermetabolism (140 vs. 137% of Harris Benedict prediction). Plasma glucose and insulin were increased in the 2 groups, while C peptide levels were higher in obese patients. The pattern of substrate oxidation differed in the 2 groups: in obese patients both net protein (22 vs. 15%) and net glucose (39 vs. 24%) oxidation were increased, while net fat oxidation was reduced (39 vs. 61%). Whole body protein turnover and protein synthesis were increased in obese patients. This was associated with increased daily nitrogen and 3-methylhistidine excretion, and decreased protein synthesis efficiency (synthesis/turnover). Daily muscle degradation was also higher in obese patients. Altogether, these results suggest that the metabolic and endocrine changes associated with obesity

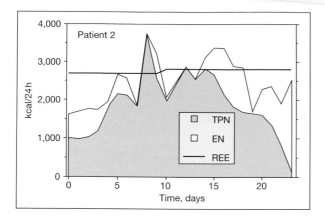

Fig. 2. Nutritional support of a 28-year-old severely obese patient (height 175 cm, admission weight 90 kg) during the first 23 days after ICU admission. The patient suffered gastrointestinal leak 12 days after bypass carried out 1 year after a gastroplasty. In the ICU he was in septic shock with respiratory and renal failure. Nutritional assessment showed severe acute malnutrition (20-kg weight loss over a year, BMI 44.1 → 29.4 kg/m^2, no nutritional support after surgery). Nutritional support was started using combined enteral (EN) and parenteral (TPN) feeding. Resting energy expenditure (REE) was determined by indirect calorimetry on days 1 and 10, amounting to 2,700 and 2,800 kcal/day, respectively. Energy delivery amounted to 65% of measured REE during the first week. Enteral support was interrupted during the 2nd week due to surgical complications and resumed thereafter, enabling TPN weaning on day 23.

modify the metabolic response to injury and further increased protein catabolism. This contrasts with the fair adaptation of healthy obese subjects to starvation: they have better nitrogen preservation than lean subjects and longer survival during hunger strike [11, 12].

Nutritional Assessment

Accurate nutritional assessment is difficult in critically ill patients [13]. This is related to the confounding effects of fluid retention on body anthropometry and to the joint effects of dilution and acute phase response on visceral protein plasma levels. BMI calculation is markedly affected by fluid retention and cannot be used to detect obesity in ICU patients [14]. Fluid therapy may induce 20–30% BW gain in patients with major burns or trauma or suffering from severe infection. In such conditions, the analysis of water balance will give more useful information than actual BMI. In patients with short-lasting illness before ICU admission, the anamnestic BMI, calculated from prehospital BW, is more accurate to assess the presence of obesity (or malnutrition).

Malnutrition and obesity may coexist [15], but the early detection of malnutrition in critically ill obese patients can be difficult, since previous malnutrition, accelerated catabolism and fluid retention may blunt nutritional assessment. In such patients, accurate nutritional assessment is not possible; it should therefore be approximate, based on history (weight loss, duration of fasting) and on simple clinical and biochemical variables.

Nutritional Requirements

Resting energy expenditure (REE) is increased in obese subjects, due to the concomitant increase in the fat mass and the metabolically active fat-free mass. In healthy nonobese subjects, accurate prediction equations have been developed and validated in large populations: REE predicted from the Harris-Benedict equations has a high correlation ($r > 0.80$) with measured REE by indirect calorimetry and a fair precision (coefficient of variation of $<10\%$). This in not the case in healthy obese subjects with BMI of $>30 \, kg/m^2$, in whom prediction based on Harris-Benedict equations overestimates REE, particularly for BMI of $>50 \, kg/m^2$.

REE is difficult to predict in all critically ill patients since it is influenced by multiple and changing factors related to the acute illness, level of stress and treatments [8]. Prediction equations have been developed for specific medical conditions, although their utility in clinical practice is controversial. Measurement with indirect calorimetry is the only validated method to accurately determine the metabolic rate of obese and nonobese critically ill patients, although prediction of 24-hour REE derived from short-time measurements (30–45 min) has a lower accuracy. Prediction equations specifically devoted to obese patients have been published, although they have not been validated on a large scale [16–19]. In obese patients with BMI of $<50 \, kg/m^2$, estimated energy requirements amount to about 20 kcal/kg ABW, although variability is substantial [19, 20]. In a study performed in 57 obese critically ill patients, the Harris-Benedict equation with an adjusted BW (mean value of actual and IBW) and a stress factor of 1.3 was the most accurate predictor of measured REE, both in mechanically or spontaneously breathing patients (bias $<200 \, kcal$, precision $\pm 120 \, ml$, 67% of patients with predicted REE $\pm 10\%$ of measured REE) [19]. This prediction performed better than the Ireton-Jones equations, and the simple rule of 21 kcal/kg ABW/day (bias 270 kcal, 24% of predictions $+10\%$ measured REE). Prediction was poor in patients with BMI >50. In another study, the Harris-Benedict equation with an adjusted BW was less accurate than a kilojoules per kilogram-adjusted BW strategy to predict REE [18]. Altogether, these studies suggest that simple rules can be used to have a rough estimate of REE in critically ill obese patients with a BMI of $<50 \, kg/m^2$. In more severely obese patients, or in those with major stress (severe sepsis or trauma, multiple organ failure), or with poor response to nutritional support, the use of indirect calorimetry is recommended, since the low accuracy of any prediction equation prevents their use to determine energy requirements.

The current literature suggests that hypocaloric nutrition should be preferred to isocaloric feeding in obese critically ill patients. If such a strategy is used, nonprotein energy requirements are calculated to cover about 50–60% of REE, amounting to about 20–25 kcal/kg ideal BW (IBW) or 13–16 kcal/actual BW (ABW) [21, 22]. It is worth reminding that estimations based on IBW tend to underestimate REE, while those based on ABW tend to overestimate it [18]. When isocaloric feeding is the goal, these figures are increased to about 35–45 kcal/kg IBW or 20–25 kcal/kg ABW [21, 22]. IBW can easily be calculated with the Hamwi equations: (1) IBW_{males} (kg) = 48 + (height (cm) − 152) × 1.06, and (2) $IBW_{females}$ (kg) = 45.4 + (height (cm) − 152) × 0.89 [23].

Current literature suggests that protein requirements are proportionally higher in obese than in nonobese ICU patients, amounting to about 2 g/kg IBW or 1.2–1.3 g/kg ABW, although the level of evidence is rather low. Such levels have been shown to be associated with positive or near zero nitrogen balance [21, 22, 24]. In hypocaloric feeding, the largest part of nonprotein energy should be covered by carbohydrates, keeping in mind that obese patients are often intolerant to glucose. The current literature suggests that hypocaloric carbohydrates are well tolerated in acutely ill obese patients. Most experts recommend reducing the administration of conventional fat solutions to a small part of total energy or to the amount necessary to cover the essential fatty acid requirements [14, 15]. This recommendation does not hold when fat is administered for a nonenergetic goal, i.e. to modulate body functions or responses, such as immunity and inflammation [25]. There is no indication in the literature that micronutrient requirements differ in obese and nonobese patients.

Nutritional Support in Obese Patients

Two reviews have recently been published on nutritional support of critically ill obese patients [14, 15]. Critically ill obese patients require artificial nutrition when it is not possible to feed them adequately by the oral route, as any other ICU patient [26]. Since their metabolic adaptation to fasting is altered during severe stress, they may require early nutritional support. During starvation, the enormous amount of energy stored in their adipose tissue does not protect them from rapid protein catabolism and accelerated malnutrition [9, 15]. Most experts recommend that indications and timing of artificial nutrition in obese patients submitted to major stress should not differ from the current recommendations applied in nonobese patients [14, 15, 26].

Most of the general aspects of nutritional support do not differ in obese and nonobese ICU patients: this is true for the indications to artificial feeding, techniques of feeding, routes and timing of nutrition. The only differences concern energy and nutrient requirements. Several conceptual and clinical arguments suggest that hypocaloric feeding could be an appropriate strategy in obese patients, even during acute illness [14, 15]. The concept is simple: protein sparing is the main objective, while energy requirements are partly covered by the large amount of fat stores [27]. Several studies suggest that such a strategy is effective in acutely ill obese patients (table 2) [21, 28–31]. Practically, 1.5–2.0 g/kg total BW protein is provided daily, while nonprotein energy supply is limited to about 50–60% of REE or 20–25 kcal/kg IBW.

Providing amino acids as the sole energy nutrient in nonstressed obese patients makes it possible to achieve nitrogen equilibrium in a situation of energy deficit. During moderate stress, such a mechanism of nitrogen sparing seems to be effective. This concept was first assessed in 1979 by Greenberg and Jeejeebhoy [27] in a nonrandomized study performed in 2 groups of 6 surgical patients described as 'having sufficient fat stores to justify intravenous hypocaloric feeding during 7 days', although no data were provided about BW. The patients received 2 different amino acid mixtures as the sole source of energy: 0.83 vs. 1.83 g/kg IBW/day. The high nitrogen solution made it possible to achieve nitrogen equilibrium (cumulated nitrogen balance + 16 ± 6.7 g after 7 days), but not the low nitrogen solution. Dickerson et al. [31] administered hypocaloric (51.5% measured resting metabolic rate), high-protein (2.1 g/kg IBW/day) total parenteral nutrition (TPN) for a prolonged period (48 ± 31 days) in 13 obese surgical patients. Such feeding was well tolerated: all patients had full tissue healing of wounds and abscess cavities, and minor metabolic complications were observed in only 1 patient. Nitrogen balance was at equilibrium or slightly positive, while serum albumin increased throughout the study. Such beneficial results occurred despite a progressive weight loss (−8.6%).

Hypocaloric versus isocaloric parenteral nutrition was compared in 2 consecutive randomized studies performed in obese patients with severe stress by the same group of authors [21, 29]. In the first study, 16 obese patients (BW >130% IBW) were randomized to receive isonitrogenous hypocaloric or isocaloric nutrition. Nonprotein energy amounted to 50 or 100% of measured resting metabolic rate. TPN was provided for 9.6 ± 3 days. The 2 regimens were well tolerated. Cumulated net nitrogen balances in both groups were positive. Changes in BW and serum albumin did not differ between the groups. In the subsequent study, protein supply was increased to 2 g/kg IBW/day, while energy supply was calculated using a fixed total energy:nitrogen ratio (75:1 vs. 150:1 kcal/g N) [29]. This eliminated the necessity to perform indirect calorimetry. Total daily energy amounted to 94 ± 21 kJ/day (22 kcal/kg/day) in the control group and to 57 ± 12 kJ in the hypoenergetic group. Mean net nitrogen balance and weight changes were similar in the 2 groups.

Table 2. Studies on hypocaloric nutrition in obese patients

Trial	Type of study	Number of patients	Patient category/ level of stress	Patient BW kg	Route	Energy supply kcal·kg⁻¹·day⁻¹	Protein supply g·kg⁻¹·day⁻¹	Length of artificial feeding, days
Greenberg et al. [27], 1979	Nonrandomized comparison trial 2 groups of patients	12 6 vs. 6	Patients with 'sufficient fat stores' Moderate stress	Not mentioned	PN	No nonprotein energy	0.83 vs. 1.83	7
Dickerson et al. [31], 1986	Prospective observational study	13	Postoperative Moderate stress	127 ± 60	PN	51.5% MREE	2.1/kg IBW	48 ± 31
Burge et al. [21], 1994	RCT Hypo- vs. isocaloric	16 9 Hypo vs. 7 Iso	Surgical patients Moderate/severe stress	90 ± 12.5 vs. 102 ± 19.9	PN	22 vs. 42/kg IBW	2.0–2.2/kg IBW	9.6 ± 3.0
Choban et al. [22], 1997	RCT Hypo- vs. isocaloric	30 16 H vs. 14 Iso	Surgical ICU patients Severe/moderate stress	97 ± 19 vs. 90 ± 17	PN	22 vs. 36/kg IBW	2.0 vs. 2.0/kg IBW	10 ± 3 vs.11 ± 2
Liu et al. [28], 2000	Retrospective study 2 groups of patients aged <60 vs. ≥60 years	30	Hospital patients Light/moderate stress	97 ± 16 vs. 84 ± 20	PN	18.2 ± 3.7 vs. 18.3 ± 2.6/kg ABW	1.5/kg ABW	13 ± 13 vs.13 ± 8
Dickerson et al. [30], 2002	Retrospective study Hypo- vs. isocaloric	40 H 28 Iso 12	Critically ill Severe stress	118 ± 41 vs. 102 ± 36	EN	16.2–22.2 vs. 21.5–29.9/kg IBW	1.14–1.53 vs. 1.29–1.85/kg IBW	15 ± 11 vs. 26 ± 15

PN = Parenteral nutrition; EN = enteral nutrition; IBW = ideal body weight; ABW = adjusted body weight; RCT = randomized controlled trial.

A recent retrospective study suggests that hypocaloric enteral feeding was as effective as isocaloric feeding in 40 critically ill obese patients [30]. The patients had weights of >125% IBW and received 7 days or more of enteral nutritional support. They were divided into 2 groups according to energy supply: isocaloric feeding, 20 kcal/kg adjusted BW/day, and hypocaloric feeding <20 kcal/kg adjusted BW/day, with adjusted BW = (ABW − IBW) × 0.25 + IBW. BW, BMI, severity of illness and protein supplies were similar in the 2 groups. Despite lower energy supply, the hypocaloric group had similar nitrogen balance and serum pre-albumin as the isocaloric group. Glycemia was not affected by energy supply. The hypocaloric group had a significantly shorter ICU stay (19 ± 10 vs. 29 ± 16 days, p < 0.03) and shorter antibiotic therapy (17 ± 12 vs. 27.4 ± 17 days, p < 0.03). Altogether, these data show that hypocaloric feeding is well tolerated in acutely ill obese patients, even when prolonged: it does not seem to be associated with increased protein catabolism, or with deleterious clinical consequences. These data seem to be in contradiction to those collected in nonobese ICU patients receiving prolonged enteral or parenteral nutritional support, since there is evidence that marked energy and protein deficits are associated with poor clinical outcome and with increased systemic complications like infections in the nonobese [32, 33]. Clearly, the safe level of energy deficit remains to be determined in different patient populations. This is particularly important when considering the actual predominance of exclusive enteral feeding.

Bariatric surgery generally does not require prolonged ICU support. It may however result in severe abdominal complications requiring artificial nutrition, like intestinal leakage and fistulae. They frequently occur during the period of maximal weight loss after surgery, i.e. during the period at risk of malnutrition. Such complications generally involve the gut, which is out of function for variable periods of time: TPN is required for life support [34]. Figures 1 and 2 show examples of such patients admitted to our surgical ICU, with the progressive introduction of enteral feeding. These patients were in septic shock due to peritonitis with acute respiratory failure on admission and required repeated surgical sessions. On admission they had acutely lost 20 and 45 kg BW, respectively, and had been fasted for many days.

Technical Problems

Vascular access can be a major technical problem in obese patients requiring anesthesia and surgery or venous access for parenteral nutrition. Peripheral veins are usually difficult to detect and consequently catheter insertion can be a worry. A more frequent use of central venous access is therefore commonly required, but internal jugular and subclavian vein catheterization may be difficult, resulting in a higher incidence of puncture complications and catheter malposition [35]. This may favor catheter-related thrombosis and infection.

Although obese patients have an increased incidence of infections, particularly postoperative wound infection, obesity per se is usually not considered as a risk factor for catheter sepsis [36]. Considering all these potential risks related to vascular access and catheter maintenance, it is rather surprising that there is no single catheter complication reported in the 6 studies of table 2 (141 patients enrolled). This may reflect the fact that many nutritionists do not insert the catheters themselves in difficult patients, such as the grossly obese, and therefore underreport the related complications.

Complications of Nutritional Support

Malnourished stressed obese patients may constitute a true challenge for the nutritionist. However, despite such difficulty there is little evidence in the literature that complications related to nutritional support are common [37].

Obese patients are prone to develop glucose intolerance or diabetes. There is, however, no indication in the literature that artificial feeding in obese ICU patients is associated with hyperglycemia requiring intensive insulin therapy or with diabetic decompensation. This may partly be explained by the administration of hypocaloric nutrition. A randomized controlled trial compared hypo- and isocaloric intravenous nutrition in obese hospitalized patients: glucose control was little affected by the amount of delivered energy and carbohydrate: there was no difference in the number of patients requiring insulin in the 2 groups [21]. However, there was a significantly higher number of days with insulin therapy in the isocaloric group and a tendency toward higher insulin requirements (daily dose 61 ± 61 vs. 36 ± 47 U/day, NS). In another study comparing the nutritional and clinical efficacy of hypo- and isocaloric enteral support in critically obese patients, plasma glucose seemed to be unaffected by the amount of nonprotein energy supply (glucose-fat mixture) [30]. Unfortunately, neither the number of patients requiring insulin therapy nor the amount of insulin was described. These data suggest that glucose control is not a major problem in obese patients with moderate or severe stress receiving either hypo- or isocaloric feeding.

Bronchopulmonary aspiration is an established risk of enteral feeding, particularly in comatose patients. Gross obesity is often mentioned as a risk factor, since gastric emptying is delayed and intra-abdominal pressure is increased compared to healthy subjects [14, 15]. However, such an assumption is not supported by the existing literature and there is presently no rationale to avoid or to delay enteral feeding in obese patients.

Perspectives

Numerous questions remain unsolved regarding the metabolic responses to critical illness and the techniques of nutritional support in obese patients including: the role of the metabolic syndrome; nutrient utilization; the optimal feeding route, and appropriate timing of nutritional intervention. Another important issue is the assessment of nutritional status which is complicated by the acute changes in body composition related to critical illness. There is actually no validated method to detect malnutrition early in the course of disease. Another interesting issue, which deserves further research, is the role of the adipose tissue in the systemic inflammatory responses, particularly regarding cytokine and mediator release.

Conclusions

Considering the increasing incidence of obesity and the paucity of the available literature dealing with the critically ill obese, solid nutritional and metabolic studies should be promoted. Obese patients submitted to severe stress are unable to adapt to prolonged starvation. Nutritional support should be provided using similar indications, routes and timing as in nonobese critically ill patients. Numerous studies suggest that hypocaloric hyperprotein feeding should be preferred in such patients.

Acknowledgements

The authors thank M.C. Cayeux (RN) for assistance in the collection of data on obesity.

References

1. Bjorntorp P. Obesity. *Lancet* 1997; 350: 423–6.
2. Groop L, Orho-Melander M. The dysmetabolic syndrome. *J Intern Med* 2001; 250: 20.
3. Björntorp P. Body fat distribution, insulin resistance, and metabolic diseases. *Nutrition* 1997; 13: 795–803.
4. Choban PS, Weireter LJ Jr, Maynes C. Obesity and increased mortality in blunt trauma. *J Trauma* 1991; 31: 1253–7.
5. Rose DK, Cohen MM, Wigglesworth DF, DeBoer DP. Critical respiratory events in the postanesthesia care unit. *Anesthesiology* 1994; 81: 410–8.
6. Choban PS, Heckler R, Burge JC, Flancbaum L. Increased incidence of nosocomial infections in obese surgical patients. *Am Surg* 1995; 61: 1001–5.
7. Engelman DT, Adams DH, Byrne JG, Aranki SF, Collins JJ Jr, Couper GS, Allred EN, Cohn LH, Rizzo RJ. Impact of body mass index and albumin on morbidity and mortality after cardiac surgery. *J Thorac Cardiovasc Surg* 1999; 118: 866–73.
8. Chioléro R, Revelly JP, Tappy L. Energy metabolism in sepsis and injury. *Nutrition* 1997; 13: 45S–51S.
9. Jeevanandam M, Young DH, Schiller WR. Obesity and the metabolic response to severe multiple trauma in man. *J Clin Invest* 1991; 87: 262–9.
10. Jeevanandam M, Ramias L, Schiller WR. Altered plasma free acid levels in obese traumatized man. *Metabolism* 1991; 40: 385–90.
11. Forbes GB, Drenick EJ. Loss of body nitrogen on fasting. *Am J Clin Nutr* 1979; 32: 1570–4.

12. Leiter LA, Marliss EB. Survival during fasting may depend on fat as well as protein stores. *JAMA* 1982; 248: 2306–7.
13. Ravasco P, Camilo ME, Gouveia-Oliveira A, Adam S, Brum G. A critical approach to nutritional assessment in critically ill patients. *Clin Nutr* 2002; 21: 73–7.
14. Heymsfield SB, Choban PS, Allison DB, Flancbaum L. Nutrition support of the obese patient. In: Rombeau J, Rolandelli R, eds. *Clinical nutrition. Parenteral nutrition*. Philadelphia: Saunders, 2001: 407–28.
15. Choban PS, Flancbaum L. Nourishing the obese patient. *Clin Nutr* 2000; 19: 305–11.
16. Ireton-Jones CS, Francis C. Obesity: Nutrition support practice and application to critical care. *Nutr Clin Pract* 1995; 10: 144–9.
17. Owen OE, Holup JL, D'Alessio DA, Craig ES, Polansky M, Smalley KJ, Kavle EC, Bushman MC, Owen LR, Mozzoli MA, Kendrick ZV, Boden GH. A reappraisal of the caloric requirements of men. *Am J Clin Nutr* 1987; 46: 875–85.
18. Cutts ME, Dowdy RP, Ellersieck MR, Edes TE. Predicting energy needs in ventilator-dependent critically ill patients: Effect of adjusting weight for edema or adiposity. *Am J Clin Nutr* 1997; 66: 1250–6.
19. Glynn CC, Greene GW, Winkler MF, Albina JE. Predictive versus measured energy expenditure using limits-of-agreement analysis in hospitalized, obese patients. *JPEN J Parenter Enteral Nutr* 1999; 23: 147–54.
20. Amato P, Keating KP, Quercia RA, Karbonic J. Formulaic method of estimating calorie requirements in mechanically ventilated obese patients: A reappraisal. *Nutr Clin Pract* 1995; 10: 229–32.
21. Burge JC, Goon A, Choban PS, Flancbaum L. Efficacy of hypocaloric total parenteral nutrition in hospitalized obese patients: A prospective, double-blind randomized trial. *JPEN J Parenter Enteral Nutr* 1994; 18: 203–7.
22. Choban PS, Burge JC, Scales D, Flancbaum L. Hypoenergetic nutrition support in hospitalized obese patients: A simplified method for clinical application. *Am J Clin Nutr* 1997; 66: 546–50.
23. Hawmi GJ. Therapy: Changing dietary concepts: In: Ts D, ed. *Diabetes mellitus: diagnosis and treatment*. New York: American Diabetes Association, 1961: vol 1, 73–8.
24. Dickerson RN, Guenter PA, Gennarelli TA, Dempsey DT, Mullen JL. Brief communication: Increased contribution of protein oxidation to energy expenditure in head-injured patients. *J Am Coll Nutr* 1990; 9: 86–8.
25. Dupont IE, Carpentier YA. Clinical use of lipid emulsions. *Curr Opin Clin Nutr Metab Care* 1999; 2: 139–45.
26. Aspen Board of Directors and the Clinical Guidelines Task Force. Guidelines for the use of parenteral and enteral nutrition in adult and pediatric patients. *JPEN J Parenter Enteral Nutr* 2002; 26: 1SA–138SA.
27. Greenberg GR, Jeejeebhoy KN. Intravenous protein-sparing therapy in patients with gastrointestinal disease. *JPEN J Parenter Enteral Nutr* 1979; 3: 427–32.
28. Liu KJ, Cho MJ, Atten MJ, Panizales E, Walter R, Hawkins D, Donahue PA. Hypocaloric parenteral nutrition support in elderly obese patients. *Am J Surg* 2000; 66: 394–400.
29. Choban PS, Burge JC, Scales D, Flanchbaum L. Hypoenergetic nutrition support in hospitalized obese patients: A simplified method for clinical application. *Am J Clin Nutr* 1997; 66: 546–50.
30. Dickerson RN, Boschert KJ, Kudsk KA, Brown RO. Hypocaloric enteral tube feeding in critically ill obese patients. *Nutrition* 2002; 18: 241–6.
31. Dickerson RN, Rosato EF, Mullen JL. Net protein anabolism with hypocaloric parenteral nutrition on obese stressed patients. *Am J Clin Nutr* 1986; 44: 747–55.
32. Bartlett RH, Dechert RE, Mault JR, Ferguson SK, Kaiser AM, Erlandson EE. Measurement of metabolism in multiple organ failure. *Surgery* 1982; 92: 771–9.
33. Bollmann MD, Berger MM, Revelly JP, Cayeux MC, Chiolero R. Impact of energy balance on clinical outcome in ICU patients – Preliminary results. *Clin Nutr* 2001; 20 (suppl 3): S3.
34. Kushner R. Managing the obese patient after bariatric surgery: A case report of severe malnutrition and review of the literature. *JPEN J Parenter Enteral Nutr* 2000; 24: 126–32.
35. Varon J, Marik P. Management of the obese critically ill patient. *Crit Care Clin* 2001; 17: 187–200.

36. Maki DG, Mermel LA. Infections due to infusion therapy. In: Bennett J, Brachman P, eds. *Hospital infections*. Philadelphia: Lippincott-Raven, 1998; 689–724.
37. Chioléro RL, Berger MM. *What are the clinical risks related to the nutritional support of obese patients?* Educational Book, 24th ASPEN Congress, Birmingham. Geneva: ASPEN Committee, 2002, in press.

Discussion

Dr. Bozzetti: The story of obese patients reminds me of the story of elderly patients. The surgical literature is full of papers stating that you can operate on patients 80, 90 years old. You can do pancreatectomy in these patients with an acceptable risk which is quite similar to that of adult subjects. In my opinion this reflects a strong selection of the patients because if you look at the morbidity and mortality of elderly patients admitted to intensive care units (ICUs) for trauma, you see a clear correlation between age, morbidity and mortality. My interpretation is not that critically obese patients have a poor tolerance of their situation but this reflects the absence of a selection, so you see that obesity is really a major aspect. The question is have you some suggestions about the water requirement? I am not speaking of patients admitted to the ICU where I expect that the water requirement follows some rules which are different from the usual, but for the usual obese patients operated, in the postoperative period, what is the rule for the water requirements?

Dr. Chioléro: This is an important question since severely obese patients do not tolerate water and electrolyte excess in contrast to other acutely ill surgical patients, for whom we prescribe a large quantity of water and electrolyte. Obviously this has to be taken into account when you prescribe the nutrition. I think your first comment is also important. For a lot of surgical procedures we can do what we have to do with the obese patients: the experience all over the world in cardiac surgery patients, a population with a lot of obese patients, shows that such patients do tolerate surgery quite well. But there is a limit as shown by the data collected in severe trauma or severely burned obese patients, demonstrating an increased rate of complications and even decreased survival rate. Bariatric surgery complicated by abdominal and septic postoperative problems is another field where we sometimes have a lot of difficulty in severely obese patients associated with a poor clinical outcome. Clearly, a lot of work should be done to identify the patients at risk and to delineate therapeutic strategies.

Dr. Labadarios: I would like to give Dr. Bozzetti's question a little bit more of a global nature. We are all concerned about this so-called pandemic of obesity and in my opinion correctly so. But we have been so preoccupied, almost in a state of panic, about addressing this emerging pandemic. Is there room for us to consider the concept of healthy obesity? I mean, you have not shown us that these people actually behave any differently from you and me. Is there room for such a concept of healthy obesity? I know our American friends would now shout me down and we can argue about the data that we have one way or the other, but have we ever spent time thinking about this concept and is there such a concept to think about?

Dr. Chioléro: I think this is an interesting comment which includes two aspects. As an intensivist I could answer that there is little problem. If you consider epidemiology, I think the point of view is different since clearly even simple overweight is associated with increased comorbidities over a long period. So it is both true and false that overweight is a problem. A normal body mass index (BMI) is required to have a maximal life expectancy. This is not true during short periods, like the postoperative period, where this epidemiological point of view is not relevant.

Dr. Moore: Your talk identifies a major problem that is not very well studied. When we ran across that Choban study, we returned to the ICU similar to you. Unfortunately in Texas there are a lot of obese patients, and we really could not document any difference in mortality. We showed the obvious: the bigger the patient is the harder it is for us to get the patient off the ventilator, and this increased ventilator-associated pneumonias, but those ventilator-associated pneumonias don't really contribute very much to mortality. You are an expert in indirect calorimetry, and we have a very difficult time using indirect calorimeter to identify how we should feed patients in the ICU, so we vary between using ideal body weight and adjusted body weight. Which one should we use?

Dr. Chioléro: It is a difficult question. I agree with you that indirect calorimetry is difficult, particularly in obese trauma patients in the ICU setting. For example I made the comment that net substrate calculation using indirect calorimetry in the ICU is particularly difficult since small errors on the respiratory quotient induce a large change in substrate oxidation. But if it will give you an idea of how much energy the patient is spending at that time, remember that we do 20- or 30-min measurements a day, a very short measurement time taking into account the 1,440-min length of the whole day. Concerning your question on the kind of body weight for nutrition prescription (actual or ideal), I would say that, except in obese patients with renal or acute liver failure, in whom protein supply should probably be reduced, I think the concept developed by Choban and Flancbaum based on ideal body weight is a clever convenient one and very simple. They prescribe energy and nutrient based on a rule consisting of giving 2 g protein/kg ideal body weight with an energy protein ratio of 50 kcal/g nitrogen. The concept of hypocaloric nutrition is well established but the optimal energy and protein supply has not been assessed. What we know is that hypocaloric feeding which is quite well tolerated, may facilitate glycemia control. It will decrease fluid supply and it is easy to use for the nutritionist.

Dr. De Bandt: There is convincing evidence of disimmunity associated with diabetes and obesity. Is there an improvement or some hint of improvement in immunological parameters during a hypocaloric diet in these patients?

Dr. Chioléro: This is certainly an important point but I have no information on this aspect since I am not a specialist in immunology. In the literature I have seen no mention of this important point.

Dr. Rosenfeld: You mentioned that syndrome X and intra-abdominal fat distribution in these patients clearly have more complications. Isn't it time for critically ill obese patients to be stratified by fat distribution? In our unit we have seen patients who had more intra-abdominal fat and higher levels of reactive C protein and more complications, more organic failure. Isn't it time to stratify patients by fat distribution?

Dr. Chioléro: I agree with your comment that fat distribution could be important in critically ill patients, remembering that waist circumference may be influenced by fluid accumulation in surgical patients or by bowel distention. Anthropometry assessment is sometimes very inaccurate in such patients, including fat distribution. Since many of these patients require CT scan for non-nutritional purposes, we could perhaps collect interesting information on fat distribution. But I am unaware of any study on this point.

Dr. Martindale: I routinely do bariatric surgery on patients over 350 kg. It is a very interesting population. As Dr. Moore mentioned, after the Choban study came out he went to the unit and looked at the complications in that population. We did the same and we very interestingly found a big dichotomy between those who came in ambulatory and those who did not. The 350-kg patient who walks into the hospital does very well. The 350-kg patient who can no longer walk because of the obesity has a tremendously long hospital stay, a tremendously long ventilator requirement and has the complications associated with hospital stay, not so much with the surgical procedure, I mean routine PE. Any nonambulatory patient over 350 kg who comes to the hospital for a bariatric procedure gets a filter because they have PE. Virtually all of them get PEs postoperatively. So I think that is a key. Looking at their premorbid conditions in the surgery is the key, and in trauma we obviously can't do that.

Dr. Chioléro: I think this is an interesting comment since organ function including muscle is related to nutritional status and is an important aim in nutritional support. A similar observation was made more than 20 years ago in patients requiring aggressive pulmonary resection. Those who are able to walk and perhaps even to climb some steps usually had an uncomplicated postoperative course, while those with more severe functional abnormalities usually had a bad postoperative evolution.

Dr. Allison: Concerning the protein metabolism of obese surgical patients, I guess you would accept that the higher nitrogen output simply reflects the fact that these people have a bigger lean mass. Elia reviewed prolonged fasts in very obese individuals, some up to a year. He showed with a prolonged fast that the obese individuals tend to protect their lean mass in a curious way. In other words even when you adjusted it for lean mass their nitrogen output was consistently 2 g/day less over the whole period of time. What you are saying is that this protective relationship, almost as if the lean mass knows what the adipose tissue reserve is, is abolished when you have an injury. So do you think this protective effect of obesity which is seen in prolonged starvation is lost with the stress response?

Dr. Chioléro: Yes, and this is not specific to the obese patients since it may be observed in all severely stressed ICU patients. There are few studies on starvation in ICU patients. Ketosis is nearly totally suppressed in critically ill obese and nonobese patients. This is an adaptation phenomenon related to the increased glucose requirements of the wounds and inflammatory cells. In such conditions there is a redistribution of the metabolic priorities. But I am unaware of data on ketosis in obese patients with prolonged hypocaloric feeding. In Dickerson's study in which there was prolonged hypocaloric feeding in surgical patients, no data on ketosis were given. I think there is a lot of work to be done on starvation in these patients.

Dr. Cynober: What about patients who undergo gastroplasty surgery in the short term and in the middle term? Are there some data especially with regard to lean body mass variations?

Dr. Chioléro: Yes, there are data coming from America. Dr. Martindale explained that he observed many patients weighing more than 350 kg being operated on the stomach or having bypasses. Bariatric surgery is a complex issue. Data on body composition after surgery were presented at the last ESPEN meeting. The patients lose weight but lean body mass seems to be preserved, provided adequate nutritional support is offered.

Dr. Martindale: I think you are right, they lose weight. They protect their lean body mass. Persons over 350 kg lose about 80% of their excess weight at 5 years, and by 10 years it is down to about 65%, and 15 years it stays about that.

Dr. Cynober: In our institution we have an important department looking at obesity and surgery and so on. For example we are looking at trace elements, vitamins, vitamin A and so on. We have the feeling that these patients are rapidly depleted in micronutrients. I don't know if in your experience you are measuring lean body mass but when you are looking with Dexa, these patients clearly become malnourished very rapidly. I don't know if you agree that there are very few studies looking very carefully at the behavior of lean body mass in these patients after surgery.

Dr. Chioléro: They need regular specialized nutritional support otherwise they will become malnourished after 1–2 years.

Dr. Labadarios: In relation to these very interesting data that Dr. Martindale mentioned, I would like to ask whether he has got any data on biomarkers between these two classes of people, the ones that are ambulatory and the ones that are not. My question is, are these, the ambulatory patients, not the ones that have really adapted to an 'unphysiological' state as opposed to those that come in bedridden? You said pulmonary embolism is common in all of them, but is it really common in all of them? Do you have any data on that specific point?

Dr. Martindale: Before we were routinely putting in filters. We have data on that just because of the poor clinical outcomes: the bigger they are, the more obese they are, and the longer they stay in bed. I think the comment about rapid malnutrition, the problem in the US is that the reimbursements for bariatric surgery are very high. So many surgeons who have no interest in obesity and no interest in nutrition are now doing bariatric surgery. To me this is criminal because they are doing it for the reimbursement, not because they care about the problems in the patients. So by 1, 2 and 5 years these patients are left by themselves with nobody following their malnutrition problems. The true studies that have been done are really only in abstract form showing that these people are all malnourished at 1 year. It is controlled undernutrition, and that exact word, control, is not in there. There is nobody controlling these people when they are left alone except in a few centers. In a few centers where vitamin levels and protein levels are routinely followed and outputs at 6 months and 1 year are routinely looked at, patients are put on a tread mill to see what their performance levels are. But nobody in the US has got any long-term studies in this area, and the problem is that there are 65,000 bariatric surgery procedures being done in the US this year. It is estimated that in 2005 it will go to 80,000, and the reimbursement for a bariatric procedure is USD 4,200, the reimbursement for a ripple procedure in the US right now is USD 2,600.

Dr. Bouletreau: Would you say in your patients that the risk is more the complications of obesity than the obesity itself?

Dr. Martindale: No, it is the complication of the obesity if you look at hypertension, glucose intolerance, sleep apnea and those things. Sleep apnea within 16 weeks is 100% cured, the diabetes is about 80% cured, and the national study health just made a comment on curing type-II diabetes with bariatric surgery in the obese population, and the President of the United States recently declared that obesity is a disease, an independent disease, not just a risk factor or comorbid factor, but a disease, and that allows the government to pay for much of the comorbidity associated with it. So we can cure the diabetes, the hypertension and sleep apnea almost 100% of the time with the operation. The problem is we are not treating. As you saw from those maps the only state in the United States that has under 15% obesity is Colorado and that is because of an education program from day 1 of starting elementary school. We have lost our benefit once we are treating the disease surgically, it is too late.

Dr. McClave: Your data would suggest that they don't have any trouble mobilizing fat. My question revolves around the concept of cyclic feeding. Is it important to have an off period where we can allow the insulin levels to drop and mobilize that fat, and if we provide enteral feeding but infuse it over 24 h do we jeopardize that?

Dr. Chioléro: Yes, if we increase the glucose supply and give insulin we are going to block the mobilization of the triglyceride from the fat stores, so clearly it is an important point considering cyclic feeding to optimize energy and nutrient utilization.

Dr. McClave: Did most of the studies you presented provide nutrition in a cyclic manner?

Dr. Chioléro: No, it was noncyclic nutrition.

Dr. Heyland: I have a question in that context, and I am talking here about not the severely obese but rather the more mild, moderately obese which is more common in the ICU, and the question is in the context of designing and interpreting clinical trials. I heard you say that the obese patient has different outcomes compared to the nonobese, and has different responses to stress compared to the nonobese. But specifically do they have a different response to nutritional support whether enteral or parenteral, so that they are randomized to a fixed diet one intervention, intervention A versus intervention B? Might I expect a different response in the obese versus the nonobese? And if so, how do I better characterize the obese patient, is it on the basis of the BMI, is it on the basis of the fat distribution or does it have more to do with insulin resistance, and do I need to characterize that better, and how would I do that?

Dr. Chioléro: This is a difficult question since even in nonobese patients it would be difficult to address your question. Clearly an important point to consider is the absolute value of the BMI, i.e. the fat deposition. Visceral fat deposition is another aspect to consider, as well as the relationship between the metabolic syndrome and the response to injury. Nobody has systematically assessed these points and I think they could be important. Unfortunately, there are very few nutritional and metabolic studies comparing the metabolic and nutritional response in obese and nonobese critically ill patients. To perform studies comparing the effects of a given nutritional intervention in obese and nonobese stressed patients would therefore be very interesting.

Dr. Bouletreau: Don't you think it is important even in hypocaloric feeding to preserve a certain amount of glucose and not to go back to the first studies, the first recommendations? What minimal level of glucose would you recommend?

Dr. Chioléro: I fully agree with your point of view, underlying the importance of glucose supply during hypocaloric nutrition. The best is probably to give the largest part of nonprotein energy as glucose, and only to give fat to avoid essential fatty acid deficiency or to exert specific systemic effects such as with fish oil. Concerning the minimal amount of glucose supply, I think there is no difference between obese and nonobese stressed patients. They clearly require a minimal amount of glucose to have the best metabolic control. Stress patients are not like unstressed patients during starvation.

Dr. Nitenberg: You showed many data about surgical patients and moderately stressed patients. Do you think that we have to consider obese patients differently in more severe aggressions such as severe burns or sepsis or other types of severe situations? Do you have any data on that or do other people in the audience have that?

Dr. Chioléro: Interesting question. We had a discussion after Dr. Allison's presentation concerning specific patient populations in the ICU, and we have presently many obese patients in our population. Unfortunately there is very little information in the literature concerning obese patients with specific critical conditions such as sepsis, trauma or burns. The only strong evidence is related to the severity of critical illness. Published studies show that obese patients tolerate a moderate level of stress well, but behave worse than nonobese patients during major stress.

Dr. Martindale: My question is on the volume of distribution of drugs. I worry very often that we are delivering nutrient based on ideal body weight in many cases, nitrogen anyway, but we don't change the delivery of our drugs, and the volume of distribution in these patients. I don't really have any data and I don't know what do you do at your place.

Dr. Chioléro: It is an important question. In the usual pharmacokinetic approach we should calculate the hydrosoluble drug prescription on the fat-free mass basis. But we have a lot of factors, at least in the ICU setting, which are going to influence drug distribution. We administer more fluid, they have fluid retention, and drug elimination may be altered by various factors such as liver, renal failure and other factors. Actually, in our practice in obese patients, we usually measure the plasma level of many drugs but we find no simple relationship with actual or ideal body weight. There is clearly no simple relationship between ideal and adjusted body weight and drug prescription.

Dr. Zazzo: Just a comment. Analogically, for prescribing antibiotics to obese patients the literature say that we calculate 40% of the difference between ideal and actual weight. I think it is perhaps a way to compare antibiotic equations or recommendations for it and energy supply.

Dr. Chioléro: In your experience, does it work?

Dr. Zazzo: Yes, in my experience it works for amino acids and bronchomycine because in clinical practice it is very difficult to get the dosage for β-lactamine.

Dr. Chioléro: Yes, but the volume of distribution of bronchomycine is not the right one, so probably it is a good example which goes with the concept.

Dr. Dechelotte: Just to add to the discussion: we should take the lipophilic severity of the drug into account. It is quite different between drugs that will accumulate in fat stores.

Dr. Chioléro: I fully agree.

Cymober J, Moore FA (eds): Nutrition and Critical Care.
Nestlé Nutrition Workshop Series Clinical & Performance Program, Vol. 8, pp. 207–221
Nestec Ltd.; Vevey/S. Karger AG, Basel, © 2003.

Nutritional Support in Acute Pancreatitis

Stephen A. McClave

Division of Gastroenterology/Hepatology, University of Louisville School of Medicine, Louisville, Ky., USA

Importance of Pancreatic Rest

That pancreatic rest and a reduction in exocrine secretion may allow a more expedient resolution of pancreatic inflammation is an important clinical precept in the management of patients with acute pancreatitis. Fortunately, the most common deleterious effect of early advancement to oral diet is an uncomplicated exacerbation of symptoms, which in one multi-center trial occurred in 21% of patients recovering from acute pancreatitis [1]. Of greater concern is a true exacerbation of pancreatitis, which occurs in less than one fifth of those patients who demonstrate an exacerbation of symptoms (or in 4.3% of patients overall) [1]. Relapse in response to early advancement to oral diet does impact patient outcome with regard to length of hospitalization. Length of hospitalization after advancement to oral diet was prolonged from 7 days in those patients who advanced successfully, to 18 days in those patients who suffered relapse [1]. Total length of hospitalization was nearly doubled from 18 to 33 days (p < 0.002), when relapse occurred in response to early advancement to oral diet [1]. The development of late complications of major peripancreatic infection in response to early dietary advancement described in early retrospective studies [2] has not been demonstrated in more recent prospective studies.

The understanding of what constitutes pancreatic rest has improved over the past decade. A reduction in the enzymatic protein portion of pancreatic exocrine secretion appears to be the most important factor in resolving the inflammatory response. While fluid volume and bicarbonate output from the pancreas are often simultaneously stimulated with increases in protein enzyme output, the three aspects of pancreatic secretion are not necessarily linked through the same stimulatory factors. Management strategies which reduce protein enzyme output with a continued output of volume and bicarbonate may be sufficient to rest the pancreas and allow resolution of inflammation [3]. A reduction in protein enzyme output to basal unstimulated levels may not be required to rest the pancreas, as a reduction to subclinical levels may be sufficient to promote convalescence. This strategy may be guided by resolution of symptoms. Very little secretion in the pancreas may occur at the height of acute inflammation. But most importantly, pancreatic rest may be achieved by early enteral feeding infused low in the gastrointestinal (GI) tract at the level of the jejunum with formulas comprised of components that minimize pancreatic stimulation.

Reduced Pancreatic Stimulation with Jejunal Feeding

The safety of early enteral feeding and the ability to reduce pancreatic stimulation with jejunal infusion of nutrients was clearly demonstrated in the first prospective randomized trial of enteral versus parenteral feeding in acute pancreatitis [4]. Patients placed on early jejunal feeding within 48 h of admission for acute pancreatitis demonstrated that there was no prolongation of the time to normalization of amylase, advancement to oral diet, length of time spent in the intensive care unit, or overall length of hospital stay [4]. Use of the enteral route did not increase nosocomial infections or affect overall mortality [4].

The ability of early enteral feedings to rest the pancreas relates to the fact that there are various levels of stimulation throughout the GI tract [5]. These levels of pancreatic stimulation include the cephalic, gastric, and intestinal phases [5]. The lower these nutrients are infused in the GI tract, the less likely they are to stimulate pancreatic secretion. Feeding low enough into the GI tract (i.e., the jejunum) may not only bypass the stimulatory factors, but ironically may stimulate a number of inhibitory polypeptides. Pancreatic inhibitory polypeptide, polypeptide YY, somatostatin, luminal proteases, and even bile acids all inhibit or reduce pancreatic secretion and may be released in response to jejunal feeding.

Specific characteristics and the degree of digestive complexity of individual nutrients have a differential effect on pancreatic secretion [5, 6]. Of the three major macronutrients, fat is the most potent stimulus of the pancreas and intraluminal carbohydrate is the least. Long-chain fatty acids appear to stimulate the pancreas more than medium-chain triglycerides [5, 6]. Intact protein stimulates the pancreas more than individual amino acids, and small peptides may be the form of protein which has the least stimulatory effect. Agents with high osmolarity may stimulate the pancreas more than agents with low osmolarity [6].

208

With a basic understanding of these concepts, the clinician may envision a scale over which the degree of pancreatic stimulation is determined by the inherent nature and method of delivery in which nutrients are administered. At one end of the scale is oral feeding, which invokes the greatest degree of pancreatic secretion. Delivery of nutrients to progressively lower levels of the GI tract (from the stomach to the duodenum to jejunum), is associated with a diminishing degree of stimulation. At the other end of the scale, parenteral infusion, in the absence of hypercalcemia or hypertriglyceridemia, has the least stimulatory effect and the lowest likelihood for relapse [5]. Similarly, with regard to components of the individual nutrients, fat would be at the end of the scale causing the greatest stimulation of the pancreas. Protein, and then carbohydrate, would be at the opposite end of the scale leading to lesser degrees of stimulation. The degree of disease severity (as determined by the presence or absence as well as the degree of pancreatic necrosis) [7] determines the maximal number of stimulatory factors that may be tolerated without relapse.

Importance of Maintaining Gut Integrity

While the tenant of pancreatic rest is of central importance in managing patients with acute pancreatitis, maintaining gut integrity is equally important. The GI tract is the largest immune organ in the body, containing 65% of immune tissue overall and up to 80% of the immunoglobulin-producing tissue of the body [8, 9]. As a result, utilization of the GI tract modulates the overall systemic immunity and leads to a dramatically favorable impact on patient outcome.

In the fed state, the normal villi, rich blood supply, and intercellular tight junctions contribute to the overall integrity of the GI tract. Propulsive contractions keep the concentration of bacteria at normal levels, and the secretion of bile salts and secretory IgA in response to luminal nutrients coat the bacteria and prevent adherence to the gut wall and subsequent translocation [10, 11]. The healthy gut acts as an important antigen-processing organ, in which bacterial antigen is presented across the M cells, stimulating the release and maturation of a population of pluripotential stem cells [12, 13]. These cells will migrate out from the Peyer's patches, through the mesenteric lymph nodes and thoracic duct, into the systemic circulation as a mature line of B- and T-cell lymphocytes. A portion of these cells returns to the GI tract as gut-associated lymphoid tissue (GALT) [11–13]. Lymphoid follicles are comprised mostly of helper T cells, which induce the production of secretory IgA by the plasma cells. Diffuse lymphoid tissue contained within the intestinal villli have a wider variety of cells, including helper T cells, cytotoxic T cells, B cells, and plasma cells [11–13]. A separate population of cells generated in the maturation of the pluripotential stem cells migrate out as mucosal-associated lymphoid tissue (MALT) to distant sites such as the lungs, genitourinary, breast and lachrymal glands [10–13].

In a situation of even brief disuse, gut integrity may deteriorate. In contrast to the fed state, fasting leads to villous atrophy, diminished blood flow, and loss of interepithelial tight junctions. This opens paracellular channels, allowing translocation of bacteria [13]. Reduced contractility promotes bacterial overgrowth [10]. Without nutrient-induced stimulation of secretory IgA and bile salts, bacteria are able to adhere to the luminal wall, promoting even greater translocation of bacteria and their secretory products (i.e., endotoxin) [10]. The mass of GALT may diminish, as does the antigen processing and buildup of MALT at distant sites.

The most important aspect of gut disuse may be the diminished blood supply to the gut, which leads to ischemia/reperfusion injury [14]. The generation of superoxide radicals in response to ischemia/reperfusion may promote the gut as a priming bed for macrophages [14, 15]. Macrophages, primed and activated at the level of the gut, may migrate out to distant sites such as the liver, lung, and kidney. There, they may diapedese into these tissues, introducing oxidative species [15]. Activated macrophages are the key step linking issues of gut deterioration with more systemic factors which adversely affect patient outcome [15, 16]. Activated macrophages initiate the arachidonic acid cascade.

Although simplified, the concepts presented point to the pivotal importance enteral nutrition plays in determining whether the gut promotes inflammation or enhances appropriate immune function in the setting of pancreatitis. Gut disuse, with or without parenteral feeding, leads to a process in which there is macrophage/neutrophil activation and a nonspecific pattern of exaggerated systemic inflammatory response with multiple organ failure [14–17]. On the other hand, utilizing the gut and infusing luminal nutrients instead leads to a different process characterized by the orderly generation of GALT/MALT, and the incidence of nosocomial infection and organ failure is reduced [11–13].

With loss of integrity, there is evidence in pancreatitis patients that the gut becomes 'leaky'. In a prospective randomized trial, Windsor et al. [18] showed that patients with pancreatitis maintained on enteral tube feeding had no change in IgM antibodies to endotoxin over a week of enteral feeding. In contrast, controls placed on total parenteral nutrition (TPN) and gut disuse demonstrated a statistically significant increase in IgM antibodies to endotoxin of 24.8% in response to a week of parenteral feeding ($p < 0.05$) [18]. Evidence that loss of integrity and a leaky gut lead to an increased generation of superoxide radicals was shown in the same study by the fact that total antioxidant capacity (as measured by an enhancement chemiluminescence assay) was shown to be reduced by 27.7% in the group placed on TPN [18]. In contrast, study patients on enteral feeding showed a statistically significant increase in antioxidant capacity by 32.6% over a similar week of enteral feeding ($p < 0.05$) [18].

The more important contribution from the leaky gut with compromised integrity relates to its effect on the overall stress response and disease severity caused by pancreatitis. In pancreatitis patients, significant increases in stress-induced hyperglycemia were seen in a control group placed on TPN and gut disuse [4]. No such increases in serum glucose levels were seen in the study group placed on enteral feeding [4]. In a separate study, C-reactive protein levels in a group of pancreatitis patients randomized to TPN did not change over a week of parenteral feeding [18]. In contrast, C-reactive protein levels decreased significantly from 156 to 84 g/dl in a study group placed on enteral feeding ($p < 0.05$) [18]. In the same study, APACHE II scores decreased significantly over a week of feeding within the enteral group, with no significant change in the group placed on TPN and gut disuse [18]. At the end of 1 week of nutritional therapy, 9 of 11 patients in the enteral group had resolved the systemic inflammatory response syndrome, contrasted with the group placed on TPN and gut disuse in which only 2 out of 12 patients resolved the systemic inflammatory response syndrome over their 1st week of therapy ($p < 0.05$) [18].

Most importantly, the issues of enteral access and maintenance of gut integrity in acute pancreatitis ultimately impact patient outcome. In a prospective randomized trial, patients with severe acute pancreatitis and necrosis on computerized tomography scans placed on enteral feeding developed significantly fewer septic complications compared to a similar group of patients placed on TPN and gut disuse (incidence of septic complications 28 vs. 50%, respectively, $p < 0.03$) [19]. Additionally, the number of infections in those patients who developed septic complications was reduced significantly as well from 1.35 in the group randomized to TPN/gut disuse, to 0.56 in the group on enteral feeding ($p < 0.03$) [19]. In fact, overall complications were reduced significantly from 75% in the group placed on TPN/gut disuse to 44% in the early enteral group ($p < 0.05$) [19].

Identifying Patients in Need of Aggressive Enteral Nutritional Support

Determining which patients need aggressive nutritional enteral support can be difficult for the clinician. Surprisingly, clinical assessment and physical examination on admission have been shown to be inferior to APACHE II scores in differentiating patients with severe pancreatitis with a higher likelihood of morbidity and mortality [20, 21] from those with mild to moderate pancreatitis and a low likelihood of complications. In two studies, the sensitivity of clinical assessment in identifying patients with severe pancreatitis was only 34–44%, whereas the sensitivity for an APACHE II score of >9 was 63 82% [20, 21] While the APACHE II score was superior to clinical assessment in predicting severe attacks on admission, the overall accuracy for clinical assessment was higher on admission because most mild attacks were correctly predicted [20, 21]. At 48 h, the sensitivity of both the APACHE II score of >9 and the Ranson criteria of >2 was greater (75–82%) in identifying patients with severe pancreatitis than clinical assessment (44–66%) [21]. The overall accuracy for clinical assessment at 48 h was 87–89%, which was slightly higher than the two scoring systems at 69–88% [20, 21]. Those patients with APACHE II scores of >9 and Ranson criteria of >2 account for 20% of hospital admissions, tend to have pancreatic necrosis on CT scan, have a 19% mortality rate, 38% incidence of complications, and are unlikely to achieve an oral intake successfully within 7 days of admission [7, 21–23]. In contrast, those patients with APACHE II scores of ≤9 and Ranson criteria of ≤2 account for 80% of hospital admissions, tend not to have necrosis on CT scan, have a 0% mortality rate, 6% complication rate, and a 81% incidence of reaching an oral diet successfully within 7 days of admission [7, 21–23]. Using these parameters, the clinician can predict the patients likely to develop severe pancreatitis who need aggressive enteral nutritional support and placement of early enteral access.

Is There a Role for TPN in Severe Acute Pancreatitis?

In the only prospective randomized trial of TPN versus no nutritional therapy, patients with predominantly mild acute pancreatitis (mean Ranson criteria of 1.1) placed on early TPN actually did worse than controls that received only intravenous fluid resuscitation without nutritional support [23]. TPN patients were hospitalized for 16 versus 10 days in the control group (p < 0.04), and the catheter-related sepsis in the TPN group was 10.5 versus 1.5% in historical controls (p = 0.003) [23]. Patients with mild to moderate disease do not require nutritional support. TPN is not a consideration in these patients unless a late complication develops. TPN should only be considered in those patients with severe pancreatitis who are intolerant for enteral feedings or in whom enteral access cannot be obtained. Extrapolation of data from other patient populations (such as burns, trauma and critical care) suggests that it may be pertinent to withhold TPN in these patients for the first 5 days until the peak inflammatory response passes [23, 24].

Do Complications or the Need for Surgery Contraindicate Enteral Feeding?

Complications such as pancreatic ascites, fistulas, or pseudocysts are part of the natural disease course of acute pancreatitis. Information from mostly retrospective case series indicates that use of the enteral route is safe and allows resolution of these complications in most circumstances [6, 25, 26]. Experience from the literature involves patients with chronic pseudocysts, fistulas, or ascites who tend to be past the peak of inflammation. These patients continue to require hospitalization, but are fed successfully by nasoenteric tube or by elemental or semi-elemental diet ingested orally. Resolution of the complication usually occurs over several weeks, with a few episodes of diarrhea as the only problem [6, 25, 26].

The need for surgery to treat hemorrhagic or infectious complications from pancreatitis give the opportunity to obtain a more definitive enteral access [27, 28]. In two studies from Europe in which patients operated on for acute pancreatitis were randomized to enteral feeding or TPN postoperatively, no differences in outcome between the two groups were seen [29, 30]. Responses in pancreatic secretory output postoperatively were similar as well [29, 30]. These studies demonstrate that enteral feeding via jejunostomy in these patients following major pancreatic surgery is safe and well tolerated.

Initiation of Feeds

In a patient determined to be a candidate for enteral feeding for severe acute pancreatitis, a nasoenteric tube should be placed endoscopically or fluoroscopically at or below the ligament of Treitz. The tube may be secured at the nose using a nasal bridle. Feeds may be started at $25 \, cm^3/h$ and advanced to goal levels (25 cal/kg/day) over the first 24–48 h.

If the tube is low enough in the GI tract, almost any formula may be successful in putting the pancreas to rest. To obtain a maximal reduction in enzyme output, however, two groups of formulas may be selected. Earlier elemental formulas that are nearly fat-free and comprised of individual amino acids may result in the least stimulation of the pancreas. Small peptide formulas in which 70% of the fat is in the form of medium-chain triglycerides may cause slightly greater stimulation of the pancreas, but this is offset by greater, more efficient absorption.

Usually partial ileus is a minimal problem, occasionally requiring a decrease in rate, but not necessarily cessation of feeds. The timing and advancement to oral diet is somewhat difficult, but in general should be considered once the patient has been pain free for 24–48 h, with levels of amylase and lipase decreasing toward normal. Criteria which may help in indicating readiness for advancement to oral diet include a total duration of painful period <6 days, serum lipase on the day prior to advancement of <3 times normal, and a CT score on pancreatic necrosis of C or better [1].

References

1. Levy P, Heresbach D, Pariente EA, Boruchowicz A, Delcenserie R, Millat B, Moreau J, Le Bodic L, de Calan L, Barthet M, Sauvanet A, Bernades P. Frequency and risk factors of recurrent pain during refeeding in patients with acute pancreatitis: A multivariate multi-centre prospective study of 116 patients. *Gut* 1997; 40: 262–6.

2. Ranson JHC, Spencer FC. Prevention, diagnosis and treatment of pancreatic abscess. *Surgery* 1977; 82: 99–106.
3. Cassim MM, Allardyce DB. Pancreatic secretion in response to jejunal feeding of elemental diet. *Ann Surg* 1974; 180: 228–31.
4. McClave SA, Greene LM, Snider HL, Makk LJ, Cheadle WG, Owens NA, Dukes LG, Goldsmith LJ. Comparison of the safety of early enteral versus parenteral nutrition in mild acute pancreatitis. *JPEN J Parenter Enteral Nutr* 1997; 21: 14–20.
5. Corcoy R, Ma Sanchez J, Domingo P, Net A. Nutrition in the patient with severe acute pancreatitis. *Nutrition* 1998; 4: 269–75.
6. Parekh D, Lawson HH, Segal I. The role of total enteral nutrition in pancreatic disease. *S Afr J Surg* 1993; 31: 57–61.
7. Banks PA. Pancreatitis for the endoscopist. ASGE Postgraduate Course, Digestive Disease Week, San Francisco, May 1996.
8. Bengmark S. Gut microenvironment and immune function. *Curr Opin Clin Nutr Metab Care* 1999; 2: 1–3.
9. Brandtzaeg P, Halstensen TS, Kett K, Krajci P, Kvale D, Rognum TO, Scott H, Sollid LM. Immunobiology and immunopathology of the human gut mucosa: Humoral immunity and intraepithelial lymphocytes. *Gastroenterology* 1989; 97: 1562–84.
10. DeWitt RC, Kudsk KA. The gut's role in metabolism, mucosal barrier function, and gut immunology. *Infect Dis Clin North Am* 1999; 13: 465–81.
11. Kagnoff MF. Immunology of the intestinal tract. *Gastroenterology* 1993; 105: 1275–80.
12. Targan SR, Kagnoff MF, Brogan MD, Shanahan F. Immunologic mechanisms in intestinal diseases. *Ann Intern Med* 1987; 106: 853–70.
13. Dobbins WO. Gut immunophysiology: A gastroenterologist's view with emphasis on pathophysiology. *Am J Physiol* 1982; 242: G1–G8.
14. Frost P, Bihari D. The route of nutritional support in the critically ill: Physiological and economical considerations. *Nutrition* 1997; 13: 58S–63S.
15. Moore EE, Moore FA. The role of the gut in provoking the systemic inflammatory response. *J Crit Care Nutr* 1994; 2: 9–15.
16. Fink MP. Why the GI tract is pivotal in trauma, sepsis, and MOF. *J Crit Illness* 1991; 6: 253–69.
17. Moore FA, Feliciano DV, Andrassy RJ, McArdle AH, Booth FV, Morgenstein-Wagner TB, Kellum JM Jr, Welling RE, Moore EE. Early enteral feeding, compared with parenteral, reduces postoperative septic complications. *Ann Surg* 1992; 216(2): 172–83.
18. Windsor AC, Kanwar S, Li AG, Barnes E, Guthrie JA, Spark JI, Welsh F, Guillou PJ, Reynolds JV. Compared with parenteral nutrition, enteral feeding attenuates the acute phase response and improves disease severity in acute pancreatitis. *Gut* 1998; 42: 431–5.
19. Kalfarentzos F, Kehagias J, Mead N. Enteral nutrition is superior to parenteral nutrition in severe acute pancreatitis: Results of a randomized prospective trial. *Br J Surg* 1997; 84: 1665–9.
20. Wilson C, Heath DI, Imrie CW. Prediction of outcome in acute pancreatitis: A comparative study of APACHE II, clinical assessment and multiple factor scoring system. *Br J Surg* 1990; 77: 1260–4.
21. Larvin M, McMahon MJ. APACHE-II score for assessment and monitoring of acute pancreatitis. *Lancet* 1989; ii: 201–5.
22. Corfield AP, Cooper MJ, Williamson RC, Mayer AD, McMahon MJ, Dickson AP, Shearer MG, Imrie CW. Prediction of severity in acute pancreatitis: Prospective comparison of three prognostic indices. *Lancet* 1985; ii: 403–7.
23. Sax HC, Warner BW, Talamini MA, Hamilton FN, Bell RH Jr, Fischer JE, Bower RH. Early total parenteral nutrition in acute pancreatitis: Lack of beneficial effects. *Am J Surg* 1987: 153: 117–24.
24. Braunschweig CL, Levy P, Sheean PM, Wang X. Enteral compared with parenteral nutrition: A meta-analysis. *Am J Clin Nutr* 2001; 74: 534–42.
25. Voitk A, Brown RA, Echave V, McArdle AH, Gurd FN, Thompson AG. Use of an elemental diet in the treatment of complicated pancreatis. *Am J Surg* 1973; 125: 223–7.
26. Bury KD, Stephens RV, Randall HT. Use of chemically defined, liquid elemental diet for nutritional management of fistulas of the alimentary tract. *Am J Surg* 1971; 121: 174–83.
27. Lawson DW, Daggett WM, Civetta JM, Corry RJ, Bartlett MK. Surgical treatment of acute necrotizing pancreatitis. *Ann Surg* 1970; 172: 605–15.

28. Kudsk KA, Campbell SM, O'Brien T, Fuller R. Postoperative jejunal feedings following complicated pancreatitis. *Nutr Clin Pract* 1990; 5: 14–7.
29. Hernandez-Aranda JC, Gallo-Chico B, Ramirez-Barba EJ. Nutritional support in severe acute pancreatitis (in Spanish). *Nutr Hosp* 1996; 11: 160–6.
30. Bodoky G, Harsanyi L, Pap A, Tihanyi T, Flautner L. Effect of enteral nutrition on exocrine pancreatic function. *Am J Surg* 1991; 161: 144–8.

Discussion

Dr. Berger: To your knowledge are there any data showing that early antioxidant therapy will bring any changes, because there are groups [1] saying that they include them in their management. There are poor quality studies using selenium saying the same [2]. Are you aware of any developments in this area?

Dr. McClave: I was at ESPEN 2 and there were some papers on selenium, but I can't remember if they were on pancreatitis patients or not, but the effects you see from total parenteral nutrition (TPN) were improved. That is why I think it will be a huge step in improving the efficacy from TPN by including those very early on.

Dr. Nitenberg: I think you did not mention the type of enteral nutrition you propose for your patients. Do you think that in this type of patient with acute pancreatitis you can use polymeric diets or do you think that you have to use an oligopeptide diet or elemental diet?

Dr. McClave: A good question and a couple of different reactions. I think if the tube is down low enough the type of formula does not matter, but to ensure that there is tolerance then I think there are two categories of formulas that will work. One would be the old elemental nearly fat-free formulas, and this is the one disease process where I think that makes sense, in which the content of fat is the greatest stimulant of exocrine secretion. The other formula would be small peptide formulas in which the fat is in the form of medium chain triglycerides (MCT) and in the small peptides. There have been two studies, one in rabbits where the pancreatic duct was ligated, and individual amino acids were not absorbed as well as if they took the individual amino acids and made a dipeptide out of them, so that would suggest that peptides are better. And then there was a study in humans with cystic fibrosis in chronic pancreatitis and their small peptide absorption was better than elemental formulas. But I think if the tube is down low enough it is not a critical issue. Once 10 years ago we had the tube 10 or 12 cm below the ligament of Treitz and every time we started feeding we had an exacerbation of pain, and these were patients in whom I would use the fat-free elemental formula.

Dr. Moore: There is the concept that arginine via nitric oxide could hurt the gut. At our trauma research center we tried to implicate nitric oxide in different injury models, and it turns out that when we create sepsis with lipopolysaccharide (LPS), nitric oxide synthetase is expressed in the ileum. If we look at shock or gut ischemia reperfusion we don't get that same induction of nitric oxide synthetase. To implicate it into reperfusion injury of the gut we have to go to very severe ischemic insult. I think that hemorrhagic shock is different from sepsis when it comes to nitric oxide synthetase. The second point I would like to make is, you are saying that you are going to assess the severity of pancreatitis by the degree of pancreatic necrosis. That would mean you get a CT scan on everybody. The third comment I have is when Dr. Kudsk and I started promoting enteral nutrition in trauma patients in the late 1980's it took a decade before it became a standard of care. So I wonder now how you are going to promote this concept.

Dr. McClave: First on the issue of sepsis versus ischemia reperfusion versus pancreatitis, I think we are all nervous with circulating LPS and endotoxin to be pounded on with arginine, but the point I was trying to make was that pure stress alone without endotoxin might be different. I am not an immunologist, but this feeding alone produces that tolerance factor and a downregulatory response, is that going to help protect us in that situation? The second issue about whether or not we need a CT scan, they are going to get it anyway. This is controversial but I think it is almost a standard of care as if pancreatic necrosis is present on CT scan that antibiotics are standard of care. I agree with that. If the scores are really low, if you have 0 Ranson criteria to an alcoholic pancreatitis and alcohol ideology tends to have milder pancreatitis than the gold standard of some other ideology, and you have 5 Apache points, it would be tough to justify a CT scan there. I wish our residents and doctors would check these scoring systems before they get the CT scan, but it is close to being a standard of care I think. The last question is how do we promote this to other doctors. We had some conversation earlier this week that is it still the gold standard to give TPN, and I would make the point that there is a difference between the gold standard and common practice. I think the evidence would suggest that the gold standard should be enteral feeding but common practice is still TPN or providing nothing, and there we just have to educate our doctors and show them the data.

Dr. Rosenfeld: Just a short comment about a study in 1991 showing that TPN that was not started until 72 h reduced morbidity and complications. Could you comment on these results, does this reduce complications and morbidity?

Dr. McClave: Was that an earlier study where the timing of TPN was looked at?

Dr. Rosenfeld: Yes, not starting TPN until 72 h reduces complications and mortality.

Dr. McClave: All right, early versus late. I think it is tough without a control group that got no TPN and without a control group that got oral feeding. I don't know what to do with those data. I just suggest the opposite that we wait later and that is because we don't have a control group from that study. I can't extrapolate from that study.

Dr. Schulz: I think we have to focus a little bit on feeding the gut in different immune system settings. We should distinguish between the small bowel and the colon. The small bowel does not usually have relevant bacterial concentrations like the colon. Looking at the immune system there is also a big difference because we find no Peyer's patches in the colon but we have millions of lymphocytes and intraepithelial lymphocytes in the colon. T-cell subtypes differ in their homing location in the intestine. From an immunological standpoint and the different physiological functions, the colon and the small bowel look like different organs. This has to be considered when we talk about feeding the gut and using fiber for the colon mucosa or immune-enhancing diets for the small bowel mucosa. My question is, do you have any data about the bacterial setting in necrotic pancreatitis? We have tried to find some, but have failed so far.

Dr. McClave: First about your comment, I would almost put the question back to you. I guess we are interested in permeability at the level of the colon because that is where all the bacteria are, pus is the setting, is the environment, is permeability determined by what is going on higher up in the small bowel where this immune tissue is, and I would think it could be the situation where what is going on in the small bowel sets the tone for the colon. You might comment on that. As far as evidence of what is in the pancreatic abscess and where they came from: usually these are multiorganisms and they tend to be enterocoliforms. There are all kinds of anecdotal data that bacteria from the gut are getting through lymphatics or micropools in the colon and then are setting the pancreas from the gut, but they are anecdotal data. But certainly those data on endotoxin exposure would suggest that you may infect the pancreas from coliforms in the gut.

Dr. Cynober: I would like further comment on the question of nitric oxide. Just to summarize the result of very simple experiments we performed in our laboratory with rats (unpublished data). We had control rats and of course no mortality occurred. We had healthy rats receiving *L*-nitro-arginine methyl ester (L-NAME) or a thiourea which are inhibitors of the constitutive nitric oxide isoform and inducible enzyme, respectively, there was no mortality with the two inhibitors. Then in another group we administered LPS from *Escherichia coli* at 10 mg/kg and there was also, no mortality. The 4th group was rats receiving both LPS and L-NAME, and we had 40% mortality. When L-NAME was replaced in another group by thiourea again we had no mortality. In my opinion we have to carefully discuss this issue because obviously in a certain number of situations the effect is not the same whether you are inhibiting nitric oxide synthetase in the endothelium or in immune cells. There are data which indicate that the nitric oxide-increased production by endothelial cells in the splanchnic area is absolutely mandatory to maintain regional blood flow, and blocking this enzyme will kill the animals. Finally from the data you presented I have not noticed any positive effect with an immune-enhancing diet, but I have also not noticed deleterious effects.

Dr. McClave: You are right, there is a dichotomy here that inhibiting nitric oxide is not, it is a double edge sort, they are good things that come from generating nitric oxide-like bacterial killing and the other thing is blood flow, but maybe that is one of the issues that maintains blood flow into the gut. I don't know what the right answer is. The bigger concern for me is do we behave differently if there is ongoing sepsis at the outset and noncirculating endotoxin versus they are just inflamed with the pancreatitis. We start our immune formula and then the patients become septic: are we obligated to stop or can we just feed through the sepsis; I don't know the answer to those questions.

Dr. Martindale: My question is on the timing of the CT – back to Dr. Moore's question. As you know if you do it at 72 h you have a 90% accuracy of picking up pancreatic necrosis, if you do it at 24 h it is only about a 50% accuracy. So I wonder if there should be a time when we resuscitate the patients, watch them, and then CT them to look for the necrosis?

Dr. McClave: I think we have to be careful. I believe in this window of opportunity and I don't know how long it is. The best thing I can do is look at the studies where the patients get enteral feeding versus they don't. When the patients don't get enteral feeding, usually by around day 5 or 6 they are starting some feeding. So you can almost look at feeding within 48 h to 5 or 6 days, and I think we are going to see benefits from the early feeding. If we wait until the 72-hour marker to let the CT scan decide for us, we may be missing opportunities, so I would go back to the scores on admission and at 48 h to determine whether we feed or not, and the time of the CT scan is usually somewhere in there. It is a great point, you can miss necrosis if the CT scan is done too early.

Dr. Carlson: One of the things that we see in surgical practice is the establishment of infected pancreatic necrosis if only for the reason that we don't know that we are into a cycle of complex high-risk surgical treatment. It is clear that there are groups of people who develop sterile necrosis who you can often treat conservatively and it takes a long time until they settle, and there is another group of patients who develop infective necrosis who very rapidly deteriorate and have a prohibitive mortality if you don't operate on them. The question I want to ask is, what are the factors in relation to intestinal microbiology which determine which people get sterile and which people get infected necrosis? Bengmark (unpublished) for example has recently done some work on synbiotics. Is this an area we should be looking at, in which we are not just talking about manipulating gut nutrition but manipulating gut microbiology simultaneously.

Dr. McClave: It is a good question and I don't know whether feeding or not changes the bacterial flora in the gastrointestinal tract. But I think an important concept is that pancreatic necrosis is not a contraindication to feeding. It is actually the feeding, if anything, that is going to protect the patient from getting that necrosis infected, and I think that is the most important part. Whether it changes the flora or not I don't know.

Dr. Déchelotte: I would like to come back to a point of pathophysiology which perhaps addresses the time of early ischemia of the pancreas itself. It is well known that in these patients there may be some splanchnic ischemia including the gut and pancreas. I can remember an experimental study in rats some years ago with chemically induced pancreatitis that was aggravated with simultaneous ischemia, the pancreas itself with an increase in the IL-8 level. We know that IL-8 is a good predictor of severity in the pancreas. There was a study by Debaux in glutamine-supplemented parenteral nutrition that nicely showed a declined the IL-8 level, and on the other hand Roth has shown negative results in pancreatitis. So my suggestion would be to think of an earlier supply of some specific nutrients to the gut and to the pancreas, at the same time protecting from this ischemic and oxidative stress injury quite early, because we generally discuss nutritional support in acute pancreatitis patients after 2 or 3 days at the best, and by then we have probably missed half of our ability to do something.

Dr. McClave: Great point and I am fascinated by the concept that enteral feeding would help promote blood flow to the pancreas and prevent ischemic damage. The second issue that this evokes is the concept of adequate resuscitation, and we have talked about the danger of overloading with salt water, but in pancreatitis they really talk about being overly aggressive to the point that your end point of adequate resuscitation is a drop in hematocrit by 10%. So I think apart from getting feeding started, there is also adequate resuscitation. These patients are obviously losing water and volume and it is a very important part, maybe just as important as feeding.

Dr. Déchelotte: Do you think it would be possible to have minimal enteral feeding in these patients, very minimal caloric supply in the very early hours, but maximal supply of the specific nutrients such as glutamine and antioxidants?

Dr. McClave: I made a comment yesterday about how much enteral feeding it takes to get the job done. I don't think trophic feeding is enough. What we are talking about is the functional opening up of those channels and I think it takes closer to 50–60% of calories to get that achieved so I think you have to get the feeding high enough or you won't get the end point you want.

Dr. Labadarios: One would accept that the enteral route is becoming increasingly the route of choice in pancreatitis. The data you presented seemed to show that there is a group or a subgroup within a population of patients with mild to moderate pancreatitis, who actually don't tolerate enteral feeding. What reasons do you think may be involved in those patients who actually do not tolerate enteral feeding?

Dr. McClave: I am not sure I understand what you are getting at there, but you may be referring to the Schneider study where they didn't know how severe the pancreatitis was and yet they tried to enterally feed the patients, which means that they tried to enterally feed patients with mild and moderate pancreatitis. Tolerance is a slippery slope and there is a tremendous variation in the local expertise and their ability to do it right, and so I think that is why we see differences in tolerance. Does that answer your question?

Dr. Labadarios: Partly yes. Perhaps I should make my question a little bit clearer. The concept that is emerging is that all patients with mild to moderate pancreatitis will tolerate enteral feeding provided you don't lose the window of opportunity, but clinical experience may actually be a little bit different.

Dr. McClave: You might be misinterpreting it. I don't think they need nutritional support unless a complication develops or they deteriorate. But if our assessment priorities are correct on admission, the mild or moderate patients will do well, the chances are they will be on an oral diet within 7 days, and the risk of complications is very low. So really you don't need to challenge them with enteral feeding. That does not mean they won't exacerbate on day 5 when you give them clear liquids, there is no guarantee, but the point is that you don't need to have aggressive artificial nutritional support in those patients.

Dr. Fusco: How can you avoid pancreatic stimulation just feeding by the intragastric route? In our experience the only way to reduce the pancreatic enzyme flow is to infuse enteral feeding after the ligament of Treitz.

Dr. McClave: I had a talk with Dr. Imrie 2 weeks ago. We had a very sick patient, who we described in our lecture, a 72-year-old man with 5 Ranson criteria, which means a 40% mortality rate, diabetic, on the ventilator with chronic renal insufficiency, BUN and creatinine of 50 and 5 on a good day, and he got into the study. We randomized the jejunal feeding and he did well for 6 days. Then on the 7th day he became very ill and his temperature went from 37.8 to 40 °C, his white count, which had decreased from 20 down to 15, shot up to 30, and he looked septic. But all our cultures were negative, the chest X-ray which already showed inflammatory respiratory distress syndrome did not change, none of the cultures were positive. I remember at 4 o'clock in the afternoon I got a call from one of my colleagues who just told me that the tube was back in the stomach. We put the tube back down into the jejunum, no other management occurred other than that, and the fever went back down and the patient did well, but it scared us to death. And that is why I comment on the Imrie study. If your institution is still trying to decide how they stand on this issue, I do not encourage intragastric feeding because a patient like this will scare everybody. But Imrie's experience tells us that we can be surprised at how many patients with severe pancreatitis will tolerate that.

Dr. Fusco: This is not our experience because usually when we put the feeding tube into the stomach, we have many problems, particularly abdominal pain and bleeding, and so on. Maybe in the intensive care unit the patients are sicker and they won't tolerate this.

Dr. McClave: Another point I would like to make is that the tube needs to be down at or below the ligament of Treitz, and it is difficult for a radiologist to do this, and certainly bedside techniques can do that. They are secured with the bridle to the nose because if we are going to spend 30 min putting it in the right place we don't want it to come out 12 h later, that is important.

Dr. Ribeiro: If the gut is the main source of infection in severe acute pancreatitis is there a place for early selective decontamination of gastrointestinal tract?

Dr. McClave: The whole concept of decontamination is a huge controversial topic and there are tons of studies. My understanding is that it does eradicate short-term infection but that concepts of factorial resistance because of huge issue. We certainly don't have any data on pancreatitis. I think we can accomplish our end points without doing that.

Dr. Maiorova: I want to attract your attention to extremely severe acute pancreatitis in children. The reason for the development of acute pancreatitis in children is usually different from adults and, on the other hand, children are not always small adults. So could you comment. Would you suggest some differences in nutritional support of small patients or children with acute pancreatitis compared with the adults?

Dr. McClave: I am an adult gastroenterologist, I just don't have any experience, I am sorry.

Dr. Martindale: Are you using immune-enhancing diets in your pancreatitis patients now?

Dr. McClave: No but I really want to bring it up because Nestlé has agreed to support a trial. We are doing a multicenter trial right now and we are going to have 3 arms in the study, TPN done correctly, extreme enteral feeding with immune formulas, and then a group that gets nothing for 5–7 days and then goes to TPN or enteral feeding. I think using immune formulas is the right way to go, but it needs to be looked at.

Dr. Déchelotte: Don't you think you should have a 4th arm with standard enteral nutrition?

Dr. McClave: Yes, that would be the ideal, to have a group that gets a standard enteral formula and a group that gets an immune-enhancing formula. But the problem is patient recruitment is tough, even with the 7 centers that we have identified.

Dr. Bouletreau: I have a question going back to gastric feeding, because from a clinical point of view it is so much easier. Do you think it would be harmless to begin with gastric feeding and test tolerance, and then switch to jejunal feeding in a second round?

Dr. McClave: I don't think it is a good idea because the patient would get sick instead of better, and if you go and put the tube down their nose and their stomach and they get worse, can you image what it is going to be like to say to them now we want to go back and use a bigger tube, an endoscope that goes further down. I think it would be problematic. But it is a great point and I think there is a percentage of patients that would tolerate it, but I don't think it is the best way to go.

Dr. Bouletreau: So what is your recommendation?

Dr. McClave: You get the tube in, you do your markers on admission. In our institution these patients are in the emergency room for 20–24 h, so by the time we are called they are well into the 2nd day. If we react immediately and get them on schedule that day, we are still barely getting the tube in within 48 h from the time they came to the hospital. So you really have to mobilize forces quickly and get the tube in.

Dr. Rosenfeld: How do you follow up tube position?

Dr. McClave: We don't have to be getting the KUB every day, we can be guided by patients' symptoms. You check amylase and lipase but you can't have a tight think about it. If the patient is on TPN and the amylase goes from 250 to 270 nobody worries because he is on TPN. If it goes from 250 to 256 he is on enteral feeding. So you use it with clinical judgment. The patient's symptoms of abdominal pain, nausea, are valid and can guide your judgment. Another thing you should pay attention to is the residual volume. If the tube is in the small bowel and everything is going well, the residual volume should be $<10\,cm^3$, it should be very low. In a patient where the tube flips back from the small bowel to the stomach the residual volume about 12 h before goes to 50 and then 80 and then 120. So patients' symptoms can guide you and if they are questionable, if there is slow resolution of the symptoms, you might check those tube positions, and certainly after you have placed the tube check it one time as your start.

Dr. Martindale: Another controversial area that I hear many questions on is the amount of fat in the diet. As you know cholecystokinin is stimulated by fat in the diet. Does a high-fat diet make this worse? The second question on this, should we withhold intravenous lipids from people that we are unable to treat enterally?

Dr. McClave: I will start with the fat content diet first. Dr. Friedman is a gastroenterologist at Harvard who has done some studies on this. His patients have chronic alcoholic pancreatitis and are in and out of the hospital. They drink a small peptide formula with medium chain triglyceride oil orally. He can keep his patients out of hospital and has better pain management just by that dietary manipulation, drinking it. The data on fat in TPN in pancreatitis are on the case report level and there are two papers. One was a horrible case report: the patient got abdominal pain, went to surgery and had complications. It turned out to be pancreatitis. He had been getting TPN, and they did not check the triglyceride levels, they just said that it could be the fat in the TPN. But in the second study by Lashner and Henauer, the patient was on 10% fat and tolerating it well. This patient had inflammatory bowel disease. They went to 20% fat and the patient got pancreatitis. He had pancreatitis, and when the fat went to 20% he flared, but when it went back down to 10% it was well tolerated. I think if your triglyceride levels are below 400 you are fine.

Dr. Déchelotte: I would like to come back to the point of gastric feeding and nasojejunal feeding. It seems to me that until now we don't have the evidence that gastric feeding would be really worse than nasojejunal feeding. We have studies in healthy volunteers showing that intragastric feeding stimulates pancreatic secretion in comparison to nasojejunal feeding which inhibits pancreatic secretion. But in these settings with rather low amounts of nutrition in the first days I think we like the evidence, and it is a very important practical point because it is time-consuming as you know to put in nasojejunal tubes. The nasogastric tube moves every time, and it has a great impact on the medical facilities and medical time in our units. We have some data from groups such as our colleagues in Budapest who reported 2 or 3 years ago in ASPEN or the European Gastroenterology Congress that they always put gastric tubes in their pancreatitis patients, even severe patients, just because they do not have nasojejunal tubes available, and they have had very good experience with tolerance. It was not a randomized trial actually, but I think this rough experience on over 300 patients fed intragastrically is quite astonishing.

Dr. McClave: It is a great point and it hits on the issue of local expertise and can we find cost-effective ways of getting the tube into the small bowel and how can we get either our radiologist or endoscopist to get this tube down the small bowel, how can we do it cost-effectively and more easily. We are working on this. We are working on things like a portable camera that has a battery-operated light source so the whole cord is not dragged down, you just work with it in your arms and slime it down quickly, a small caliber tube that goes to the nose so you have to sedate the patient. Those are some moves in the right direction. But you have a good point about intragastric feeding, that a lot of patients are going to tolerate it, but I think you are playing with fire. Physiologically all that stimulation is right there, there are three levels but the big one is right there in the proximal duodenum. So I would rather work on expeditious low-cost ways to get into the small bowel.

Dr. Schultz: When you talk about enteral nutrition do you mean enteral nutrition with or without fiber? Are there any arguments against increased fiber contents?

Dr. McClave: I would be interested to see that but I have no data and I am not even sure what results I would expect. But it is very important and it should be investigated. That is why I said we have a lot of questions still to be answered in this area.

References

1. McCloy R. Chronic pancreatitis at Manchester, UK – Focus on antioxidant therapy. *Digestion* 1998; 59 (Suppl 4): 36–48.
2. Schoenberg MH, Buchler M, Younes M, Kirchmayr R, Bruckner UB, Beger HG. Effect of antioxidant treatment in rats with acute hemorrhagic pancreatitis. *Dig Dis Sci* 1994; 39: 1034–40.

Cynober L, Moore FA (eds): Nutrition and Critical Care.
Nestlé Nutrition Workshop Series Clinical & Performance Program, Vol. 8, pp 000–000,
Nestec Ltd.; Vevey/S. Karger AG, Basel, © 2003.

Nutritional Support in Sepsis and Multiple Organ Failure

Gérard Nitenberg

Department of Anesthesia, Intensive Care and Infectious Diseases,
Institut Gustave-Roussy, Villejuif, France

The scope of this review is to provide practical guidelines for nutritional management of critically ill patients with sepsis with or without multiple organ failure (MOF). Basically, any nutritional intervention must be based on a better understanding of septic 'autocannibalism' [1]. Clearly, sepsis causes much the same metabolic disturbance as trauma or injury, but it must be stressed that sepsis is more often complicated by subsequent insults, which explains why in some instances nutritional or metabolic support should be modulated according to different post-inflammatory states, now termed systemic inflammatory response syndrome (SIRS), compensatory anti-inflammatory response syndrome and mixed adapted response syndrome. Finally, present definitions of sepsis, SIRS and septic shock are too broad and insufficiently specific: instead, mechanistic definitions should provide more homogeneous groups of patients [2] and favor the development of new modalities on nutritional and metabolic support.

What Is the Goal of Nutritional Support in Sepsis?

As long as the hemodynamic and respiratory status remains unstable, it is probably harmful to start complex nutritional support: the nutrient supply can consist simply of sufficient glucose (200–300 g/day) to meet the requirements of glucose-dependent tissues, and of 'critical' electrolytes and vitamins, such as phosphorus and folinic acid.

When the initial sepsis does not rapidly lead to death and the patient has stabilized, it seems reasonable to begin nutrition, thereby avoiding the onset of severe metabolic disorders and/or nosocomial infections which can engender

Table 1. Nutritional or metabolic support in sepsis: A dynamic approach

Condition	Duration	Treatment
Early acute phase of stress[1] Treat the cause of sepsis Support vital functions	1–4 days	Glucose 200–300 g/day
Prolonged hypermetabolism High cardiac output state Hypercatabolism	≥5 days	Nutritional/metabolic support (immunonutrition?)
Recovery phase	weeks	Anabolic nutrition (hormonal adjunctive treatment?)
Irreversible ARDS or MODS		Nutrition is useless

ARDS = Acute respiratory distress syndrome; MODS = multiple organ dysfunction syndrome.

[1] In case of preexisting malnutrition, minimal nutritional support may be initiated immediately.

irreversible multiple organ dysfunction syndrome (table 1). Nutritional (metabolic) support is aimed at preventing or limiting the processes of malnutrition and immunosuppression which can be cofactors in the morbidity and mortality associated with sepsis states. However, nutritional support is at present one useful tool among others to help recovery in these patients in whom outcome clearly results from the combined effects of optimal therapeutic measures.

Energy Supply in Sepsis: Is More Better?

The estimation of resting energy expenditure (REE) by standard formulae (e.g., the Harris-Benedict equations corrected by stress factors) cannot be easily extrapolated to septic patients because of fluctuations according to fever, sedation, mechanical ventilation, etc. The measurement of REE by indirect calorimetry is possible, even in patients under mechanical ventilation if the inspired oxygen concentration is lower than 0.6–0.7, giving reasonable accuracy in the order of 5% [3]. Total energy expenditure (TEE) is generally no more than 1.2–1.5 higher than REE in patients with septicemia or peritonitis during 7–10 days, but progressively increases in severely septic surgical patients up to 1.7–1.8 higher than REE after 1 week [4], a fact that correlates with the results obtained during recovery from sepsis syndrome or septic shock. Calculation of VO_2 using a Swan-Ganz catheter does not correlate well with indirect calorimetry, owing to the arbitrary choice of a fixed respiratory quotient, especially in unstable patients where underestimation of VO_2 by the Swan-Ganz method can reach 20–30%.

Table 2. Proposed nutritional support for the septic patient

Energy requirements
    25–35 kcal/kg/day (acute phase)
    35–50 kcal/kg/day (recovery phase)? (see text)
Energy sources
    Glucose <6 g/kg/day
    Lipids (LCT or MCT/LCT) 0.5 g/kg/day to 1 g/kg/day
    Continuous administration over 24 h recommended
Amino acids or proteins
    1.2–2 g/kg/day (0.20–0.35 gN/kg/day)
    Adaptation according to level of catabolism (BUN, nitrogen balance)
    Conventional crystalline amino acid solutions (PN)
    Polymeric diets (EN)
Vitamins
    Standard balanced formulas (PN)
        +Vitamin K (10 mg/day)
        +Vitamin B_1 and vitamin B_6 (100 mg/day)
        +Vitamins A, C and E (antioxidants?)
Trace elements (provided normal renal function)
    Complete standard solutions
        +Zn (15–20 mg/day plus 10 mg/l of liquid stool)
        +Se (120 mg/day)
Electrolytes
    Based on daily plasma concentrations (Na^+, K^+, Ca^{2+})
        +P^{2-} (>16 mmol/day)
        +Mg^{2-} (>200 mg/day)

LCT = Long-chain triglycerides; MCT = medium-chain triglycerides;
PN = parenteral nutrition; EN = enteral nutrition.

In practice, total energy requirements in the septic patient are in the order of 25–35 kcal/kg/day (table 2). In the context of sepsis, the most important concern is not to do harm. Therefore, it is preferable to avoid excess, which cannot prevent the intense protein catabolism associated with sepsis and has well described detrimental effects [5]. However, during the recovery phase, it could be advisable to increase this amount to achieve energy balance, thus preserving endogenous fat stores.

A Classical Dilemma: Glucose or Lipids as Optimal Energy Source?

We think this question should be addressed in terms of anabolic drive in septic patients [6], but few studies have been dedicated to this problem.

Taking into account that a prevalent glucose system (70–80%) seems to be the most efficient tool to optimize protein metabolism [6, 7], glucose infusion can be progressively increased to maximal tolerance in so far as, during sepsis, the defect is not in glucose oxidation (providing endogenous release of insulin is adequate), but rather in declined nonoxidative disposal of glucose. The maximum rate of glucose oxidation is in the order of 5–6 mg/kg/min, therefore, the recommended supply of glucose for septic patients is about 3–5 g/kg/day [7].

The maximal effectiveness of insulin is decreased to approximately 50% below normal in sepsis [7]. Therefore, the addition of insulin when the endogenous blood insulin is elevated does not appear to be justified, except for avoiding hyperglycemia and osmotic polyuria. Hyperglycemia is common in critically ill patients, and this situation can predispose to nosocomial infections [8]. In a recent study by Van den Berghe et al. [9], at the time of admission to the intensive care unit (ICU) surgical patients were randomly assigned either to strict normalization of blood glucose (4–5.5 mmol/l) with intensive insulin therapy or to conventional treatment in which insulin was given only when the blood glucose level exceeded 11 mmol/l. Mortality in the group assigned to intensive insulin therapy was lower than that in the control group (4.6 vs. 8.0%; $p < 0.04$). Benefit was achieved mainly through a reduction in the incidence of MOF with a proven septic focus. In-hospital mortality and morbidity were also lower in this group. However, the value of these impressive results is restricted to patients undergoing surgery (most often cardiac surgery) at a single institution. Further studies in other groups of critically ill (septic) patients is essential to confirm its benefits. Until then, widespread adoption of this treatment would be premature.

Although there is theoretically no impairment in the ability to oxidize fatty acids during sepsis, the oxidation and clearance rates of lipids from the blood fall rapidly as the severity of sepsis increases, further suggesting poor utilization and peripheral adipose tissue storage. In addition, controversy remains surrounding the possible immunosuppressive effect of lipids in the septic patient because long-chain triglycerides (LCT) reduce the functions of the reticuloendothelial system, neutrophils, and the ratio of T-helper to T-suppressor cells. Finally, alterations in alveolar macrophages could partially explain the transient desaturation seen during intermittent infusion of lipid emulsions. However, Druml et al. [10] found no side effects in septic patients, with or without hepatic failure, during a low-rate LCT lipid infusion, suggesting that the deleterious effects of LCT emulsions are unlikely as long as the infusion rate is not excessive.

With regard to these problems, medium-chain triglycerides (MCT) have been proposed because of their potential advantages in septic patients, i.e. more even balance of n-3 and n-6 fatty acids, rapid clearance from the plasma, limited storage, and more rapid oxidation than LCT. However, recent clinical data are inconsistent and suggest that MCT-LCT emulsions do not offer clear-cut advantages over LCTs in terms of the lipid oxidation rate [11], pulmonary hemodynamics and gas exchange in septic acute respiratory distress syndrome (ARDS) [12], and do not support the systematic use of such emulsions in septic patients.

In practice, lipids can safely contribute 20–35% of nonprotein calories in septic patients or even less in patients who are very seriously septic (table 2). In any event, it is best to give a continuous 24-hour infusion, for example, with a glucose-lipid-protein mix.

Low or High Nitrogen Supply?

In the context of sepsis, equilibrium or positivity of nitrogen balance is not the goal and can even be detrimental if it leads to a rise in the metabolic stress. Correctly adapted nitrogen supply can, however, reduce the myofibrillar breakdown and stimulate synthesis of certain proteins, especially hepatic proteins involved in immune defenses. Ishibashi et al. [13] suggested that even the current recommendation of 1.2–2.0 g protein/kg/day does not take the over-hydration (up to 15 liters) of resuscitation into account, and proposed 1.0–1.2 g protein/kg/day as a fair approximation of optimal protein requirements. Interestingly, the same group showed that, despite an adequately mixed energy intake, patients lost about 13% of their total body protein over the 3 weeks following peritonitis, and this loss occurred early from the skeletal muscle, and later from visceral organs, likely leading to some loss of function.

In practice, a nitrogen supply of 200–300 mg/kg/day, i.e. 1.2–1.8 g protein/kg/day appears to be adequate (table 2), so that the ideal nonprotein calorie to grams of the nitrogen ratio in septic patients is about 100–120:1 rather than the 'classical' 150:1. An increase in nitrogen supply does not improve nitrogen balance or decrease net protein breakdown, and leads to a significant increase in energy expenditure, urea accumulation and CO_2 production.

Micronutrients and the 'Antioxidant' Concept

Iron administration is a matter of debate in septic patients. For some, any attempt at iron replacement could facilitate its availability to microorganisms. For others, severe iron deficiency impairs resistance to infection and should be corrected [14]. Deficiencies in zinc can lead to the persistence, and even the onset, of sepsis due to immune deficiency, and requirements are increased to up to 20–30 mg/day when exogenous amino acids are administered. The clinical value of trace element supplementation was elegantly proven by Berger et al. [15] in burn patients: this supplementation of copper, zinc and selenium led to a significant decrease in the number of bronchopneumonia infections and a shorter hospital stay.

It is clear that oxidative stress is increased in patients with sepsis or at risk of sepsis. Plasma concentrations of potential antioxidants, such as selenium and some vitamins (C, E, and β-carotene) are reduced in critically ill patients. Although results from many animal studies and from one clinical pilot trial [16] are encouraging, trials of early administration of antioxidants have produced uneven results, especially in the settings of reperfusion injury and ARDS after sepsis. Additionally, β-carotene and vitamin C also have pro-oxidant properties [17]. The debate is going on, and meanwhile the only certainty is that septic patients should not be deficient in micronutrients (table 2).

(Early) Enteral Nutrition: A Fashion or a Dogma?

Here I will focus on new (and frequently conflicting) data relevant to the specific field of sepsis and MOF, where definite evidence of the superiority of enteral nutrition (EN) over parenteral nutrition (PN) is still lacking [8, 18].

The Significance of Bacterial Translocation in Septic Patients

Animal studies have shown that loss of the gut-barrier function may result in bacterial (and endotoxin) translocation and, in some instances, in systemic septic complications. In humans, the three main factors promoting bacterial translocation are present in sepsis: increase in intestinal permeability (not synonymous of translocation); decreased host immune defenses, and alterations in gut ecology. However, translocation has been shown to occur in a variety of conditions, such as surgery and intestinal obstruction [19, 20], but excluding sepsis. Thus, there is little evidence in this context that bacterial translocation acts either as a promoter or an initiator of generalized sepsis or MOF, especially when no source of infection is identifiable. This failure cannot be accounted for by inadequate technology, since DNA fragments can now be detected by molecular biology and polymerase chain reaction in the blood of patients [21].

Moreover, there is limited evidence to support the view that bacterial translocation is reduced by the use of EN or increased in patients receiving short-term PN. Thus, the increased incidence of sepsis apparently associated with total parenteral nutrition (TPN) may simply reflect the detrimental effects of overfeeding and hyperglycemia. To summarize, PN is not guilty of mucosal atrophy, altered gut-barrier function, and septic complications. Moreover, EN can cause severe problems in septic patients (see below), so that optimal nutritional care demands the use of both methodologies, often simultaneously [19].

Apart from the use of complex immune-enhancing diets, enrichment in glutamine has been shown to reduce the incidence of endotoxinemia and mortality in various animal models of gut failure, but low-dose glutamine

(20 g/day) does not obviously affect bacterial translocation. The enteral administration of short-chain fatty acids, the preferred fuel for the colonocyte, appears to reduce the atrophy of the colonic mucosa. However, in the future, the optimal therapy to maintain or restore intestinal mucosal structure and function may be a combination of specific enterally administered nutrients and mucosal trophic factors [22].

Practice and Risks of Enteral Nutrition in Septic Patients

Good reasons for the increased use of EN in ICU septic patients are numerous. EN is supposed to preserve intestinal-barrier status, to maintain secretory immunoglobulin A and gut-associated lymphoid tissue (which plays a major role as a barrier against intestinal translocation) [23], but also to enhance splanchnic blood flow and mesenteric oxygen utilization in sepsis.

Thus, to institute EN as soon as possible in ICU patients is probably justified, although problems linked to EN and more pronounced in ventilated septic patients, such as gut failure, bacterial overgrowth, and nosocomial pneumonia, cannot be forgotten [24]. Exclusive EN is precluded in unstable patients at the early stage of sepsis, because of the risk of exacerbating intestinal ischemia and of favoring the ischemia-reperfusion phenomenon. However, minimal EN (to preserve the immunologic function of the gut?) could be implemented early, in conjunction with PN, and gradually increased at the expense of intravenous intake [25], underlining that dichotomy between EN and PN is an obsolete controversy.

Once the hemodynamic and respiratory status has stabilized, the two major risks of EN are aspiration pneumonia and diarrhea. In most septic patients, EN intolerance can be controlled by the judicious use of prokinetics [26]. Only when gastroparesis persists, should postpyloric administration of EN be considered, although this does not seem to effectively reduce the incidence of aspiration and pneumonia. Diarrhea can usually be controlled by reducing the flow rate of the mixture, and by providing sufficient intraluminal sodium (above 80 mmol/l of diet), but the danger is to overlook a 'silent' gut failure with underlying ischemia with a high risk of entry into a MOF state. Therefore, EN may be considered a 'stress test': persistent symptoms of gut failure usually indicate a poor prognosis, and are a formal indication for withholding or withdrawing EN [27] (fig. 1).

Is Parenteral Nutrition Associated with a Higher Morbidity than Enteral Nutrition?

There is in fact reasonable evidence that TPN is associated with a higher incidence of septic morbidity in critically ill patients with severe burns and patients with blunt or penetrating trauma [8, 28]. However, there is no consistent evidence that in sepsis EN is associated with improved clinical outcome when compared with TPN.

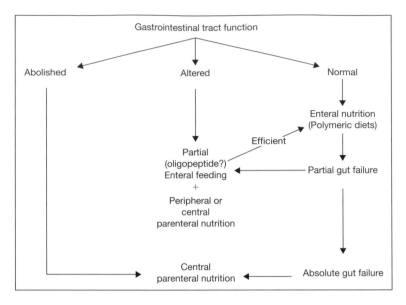

Fig. 1. Example of a decision tree for selecting the type of nutritional support in sepsis. It must be kept in mind that at least a part of the nutrition can be delivered by the enteral route in almost all the cases.

Does the Timing of Enteral Nutrition Administration Affect Infectious Morbidity and Mortality?

Again this question has never been well studied in septic patients. Based on experimental studies showing that early EN is associated with a decreased cytokine and catabolic response to sepsis, starting EN as soon as possible could be an essential prognostic factor, but results of well-designed studies are somewhat inconsistent, or even worrisome [29]. Clearly, further studies are required before firm conclusions may be made.

To sum up, EN can improve the outcome of (severely?) septic patients when nutrition is initiated at an early stage, within 24–48 h after the initial septic event. After the 2nd or 3rd day, EN and PN appear to give similar results. EN seems to be accompanied by an increased incidence of gastrointestinal side effects and a higher failure rate in achieving targeted nutrition support goals [30], so my experience and my personal recommendation is to institute early partial EN with the goal of exerting beneficial effects on the gut, and to carefully increase the delivery rate to avoid splanchnic hemodynamic impairment.

'Immunopharmacology' in Sepsis

During the last decade, new specific substrates now termed 'immuno-nutrients' or 'nutraceuticals' have been used with the aim of preserving intestinal

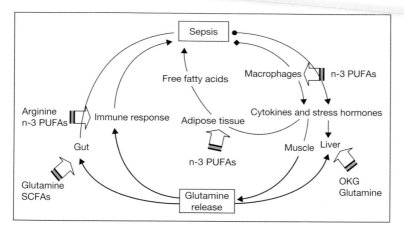

Fig. 2. Potential roles and sites of action of immunonutrients in sepsis. The optimal dosage, route and timing of administration of each nutraceutical (alone or in combination) is unknown. OKG = Ornithine α-ketoglutarate; SCFAs = short-chain fatty acids; PUFAs = polyunsaturated fatty acids.

barrier function, maintaining antioxidant defenses, and correcting specific metabolic and/or immunologic disturbances, which are partially dependent on cell activation induced by mediators (fig. 2).

New Lipids

Conventional intravenous lipid emulsions and enteral diets are relatively rich in n-6 polyunsaturated fatty acids (PUFAs), and are poor in n-3 PUFAs (fish oil) whose degradation leads to 10- to 100-fold less platelet activation and thrombogenesis compared to n-6 PUFAs. Thus, reducing the n-6/n-3 PUFA ratio makes sense within the setting of severe sepsis and MOF [31]. However, there are some restrictions to this stimulating concept [32]: the suppression of T-cell-mediated immune function has an adverse effect of fish oil supplementation, and the suitable action of fish oils on mediators may depend on the timing of administration, i.e. during the acute sepsis syndrome or later, when 'chronic sepsis' is established. Additionally, the metabolic fate of n-3 PUFAs is markedly dependent on the route of administration, either enteral or parenteral. One randomized study was specifically focused on the effect of EN enriched with eicosapentaenoic acid, γ-linolenic acid and antioxidants on the post-injury response in 146 mechanically ventilated patients with ARDS [33]. In the 98 evaluable patients, mainly those in whom a feeding period of 4–7 days could be completed, the specialized diet had beneficial effects on gas exchanges, the need for mechanical ventilation and ICU care, and significantly reduced the onset of new organ failures. However, in the intention-to-treat analysis, there was no difference between the groups in terms of infectious morbidity, hospital stay, and mortality. Future studies are now needed to elucidate the molecular mechanisms modified by fish oils to improve dietary strategies in sepsis and MOF.

Is Qualitative Manipulation of Nitrogen Substrates Useful In Septic States?

Glutamine becomes an essential amino acid in inflammatory conditions such as injury and sepsis, and is the preferred fuel and precursor of purines and pyrimidines for rapidly dividing cells such as lymphocytes, macrophages and enterocytes. It is involved in inter-organ nitrogen transport and in glutathione synthesis, thus offsetting free radical generation. Moreover, glutamine requirements increase considerably during inflammatory states, and relative tissue glutamine deficiency may thus occur [34]. As with other pharmaconutrients, data gathered from studies carried out in heterogeneous populations of critically ill patients should be carefully extrapolated to septic ICU patients [35]. In addition, dose-effect studies aimed at determining the optimal dosage of glutamine are lacking.

In a randomized, controlled trial of 84 ICU patients, including a large subset of septic patients [36], survival at 6 months was improved in the group of patients receiving glutamine-supplemented (20 g/day) TPN (p = 0.049), owing to late deaths in the control group, which were unlikely related to nutrition. Costs and length of hospitalization were also reduced in the patients receiving glutamine. It is noteworthy that the author himself has indicated that these results 'seem too good to be true' and are only applicable 'to a very small subset of very sick septic ICU patients with gut failure'. This is in agreement with the global negative results of the largest trial of glutamine supplementation (20 g/day) of PN in 170 hospitalized patients [37], although subgroup analyses suggest that supplementation may have advantages in selected populations, such as septic patients, patients with MOF and those with hematologic malignancies.

Two randomized studies of glutamine-supplemented EN in critically ill patients have also been reported. The first compared a glutamine-enriched (10 g/l) diet with an isonitrogenous glycine-enriched control diet in 78 ICU patients [38], and was unable to show any difference in mortality or the length of ICU and hospital stay between the 2 groups, but showed reduced costs in the glutamine group. The other compared a diet based on strong enrichment in glutamine (30.5 g/100 g of protein) and a large percentage of arginine (8.5 g%), with a control isocaloric, isonitrogenous enteral diet in 72 multiple trauma patients [39]. There was a significantly lower incidence of pneumonia and bacteremia in patients fed glutamine. However, the duration of mechanical ventilation and the length of hospital stay were not different, and the mortality rates (probably low) were not reported.

In sum, although the body of evidence suggesting clinical benefits from the utilization of glutamine is growing, the available data are not sufficient to recommend its routine use, either by the enteral or the parenteral route, in critically ill septic patients. Further trials are clearly required to establish firm dose recommendations, to identify whether the enteral route for glutamine administration should be preferred for patients with mild infection, and to confirm whether a reduction in mortality is effective in severe sepsis.

The anabolic properties, the anticatabolic properties (stimulation of glutamine, arginine and proline synthesis), and the immunomodulatory capabilities of ornithine α-ketoglutarate (OKG) are well adapted to ICU septic patients. Moreover, ornithine is a precursor of polyamines, which are essential for cell multiplication in the intestinal mucosa. Indeed, enteral administration of OKG in severely burned patients has shown favorable results in terms of both metabolic parameters and morbidity [40]. However, no study demonstrating the effect of this nitrogen compound in septic patients is presently available.

Arginine is a conditionally essential amino acid in adults and becomes essential in hypermetabolic and septic states. Arginine enhances T-lymphocyte proliferation and activation, and significantly increases hepatic protein synthesis in various models of gram-negative sepsis [41]. In addition, arginine may contribute to the complex cellular interactions evoked in septic animals or patients via increased production of reactive nitric oxide [42]. However, administration of arginine-enriched enteral diets raises certain conceptual problems in sepsis, on one hand, because the metabolic interactions between arginine and glutamine (in diets containing both substrates) are complex and potentially detrimental, and on the other hand, because its bioavailability is strongly decreased after enteral administration in severe infection. There is an urgent need to better define the value and the optimal level of enteral supplementation in arginine for critically ill septic patients, as certain animal data suggest that an excessive concentration could be harmful [43].

Do Immune-Enhancing Diets Improve the Outcome of Septic Patients?

The concept of nutritional immunopharmacology has become the rationale for the marketing of specific enteral formulas aimed at modulating the inflammatory and immune response injury in immunocompromised patients. All the recent systematic reviews confirm that these diets reduce the rate of infective complications and the length of hospital stay after major surgery and in trauma patients [44, 45]. But whether they are likely to improve the clinical outcome of ICU septic patients remains questionable. Well-designed randomized, controlled studies have been carried out recently in heterogeneous populations of ICU patients, some of them being septic, but only one study specifically addressed the question in septic patients (table 3).

In a multicenter double-blind, randomized study involving 326 ICU patients (mostly young and traumatized), the patients received early EN with either Impact or an isocaloric nonisonitrogenous diet [46]. The only objective, paradoxical result of the intention-to-treat (ITT) analysis is that mortality was higher in the Impact group than in the control group (23/147 vs. 10/132;

Table 3. Prospective randomized controlled trials of immune-enhancing diets in septic and nonseptic ICU patients

Reference	Patients (n) Diet(s)	Isocaloric isonitrogenous	Results Statistical significance	Efficacy? Comments
Bower et al. [46], 1995	ICU (n = 326) Impact vs. Osmolite	No (IED > Std) No (IED > Std)	⇑ Mortality with Impact(!) ⇓ Infections (NS) ⇓ LOS (p < 0.05) In the 'septic' subgroup	No Complex and questionable post hoc stratification Marginal and partial benefit for septic patients
Atkinson et al. [47], 1998	ICU (ITT, n = 398; 'successful early nutrition', n = 101) Impact vs. Std	Yes	Identical mortality (48 vs. 44%) in ITT ⇓ Duration MV, LOS, SIRS (all p < 0.05) in the 'successful early nutrition' subgroup	Yes ? 'early nutrition' subgroup defined a priori, but unchanged mortality and morbidity Waiting for the medico-economic study
Jones et al. [38], 1999	ICU patients (n = 78) Gln-enriched EN vs. Std	Yes	No difference in late (6 months) mortality, ICU and hospital LOS ICU and hospital costs (p = 0.036) in the treated group	No Per protocol analysis (50 'successful EN' patients) Interesting cost-efficacy evaluation
Gadek et al. [33], 1999	ICU patients with or at risk of ARDS (n = 142) n-3 and vitamin E-enriched diet vs. Std	Yes	⇑ PaO_2/FiO_2 (p < 0.05) Duration MV and ICU LOS (p < 0.05) in the treated group	± Per protocol analysis (n = 98) Mortality and hospital LOS not improved Intrinsic role of antioxidants on lung?
Galban et al. [48], 2000[1]	ICU, septic patients (n = 176) Impact vs. Precitene HN	Yes	⇓ Mortality (19 vs. 32%; p < 0.05) Nosocomial Infections (p = 0.01) and bacteremias (p = 0.01) in the Impact group	Yes No difference in LOS and duration of MV Beneficial effect of the IED more pronounced in less severe patients (10 < Apache II < 15)

IED = Immune-enhancing diet; LOS = length of stay; ITT = intention-to-treat; SIRS = systemic inflammatory response syndrome; Gln = glutamine; MV = mechanical ventilation; EN = enteral nutrition.
[1] Nonblinded study.

p = 0.051 in the χ^2 test)! The post hoc allocation of the patients to 4 subgroups according to the food actually received is a flawed use of baseline data, as the statistical power of the study was insufficient, and it is based on the assumption that treatment has no influence on the result. To make a long story short, the incidence of infections was not different between the 2 groups, and the shorter median length of stay in the Impact subgroup of 89 patients with sepsis (18 vs. 28 days; p < 0.05) was no doubt explained by the excess deaths!

The study of Atkinson et al. [47] evaluated the clinical effects of Impact and a control diet in 398 mechanically ventilated ICU patients. In the ITT analysis there was no difference between the 2 groups in terms of mortality, infectious morbidity, or the ICU/hospital length of stay. However, in the 'early effective nutrition' subgroup (those receiving more than 2.5 liters of EN in the first 72 h), Impact yielded a significant reduction in the duration of mechanical ventilation, the length of ICU stay and hospital stay, as well as the average duration of SIRS (p < 0.05 for all these markers). These results strongly suggest that immunomodulating diets are clinically effective in those ICU patients who can receive early and complete EN, but the key problem is that we are unable to identify this subpopulation a priori. Are septic patients the best candidates? Is it worthwhile offering this type of nutrition to all ICU patients, and then to select probable responders according to EN tolerance?

The most relevant study by Galban et al. [48] was a multicenter, nonblinded, prospective, controlled trial involving 181 ICU septic patients who were randomly assigned to receive Impact or an isonitrogenous, but not isoenergetic, diet. The most striking result was that mortality was reduced in the Impact group of these 'true' septic patients, and in post hoc analysis this reduction was even more significant in the subgroup with less severe illness (APACHE II score between 10 and 15). However, the length of hospital stay and duration of mechanical ventilation (after censoring for the mortality rate) were not different between groups, nor was different the number of nosocomial infections. The more favorable effect in the less severely septic patients suggests that this subset of patients, close in terms of severity to surgical and trauma patients, may be more responsive to nutraceuticals.

For the Future, Is It Really Alimentary?

The clear ambition of immunopharmacological (enteral) nutrition in (septic) critically ill patients is to improve the outcome of patients. The counterpart is that proof of clinical efficacy must be shown in trials with the same methodologies as those used for new drugs (e.g. antibiotics).

This crucial question has been analyzed in several articles on the effects of supplemented enteral nutrition in critically ill patients [44, 45], but not specifically in septic patients. For septic patients in the ICU, the correct mortality and length-of-stay endpoints depend on a variety of factors related to the severity of illness, primary disease, reason for admission to the ICU, the nature of nutritional treatment, etc. Survival analysis techniques should be

235

used to avoid the influence of practice patterns on the interpretation of mortality, and to censor the effects of death on the length of ICU or hospital stay. To avoid the problem of competing mortality, another solution might be to calculate life-support-free days (e.g. the number of days without mechanical ventilation), a measure that combines mortality and morbidity. In addition, some discrepancies among efficacy analyses of immune nutrition can be explained by the different methodological approaches of the individual studies: ITT analyses, efficacy analyses, and compliance analyses. Despite the progress borne to our practice by evidence-based medicine, we must never forget that truth has variable geometry in medicine, that recommendations are not rules, and that each medical decision relies on outcome trials but should be highly individualized [44].

My personal opinion is that infective morbidity and, presumably, length of hospital stay are reduced by immune EN in multiple trauma patients, and in major surgery. However, such clear-cut evidence is lacking for ICU patients, and especially septic ICU patients, who are too often intolerant to (early) enteral nutrition despite the extensive use of prokinetics. Another subsidiary problem is that we cannot yet determine which nutraceutical(s) is (are) responsible for the improved clinical outcomes, so we have to blindly arbitrate between individual immunonutrients (glutamine, n-3 fatty acids, OKG, etc.), and between the different immune-enhancing diets.

Hormonal Interventions

Recombinant human growth hormone (GH) has the strongest anabolic properties, including stimulation of muscle-free glutamine retention, and plays a role in the enhancement of antioxidant defenses and in the control of proinflammatory cytokine production. Unfortunately, in severely stressed patients, such as those with sepsis, added GH may not be biologically active or could even be harmful. Thus, in two well-designed parallel randomized studies involving a total of 532 ICU patients (in which we concede the subset of septic patients was not clearly stated), in-hospital mortality was significantly higher in the GH groups and persisted at the 6-month follow-up, whatever the type of stratification [49]. Among the potential reasons for such an apparently paradoxical result, the unusual underfeeding of the patients and the very high doses of GH that were used in the trial (0.10 mg/kg/ – 1 mg = 3 IU) must be underlined. In summary, the use of GH in ICU septic patients cannot presently be recommended.

A large number of the physiologic actions of GH are mediated at the tissue level by IGF-1 that is released in response to GH. The lack of response to GH could be due to a blunted response of IGF-1 to GH, a consistent finding in sepsis [50]. IGF-1 is a short-acting compound, which reduces protein breakdown, increases protein synthesis, but causes abrupt and severe hypoglycemia.

Preliminary results of recombinant human IGF-1 use in catabolic patients are encouraging, but the effects are transient, so additional studies are needed to determine if this concept is valid in critically ill septic patients.

It has become evident that male and female sex steroids are involved in the regulation of immune responses and in the development of cell and organ dysfunction after acute stress. Knoferl et al. [51] have nicely explored this approach in different animal models with exciting preliminary results. In a recent study [52], 60 multiple trauma patients were randomized to receive either 10 mg oxandrolone twice daily or placebo (thiamine, 50 mg) in addition to the same immune-enhancing diet for 28 days. No differences were seen in body cell mass changes, length of ICU and hospital stay, and incidence of septic events or MOF. Therefore, whether anabolic steroids play a role in selected (septic?) subsets of catabolic ICU patients is yet to be elucidated.

Conclusions

The primary goal in the initial phase of sepsis is to implement aggressive measures to preserve the hemodynamic and respiratory status, while searching for and treating the cause of sepsis. Nutritional support is useless and potentially detrimental, until the patient's condition has stabilized. When this is achieved, nutrition must begin without any delay in order to prevent severe post-insult malnutrition, but the role of nutrition (enteral or parenteral) as a life-support modality remains controversial in these instances. Some principles are now considered as 'gold standards' for conventional nutrition, such as the dangers of overfeeding, the restriction of lipids and to a lesser degree carbohydrates, a careful increase in nitrogen supply, and special attention must be paid to micronutrient supply. However, we have to remain open minded about unsolved debates: the actual benefit of (early) enteral nutrition, the adequate amount and nature of the nitrogen supply, the optimal lipid/carbohydrate ratio in severe sepsis, or the clinical relevance of antioxidant therapy. In these times of cost containment, we have to bring proof of the clinical efficacy of the concept of 'immunopharmaconutrition', before the use of nutraceuticals, individually or in combination, enterally or parenterally, can be proposed as a standard of care. The conception, realization and interpretation of well-conducted prospective clinical trials in ICU/septic patients, characterized by the highest risk of development of multiple organ dysfunction, are our challenges for the next years.

References

1. Nitenberg G, Gachot B, Antoun S. Metabolic response to sepsis. In: Thijs L, Dhainaut J, eds. *Sepsis*. London: Blackwell, 2000; 327–36.
2. Abraham E, Matthay MA, Dinarello CA, Vincent JL, Cohen J, Opal SM, Glauser M, Parsons P, Fisher CJ Jr, Repine JE. Consensus conference definitions for sepsis, septic shock, acute lung

injury, and acute respiratory distress syndrome: Time for a reevaluation. *Crit Care Med* 2000; 28: 232–5.

3. McClave SA, Kleber MJ, Lowen CC. Indirect calorimetry: Can this technology impact patient outcome? *Curr Opin Clin Nutr Metab Care* 1999; 2: 61–7.

4. Uehara M, Plank LD, Hill GL. Components of energy expenditure in patients with severe sepsis and major trauma: A basis for clinical care. *Crit Care Med* 1999; 27: 1295–302.

5. Klein CJ, Stanek GS, Wiles CE 3rd. Overfeeding macronutrients to critically ill adults: Metabolic complications. *J Am Diet Assoc* 1998; 98: 795–806.

6. Iapichino G, Assi E, Minuto A, Pasetti G, Zaniboni M. Which metabolic strategies in the early phase of injury? *Minerva Anestesiol* 1999; 65: 455–63.

7. Wolfe RR. Sepsis as a modulator of adaptation to low and high carbohydrate and low and high fat intakes. *Eur J Clin Nutr* 1999; 53 (suppl 1): S136–42.

8. Jeejeebhoy KN. Total parenteral nutrition: Potion or poison? *Am J Clin Nutr* 2001; 74: 160–3.

9. Van den Berghe G, Wouters P, Weekers F, Verwaest C, Bruyninckx F, Schetz M, Vlasselaers D, Ferdinande P, Lauwers P, Bouillon R. Intensive insulin therapy in the critically ill patients. *N Engl J Med* 2001; 345: 1359–67.

10. Druml W, Fischer M, Ratheiser K. Use of intravenous lipids in critically ill patients with sepsis without and with hepatic failure. *JPEN J Parenter Enteral Nutr* 1998; 22: 217–23.

11. Delafosse B, Viale JP, Pachiaudi C, Normand S, Goudable J, Bouffard Y, Annat G, Bertrand O. Long- and medium-chain triglycerides during parenteral nutrition in critically ill patients. *Am J Physiol* 1997; 272: E550–E5.

12. Smirniotis V, Kostopanagiotou G, Vassiliou J, Arkadopoulos N, Vassiliou P, Datsis A, Kourias E. Long chain versus medium chain lipids in patients with ARDS: Effects on pulmonary haemodynamics and gas exchange. *Intens Care Med* 1998; 24: 1029–33.

13. Ishibashi N, Plank LD, Sando K, Hill GL. Optimal protein requirements during the first 2 weeks after the onset of critical illness. *Crit Care Med* 1998; 26: 1529–35.

14. Brock J. Benefits and dangers of iron during infection. *Curr Opin Clin Nutr Metab Care* 1999; 2: 507–10.

15. Berger MM, Spertini F, Shenkin A, Wardle C, Wiesner L, Schindler C, et al. Trace element supplementation modulates pulmonary infection rates after major burns: A double-blind, placebo-controlled trial. *Am J Clin Nutr* 1998; 68: 365–71.

16. Tanaka H, Matsuda T, Miyagantani Y, Yukioka T, Matsuda H, Shimazaki S. Reduction of resuscitation fluid volumes in severely burned patients using ascorbic acid administration: A randomized, prospective study. *Arch Surg* 2000; 135: 326–31.

17. Halliwell B. The antioxidant paradox. *Lancet* 2000; 355: 1179–80.

18. Lipman TO. Nutrition support for the critically ill: Parenteral, enteral, or none? In: Nitenberg G, Chioléro R, Leverve X, eds. *Nutrition artificielle de l'adulte en réanimation.* Paris: Elsevier, 2002; 135–50.

19. MacFie J. Enteral versus parenteral nutrition: The significance of bacterial translocation and gut-barrier function. *Nutrition* 2000; 16: 606–11.

20. Kanwar S, Windsor AC, Welsh F, Barclay GR, Guillou PJ, Reynolds JV. Lack of correlation between failure of gut barrier function and septic complications after major upper gastrointestinal surgery. *Ann Surg* 2000; 231: 88–95.

21. Teba L. Polymerase chain reaction: A new chapter in critical care diagnosis. *Crit Care Med* 1999; 27: 860–1.

22. DeWitt RC, Wu Y, Renegar KB, King BK, Li J, Kudsk KA. Bombesin recovers gut-associated lymphoid tissue and preserves immunity to bacterial pneumonia in mice receiving total parenteral nutrition. *Ann Surg* 2000; 231: 1–8.

23. Zarzaur BL, Kudsk KA. The mucosa-associated lymphoid tissue structure, function, and derangements. *Shock* 2001; 15: 411–20.

24. Montejo JC. Enteral nutrition-related gastrointestinal complications in critically ill patients: A multicenter study. The Nutritional and Metabolic Working Group of the Spanish Society of Intensive Care Medicine and Coronary Units. *Crit Care Med* 1999; 27: 1447–53.

25. Omura K, Hirano K, Kanehira E, Kaito K, Tamura M, Nishida S, Kawakami K, Watanabe Y. Small amount of low-residue diet with parenteral nutrition can prevent decreases in intestinal mucosal integrity. *Ann Surg* 2000; 231: 112–8.

26. Booth CM, Heyland DK, Paterson WG. Gastrointestinal promotility drugs in the critical care setting: A systematic review of the evidence. *Crit Care Med* 2002; 30: 1429–35.

27. Wolf SE, Jeschke MG, Rose JK, Desai MH, Herndon DN. Enteral feeding intolerance: An indicator of sepsis-associated mortality in burned children. *Arch Surg* 1997; 132:1310–4.
28. Marik PE, Zaloga GP. Early enteral nutrition in acutely ill patients: A systematic review. *Crit Care Med* 2001; 29: 2264–70.
29. Ibrahim EH, Mehringer L, Prentice D, Sherman G, Schaiff R, Fraser V, Kollef MH. Early versus late enteral feeding of mechanically ventilated patients: Results of a clinical trial. *JPEN J Parenter Enteral Nutr* 2002; 26: 174–81.
30. De Jonghe B, Appere-De-Vechi C, Fournier M, Tran B, Merrer J, Melchior JC, Outin H. A prospective survey of nutritional support practices in intensive care unit patients: What is prescribed? What is delivered? *Crit Care Med* 2001; 29:8–12.
31. Mayer K, Grimm H, Grimminger F, Seeger W. Parenteral nutrition with n-3 lipids in sepsis. *Br J Nutr* 2002; 87 (suppl 1): S69–S75.
32. Furst P, Kuhn KS. Fish oil emulsions: what benefits can they bring? *Clin Nutr* 2000; 19: 7–14.
33. Gadek JE, DeMichele SJ, Karlstad MD, Pacht ER, Donahoe M, Albertson TE, Van Hoozen C, Wennberg AK, Nelson JL, Noursalehi M. Effect of enteral feeding with eicosapentaenoic acid, gamma-linolenic acid, and antioxidants in patients with acute respiratory distress syndrome. Enteral Nutrition in ARDS Study Group. *Crit Care Med* 1999; 27: 1409–20.
34. Jackson NC, Carroll PV, Russell-Jones DL, Sonksen PH, Treacher DF, Umpleby AM. The metabolic consequences of critical illness: Acute effects on glutamine and protein metabolism. *Am J Physiol* 1999; 276: E163–E70.
35. Neu J, DeMarco V, Li N. Glutamine: Clinical applications and mechanisms of action. *Curr Opin Clin Nutr Metab Care* 2002; 5: 69–75.
36. Griffiths RD, Jones C, Palmer TE. Six-month outcome of critically ill patients given glutamine-supplemented parenteral nutrition. *Nutrition* 1997; 13:295–302.
37. Powell-Tuck J, Jamieson CP, Bettany GE, Obeid O, Fawcett HV, Archer C, Murphy DL. A double blind, randomised, controlled trial of glutamine supplementation in parenteral nutrition. *Gut* 1999; 45: 82–8.
38. Jones C, Palmer TE, Griffiths RD. Randomized clinical outcome study of critically ill patients given glutamine-supplemented enteral nutrition. *Nutrition* 1999; 15: 108–15.
39. Houdijk AP, Rijnsburger ER, Jansen J, Wesdorp RI, Weiss JK, McCamish MA, Teerlink T, Meuwissen SG, Haarman HJ, Thijs LG, van Leeuwen PA. Randomised trial of glutamine-enriched enteral nutrition on infectious morbidity in patients with multiple trauma. *Lancet* 1998; 352: 772–6.
40. Coudray-Lucas C, Le Bever H, Cynober L, De Bandt J, Carsin H. Ornithine alpha-ketoglutarate improves wound healing in severely burn patients. A prospective randomized double-blind trial versus isonitrogenous controls. Crit Care Med 2000; 28: 1772–6.
41. Efron D, Barbul A. Role of arginine in immunonutrition. *J Gastroenterol* 2000; 35 (suppl 12): 20–3.
42. Bruins MJ, Soeters PB, Lamers WH, Meijer AJ, Deutz NE. *L*-Arginine supplementation in hyperdynamic endotoxemic pigs: Effect on nitric oxide synthesis by the different organs. *Crit Care Med* 2002; 30: 508–17.
43. Suchner U, Heyland DK, Peter K. Immune-modulatory actions of arginine in the critically ill. *Br J Nutr* 2002; 87 (suppl 1): S121–S32.
44. Nitenberg G, Raynard B, Antoun S. Enteral immunonutriton in critically ill patients: A critical approach. In: Pichard C, Kudsk K, eds. *From nutritional support to pharmacologic nutrition in the ICU*. Berlin: Springer, 2000; 384–408.
45. Heyland DK, Novak F, Drover JW, Jain M, Su X, Suchner U. Should immunonutrition become routine in critically ill patients? A systematic review of the evidence. *JAMA* 2001; 286: 944–53.
46. Bower RH, Cerra FB, Bershadsky B, Licari JJ, Hoyt DB, Jensen GL, Van Buren CT, Rothkopf MM, Daly JM, Adelsberg BR. Early enteral administration of a formula (Impact) supplemented with arginine, nucleotides, and fish oil in intensive care unit patients: Results of a multicenter, prospective, randomized, clinical trial. *Crit Care Med* 1995; 23: 436–49.
47. Atkinson S, Sieffert E, Bihari D. A prospective, randomized, double-blind, controlled clinical trial of enteral immunonutrition in the critically ill. Guy's Hospital Intensive Care Group. *Crit Care Med* 1998; 26: 1164–72.
48. Galban C, Montejo JC, Mesejo A, Marco P, Celaya S, Sanchez Segura JM, Farre M, Bryg DJ. An immune-enhancing enteral diet reduces mortality rate and episodes of bacteremia in septic intensive care unit patients. *Crit Care Med* 2000; 28: 643–8.

49. Takala J, Ruokonen E, Webster NR, Nielsen MS, Zandstra DF, Vundelinckx G, Hinds CJ. Increased mortality associated with growth hormone treatment in critically ill adults. *N Engl J Med* 1999; 341: 785–92.
50. Dahn MS, Lange MP. Systemic and splanchnic metabolic response to exogenous human growth hormone. *Surgery* 1998; 123: 528–38.
51. Knoferl MW, Angele MK, Schwacha MG, Bland KI, Chaudry IH. Preservation of splenic immune functions by female sex hormones after trauma-hemorrhage. *Crit Care Med* 2002; 30: 888–93.
52. Gervasio JM, Dickerson RN, Swearingen J, Yates ME, Yuen C, Fabian TC, Croce MA, Brown RO. Oxandrolone in trauma patients. *Pharmacotherapy* 2000; 20: 1328–34.

Discussion

Dr. Bozzetti: Are you suggesting that side effects from long-chain triglycerides were mainly caused by fast infusion, and if followed as low infusions they can be given cyclically?

Dr. Nitenberg: I think it is a complex situation as usual. In terms of hemodynamic status and also in terms of the properties of polymorphonuclears, such as chemotaxis and phagocytosis. We showed 10 years ago that when you administer the usual lipid emulsion, 20% intralipid, over more than 8 h without exceeding 500 ml in 8 h, you do not modify the chemotactic and phagocytic properties of the cell. In the same way we and others have shown that in fact the modification of intrapulmonary shunting and pulmonary circulation is very small, very marginal and over a very short time. One hour after the end of the infusion you have no effect, and when you administer lipids over 24 h you have absolutely no effect. This has been proven, and I remember it was also shown by your group a few years ago.

Dr. Rosenfeld: We are now going into a new area with new methods of depuration in the critical illness setting, such as plasma absorption for sepsis and hepatic dialysis. Are there any recommendations or work going on about this subject?

Dr. Nitenberg: In the setting of nutritional support I am sure there are none, unless you are aware of any work on this topic. In general about the intensive care unit (ICU) population, there are many studies about blood purification, I don't like the term blood purification. There are stimulating studies about the idea that when you perform depuration of cytokines at the right moment in the right people, which is very difficult to achieve, you can perhaps modify the course of severe sepsis. But to date, to my knowledge, there is no study at all in the ICU population about this type of intervention. But obviously it is one of the future goals of support to septic patients in the ICU.

Dr. Déchelotte: I would like to come back to the first part of your presentation on conventional parenteral nutrition in septic patients. I find it quite interesting that 10 or 30% lipids do not make any difference in the outcome of the patients. But it would be very interesting to know what difference the 10% makes in comparison to 45 or 50%, because many commercially available free-component total parenteral nutrition (TPN) diets do provide about 40 and even 45% lipids, and are routinely used in many ICU units. So I think it would be wise to check whether 10% lipids would be enough for essential fatty acid supply and provide energy with only glucose on the other hand.

Dr. Nitenberg: I totally agree with you. Until recently I wasn't sure that the administration of lipids or standard lipid emulsions in ICU patients was really dangerous. Now my opinion has changed a lot and I do agree. Probably until the threshold of 30 or 40% lipids in the amount of calories you administer to the patients, there is no clear difference in the outcome of these patients. If you go beyond this point to 50 or 60%, as you can see in some bags, it could be dangerous and it could also be metabolically dangerous because you provoke fatty infiltration and you have other problems that have been demonstrated for example by Tappy and Chioléro in Lausanne. That is the reason why in my unit we don't use these bags in ICU patients. We do not use triple solutions, only glucose protein solution in bags and we add lipids after that at various quantities, not exceeding 25–30% of the amount of calories. Sometimes in very sick patients we only administer lipids two times a week. So I totally agree with your opinion.

Dr. Berger: You were advocating early TPN especially if enteral nutrition was failing, but then we are far away from early TPN because we don't know if enteral nutrition will fail clinically before the 3rd or the 4th day if we have managed to reach the targets. So we are actually talking about medium TPN, my question is, do we know of any evidence that there are early high requirements for energy in sepsis? I am not aware of any trial in that sense.

Dr. Nitenberg: In the beginning of the sepsis, it depends on what sepsis you are talking of. In septic shock nutrition is not a problem so you have to concentrate on other therapeutic measures. In several forms of sepsis during the phase of resuscitation the need for nutrition probably does not exist, and it was suggested in old work by Payen that it could be deleterious, especially on the splanchnic bed. That study was performed in rabbits but it could perhaps be translated to patients, although I am not sure of that. In severe sepsis you really have to wait until the beginning of nutritional support. How long you have to wait, nobody knows.

Dr. Heyland: I feel the need to clarify or respond to the immunonutrition data that were presented and are limited to the sepsis population. But I think there are two other studies that contribute to this debate on the value of immunonutrition in the septic population. They are unpublished studies but they demonstrate an increased mortality in patients with infections and patients with sepsis. One of those was a study by Ross that it is coming to press at least in abstract form at an upcoming meeting. In that study there was a subgroup of patients with pneumonia which explained all the excess mortality. There is another study which compared parenteral nutrition to an immune-enhanced diet and was stratified on the basis of sepsis, similar to the Bauer study, and they found excess mortality in the septic population so they stopped enrolment of patients with sepsis in the study. So there is an emerging signal that immune stimulation in this septic population has a potential for doing considerable harm. Now on the contrary, there is the Golban study which is very challenging to interpret because the definition of sepsis was extremely loose. It certainly would not meet the same criteria as the other studies with severe sepsis, basically in positive culture and treatment with antibiotics to get into the study. All the treatment effect was observed in the least sick patients, patients with an Apache score of 10–15. Our average Apache score for patients on enteral feeding is in the 20s. So I don't know who these patients are but they don't represent severely septic patients. There are a lot of methodological limitations with that study and that leads me to why we differ in our interpretation of the literature. If you look at intention-to-treat analysis and if you look at all the studies on critically ill patients you see different signals. If you combine the experience in elective surgical patients, in obese patients, you are going to see a different picture, but if you look strictly at what is happening in critically ill patients then you look at the intention-to-treat analysis, you see a lack of signal of any benefit, but a signal of harm in the critically ill septic patients.

Dr. Nitenberg: I took that from your recent work and I put the question to the audience and to you: what is deleterious, what could be deleterious in the early phase of sepsis for these patients? Is it glutamine, is it arginine, is it n-3 fatty acids or is it only enteral nutrition by itself perhaps? I think this is a key point because we can't respond to this problem using your analysis.

Dr. Heyland: That is true. You are not going to answer that question looking at a meta-analysis, there are not sufficient details there. I don't think it is enteral nutrition by itself because both groups got enteral nutrition, so it has to be the additives in the immune-enhancing diet. Which one, I don't know. It is plausible, and I still believe that it is arginine as a precursor of nitric oxide synthetase in this population. But that is just a postulate, I don't know.

Dr. Cynober: I come back to a detail which in my opinion is not a detail. I was puzzled by your statement that, and I refer to the study of Griffiths et al. [1], there was a slightly significant difference. What is the difference between 'a slightly significant difference' and an 'interesting trend'. I think you are misusing the statistics because the principle of the statistics is the fact that you accept to be wrong at a certain risk, no more, no less, but once you have accepted this risk the things become significant or not. I think that it is very important to comply with this simple rule, otherwise we are in the situation of a recent meta-analysis discussing interesting trends [2], whereas other trends are considered as not interesting. Finally nobody understands what the final conclusion of the whole statistics together is.

Dr. Nitenberg: You can use statistics anyway you want to use them, that is the problem. Evidence-based medicine, which is sometimes called evidence-biased medicine, is a hard part of our work. I really think it helps you to understand how it is in our patients. But we have to think about statistics and we have to see what is clinically relevant and what is statistically significant. Sometimes it is statistically significant but not clinically relevant, and sometimes on the contrary it is not statistically significant but it is clinically relevant. We have to mix what is our experience and what is statistics. To come back to the interpretation of the 0.049 result of Griffiths et al. [1]. Of course this is the result and this is statistically significant. I said yesterday I don't know how 5 days of glutamine administration could influence the occurrence 4 months later of 1 myocardial infarction and 1 pulmonary embolism, which is the difference. In fact the outcome of only 1 patient could lead to nonstatistically significant results. So I think we have to think about that, not to say that the study is incorrect, this is a remarkable study. I won't say anything else. To come back to what you said about tendency, what is tendency? If I follow you it is significant or not. There is no tendency, there is only tendentious interpretation of the results.

Dr. Carlson: Just a comment and a question. The comment really relates to what Dr. Heyland just said about the difficulties in interpreting some of the studies of immune-enhanced diets. The problem is that you are not even comparing apples with oranges, you are potentially comparing apples with oranges at different stages of the development of the fruit on the tree, if I can use that analogy. One of the concerns relates to the effect of arginine on nitric oxide production. There is also quite old, I think from the lates 1970s, animal data suggesting that if you load animals with arginine before you give them endotoxin you produce a much bigger TNF response than that of endotoxin alone. So I guess one of the concerns that I have is that you may get different effects according to the time frame in the systemic inflammatory response syndrome (SIRS), compensatory anti-inflammatory response syndrome response, and perhaps if you treat people after the acute inflammatory episodes started to subside you may get beneficial effects. Certainly a lot of early deaths are actually from treatment very early in the SIRS episodes with immune-enhanced diets. That is the comment. The question I have is that you showed data which suggest that there are no adverse effects on infection rates using long chain triglyceride-based TPN. The concern I have is that bone marrow transplant patients have a fairly naked immune system, and therefore it could be argued that they are not a particularly useful group in which to compare the effect of lipid emulsion. If you look at the data from Okada et al. [3] on neonates, they found a significantly higher incidence of bacteremia in neonates fed intravenous fat compared with intravenous glucose, and in the TPN group there was impaired monocyte tumor necrosis factor (TNF) production and in vitro bacterial killing was found in the intravenous lipid-fed group. So the question I have is do you really believe that in the real world as opposed to in a test tube, giving large doses of intravenous fat is safe in an immuno-compromised septic patient?

Dr. Nitenberg: No, I did not say that. I think when I responded to the question from Dr. Déchelotte, I said that it could be hazardous to go over 30% of the energy amount in terms of lipids because we have some concern about the immunosuppressive risk of intravenous feeding with large amounts of lipid emulsion. However, if you look carefully at the literature, we have no clear proof of that. We have many suggestive data but we have no study proving that clearly, not only in septic patients but even in ICU patients. We have not yet done these experiments. We have to do that. I turn to Dr. Neu, is it true that lipid emulsions are really dangerous? When you showed your data you said that finally nobody knows clearly and you are increasing the amount of lipids you are giving.

Dr. Neu: That is the only study that I am aware of that really suggests this. I think in that particular population we really have to weigh the risks against the benefits. If you need a certain amount of calories to maintain these babies and also to provide for growth and to keep them from having denutrition during a very critical period of time, the balance still weighs toward giving the lipids.

Dr. Chioléro: I would like to make a comment on hemodynamically unstable septic patients since we all agree that during the septic shock phase is not the time to administer nutritional support. But during the subsequent phase when the patients have had noradrenaline but are unstable, we have collected some experience in Lausanne on enteral feeding giving them at least half or two thirds of the nutritional requirement by the enteral route. At the last ESPEN meeting Dr. Berger provided information on 70 cardiac surgery patients, a third of them had aortic counter pulsation, most received catecholamines. We were able to feed them enterally quite successfully. So in hemodynamically unstable patients, we believe there is no reason that enteral feeding should not be given.

Dr. Nitenberg: Really I don't know. I was surprised by the publication by Moore et al. about small bowel absorption, and finally I found two other examples in the literature. In my experience, in the very severe patients we have in our unit, I did not have this problem. So as you said, I think it is a late complication of enteral feeding in fact, not an early complication of enteral feeding. It is very interesting that when patients are hemodynamically unstable we have in fact not observed this type of necrotizing enteritis, unless we missed it. It is possible in very critically ill patients. There is one study from Russell et al., I think in 1995, in septic rats under mechanical ventilation showing that even when the hemodynamic status of the rats was restored, there was an incredible decrease in splanchnic perfusion and splanchnic extraction of oxygen, and when they added some amount of enteral feeding in these very severely septic rats they completely restored the oxygen extraction and the hemodynamic perfusion. Maybe small amounts of enteral nutrition in this critical period could be more beneficial than harmful, but we have to test this hypothesis.

Dr. Chioléro: We have tested giving enteral feeding with arginine and it was recently published in *Intensive Care Medicine*. The formula was Impact® which was administered over 6 h in cardiac surgery patients receiving high doses of catecholamine. Cardiac output increased, intramucosal pH was stable and the extraction of cardiogreen increased, so there was no sign of gut ischemia in these patients.

Dr. Moore: Nonocclusive bowel necrosis is a late event. In most patients it is due to enteral diets. One notable example was a patient who had recovered from multiple organ failure, and was on continuous hemofiltration. He was switched to intermittent dialysis. At the same time, he developed a septic event. Due to too much volume being removed during dialysis, the blood pressure dropped. Vasopressor agents were started.

The second notable case was a man who had a massive facial fracture and nearly exsanguinated. He survived but developed multiple organ failure. He was ultimately advanced to full dose jejunal feeding. After 12 days he was taken to the OR for a 10 hour reconstruction of his face. This was complicated by some excessive bleeding and his blood pressure dropped. The operating room staff didn't know that they should stop the feeding, and a day and half later he died. Critically ill patients are at risk for recurrent episodes of ischemia reperfusion, and we just have to be cautious to turn off the feeding when they get sick or something bad happens to them.

Dr. Kudsk: I want to compliment you on your brilliant presentation. There are not many studies in which patients with sepsis are generally randomized. I clearly remember that in both Dr. Moore's and my studies we showed a benefit. My study was in a group of very highly injured patients, Dr. Moore's was in a broader group. We did show a reduction in intra-abdominal abscess and septic complications and multiple organ failure. The second point is the Ross study (unpublished data) and I think that the population at risk was elderly septic patients with pneumonia. If one focuses on elderly septic pneumonia patients, I think it should be tested in another study whether there really is going to be an increase in mortality in this patient population. If it can be confirmed in a second study, I would clearly agree that in elderly septic pneumonia patients you should not use immuno-enhancing diets.

Dr. Nitenberg: I know your work and the work of Dr. Moore about trauma patients. The studies are very interesting but they only refer to multiple trauma patients in the States. We do not have that type of patient, they are very severely ill patients. If I remember correctly in the discussion of your paper you stated that your experience in fact concerns only 7% of your trauma patients included in the study. So I think the generality of this result is not obvious. That is my only comment.

Dr. Kudsk: Again it is only 7%, but with 4,500 admissions, many were people who came with isolated femoral fractures and we did not feed them enterally. Some of the patients, who we also did not feed, came in with gun shot wounds to the calf. So that is the whole population, but there was a much higher use in people who were admitted to the ICU.

References

1. Griffiths RD, Jones C, Palmer TE. Six-month outcome of critically ill patients given glutamine-supplemented parenteral nutrition. *Nutrition* 1997; 13: 295–302.
2. Cynober L. Immune enhancing diets in injured patients: An analysis of the analysis. *Metab Care* 2003; 6: in press.
3. Okada Y, Klein NJ, van Saene HK, et al. Bactericidal activity against coagulase-negative staphylococci is impaired in infants receiving long-term parenteral nutrition. *Ann Surg 2000;* 231: 276–81.

Cynober L, Moore FA (eds): Nutrition and Critical Care.
Nestlé Nutrition Workshop Series Clinical & Performance Program, Vol. 8, pp. 245–264,
Nestec Ltd.; Vevey/S. Karger AG, Basel, © 2003.

Nutraceuticals in Critical Care Nutrition

Hank Schmidt and Robert Martindale

Department of Surgery, Medical College of Georgia, Augusta, Ga., USA

The importance of nutritional support in surgical patients cannot be overstated, particularly in the realm of intensive care settings. Prevention of mucosal atrophy and stimulation of the gut-associated lymphoid tissue (GALT) by early enteral feeding in postoperative surgical patients has only recently become part of our standard of care. Feeding the gut is clearly a stimulant for the immune system, and plays a key role in lower infection rates measured in patients receiving enteral as opposed to parenteral nutrition. This association between nutrition and infection has been known for centuries. The World Health Organization report in 1968 clearly defined this association and began to set goals in clinical nutrition [1]. The understanding of the gastrointestinal (GI) tract as a major component of the human immune system and a key modulator of the organism's response to stress and injury has subsequently opened the door to an exciting new field of specialized enteral preparations sometimes referred to as nutraceuticals. The recent expansion of our understanding of stress metabolism and the systemic inflammatory response has influenced critical care nutrition on two levels. First, as stated above, is the importance of the provision of enteral macronutrients, namely a patient's requirement for protein, carbohydrate, and lipids. Secondly, research in nutraceuticals seems to have focused on various combinations of micronutrients and 'conditionally' essential nutrients. Nutraceuticals are felt to function in cellular metabolic pathways where increased demands associated with the stress response benefit from supplementation. These nutrients may be the key to fine-tuning enteral formulas for specific clinical scenarios.

For centuries, man has sought the therapeutic benefits of naturally occurring substances as components of the human diet, acknowledging the connection between health and nutrition. With the explosion of knowledge and analytical techniques in biochemistry and molecular biology, investigators may now pinpoint the specific role of many of these elements in human metabolism. This same knowledge has also produced a far greater understanding of the systemic response to stress, effected by severe catabolism and loss of lean body mass [2]. Historically, nutritional support in critically ill patients has sought to provide adequate calories and protein to induce nitrogen balance, preventing peripheral muscle breakdown. However, we have learned that provision of adequate protein and calories does not prevent loss of lean body mass in the critically ill patient. Our attention has therefore turned to supplementation of caloric requirements with specific nutrients designed to impact critical metabolic pathways. One of the earliest clinical studies evaluating such selective supplementation randomized burn patients to receive a modular tube feeding recipe (MTF), or one of two other enteral nutritional regimens traditionally used in this population. The MTF consisted of a high-protein, low-fat formulation enriched in n-3 fatty acids, arginine, cysteine, histidine, zinc, vitamin A, and ascorbic acid. Significant benefits were observed in MTF-fed patients who had lower infection rates and shorter length of hospital stay [3].

Since the first recognition of enteral nutrition as an immunomodulatory phenomenon, investigators have been challenged to find 'the right mix' for any given patient or clinical scenario. This knowledge has also essentially created a market to drive pharmaceutical research in this direction (table 1). We are now faced with the challenge of optimizing specific preparations through indepth analysis of micronutrients and their individual roles in human metabolism. A wealth of in vitro, in vivo, animal and human data has been produced in the process of examining the physiology of dietary

Table 1. Immune-modulating enteral formulas

Formula	Manufacturer	Major additives
Crucial®	Nestlé	Marine oil, arginine
Immun-Aid®	Braun	Arginine, glutamine, BCAA, nucleic acids
Impact®	Novartis	Arginine, fish oil, RNA
Impact Glutamine®	Novartis	Arginine, fish oil, RNA, glutamine
Impact with Fiber®	Novartis	Arginine, fish oil, RNA, fiber
Impact 1.5®	Novartis	Arginine, fish oil, RNA
Oral Impact	Novartis	Arginine, fish oil, fiber
Intensical®	Meade/Johnson	Arginine, canola oil, fish oil
Optimental®	Ross	Arginine, structured lipid, fish oil, canola oil
Oxepa®	Ross	Sardine, borage oil, canola oil
Alitraq®	Ross	Glutamine, arginine
Perative®	Nestlé	Arginine, canola oil

nucleic acids, arginine, glutamine, n-3 fatty acids, and an array of other less studied nutrients.

Arginine

Arginine, like glutamine, is classified as a nonessential amino acid in unstressed conditions since the body synthesizes adequate arginine for normal maintenance of tissue metabolism, growth and repair [4]. During major catabolic insults such as trauma or surgery, an increase in urinary nitrogen, excreted largely as urea, represents the end products of increased lean body tissue catabolism and reprioritized protein synthesis. Arginine during these stress situations becomes conditionally essential in that demand is greater than endogenous supply.

Numerous animal and human studies indicate that supplemental dietary arginine is beneficial for accelerated wound healing, enhanced immune response, and acceleration in attainment of positive nitrogen balance [5]. The exact mechanisms for these benefits are yet to be entirely understood but may in part be the result of arginine's role as a potent anabolic hormone secretagogue. Growth hormone, glucagon, prolactin, and insulin release are all increased with supplemental arginine. Arginine is also the substrate for production of nitric oxide and citrulline by nitric oxide synthase. Nitric oxide is a ubiquitous molecule with significant roles in the maintenance of vascular tone, coagulation cascade, immunity, stimulation of angiogenesis, modulation of the effects of endotoxin, and regulation of GI tract absorptive and barrier function [6]. Nitric oxide has also been implicated as a participant in numerous disease states as diverse as sepsis, hypertension, and cirrhosis. Arginine is also the substrate for the enzyme arginase with end products urea and ornithine. Through the production of ornithine and urea, arginine promotes proliferation of fibroblasts and collagen, both essential for later stages of wound healing. Arginine and its metabolite ornithine also serve as precursors for polyamine biosynthesis. Polyamines play a pivotal role in cell division, and DNA synthesis [7]. By supplying the amidino group for creatine synthesis, arginine is important in maintaining the reserve of high-energy phosphate required for ATP generation in muscle.

In animal models arginine supplementation has been associated with improved wound healing with increased wound tensile strength and collagen deposition [5]. Animal studies using arginine supplementation have shown improved survival in burns, intraperitoneal bacterial challenge, cecal ligation and puncture, and tumor implantation models [6].

The majority of human studies have included arginine in combination with other so-called 'immune modulating' elements making it impossible to define the specific arginine influence. While supplemental arginine has been shown to improve survival in various animal models as well as a number of in vitro

247

measures of immune function in animals and humans, the benefit of arginine supplementation alone needs further large scale studies to confirm its benefits in the clinical setting. Certainly the early data suggest that arginine upregulates immune function, modulates vascular flow patterns, and supports nitrogen balance [8, 9].

Glutamine

Glutamine is the most abundant amino acid in the body and makes up greater than 50% of the free amino acid pool [10]. Containing 5 carbons and 2 nitrogen moieties makes glutamine the major interorgan donor of nitrogen and carbon. Glutamine is now considered conditionally essential, meaning that during major catabolic insults, demand for glutamine is greater than supply. Glutamine is the primary fuel for many rapidly dividing tissues such as the small bowel mucosa and proliferating lymphocytes [11]. Glutamine has numerous metabolic roles including maintenance of acid-base status, as a precursor of urinary ammonia, as the primary fuel source for enterocytes, as fuel source for lymphocytes and macrophages, and as a precursor for nucleotides, arginine, glutathione, and glucosamine [12]. Glutamine is also a major contributor to gluconeogenesis and is the primary substrate for renal gluconeogenesis in humans. Recent reports also support a role for glutamine in decreasing peripheral insulin resistance in stress models [12]. Major surgery or trauma have been reported to cause a rapid decrease in serum and intracellular free glutamine levels. During catabolic illness glutamine uptake by the small intestine and immunologically active cells may exceed glutamine synthetic rates and release from skeletal muscle, making glutamine, like arginine, a conditionally essential amino acid [10, 13].

There is an abundance of human data regarding the use of glutamine supplementation both enterally and parenterally [4]. The majority, estimated at 70–80% of luminally supplied glutamine, is metabolized by the enterocyte, minimizing access to the systemic circulation. Clearly the target for enterally supplied glutamine is the splanchnic bed and GALT. In animal models, supplemental glutamine has been shown to enhance intestinal adaptation after massive small bowel resection [14], to attenuate intestinal and pancreatic atrophy [4], to improve survival after gut ischemia/reperfusion [15], and to prevent hepatic steatosis associated with parenteral and enteral feeding [12]. Glutamine appears to maintain GI tract mucosal thickness, maintain DNA and protein content, reduce bacteremia and mortality after chemotherapy, and reduce bacteremia and mortality following sepsis or endotoxemia [12].

In humans undergoing surgical stress, glutamine-supplemented parenteral nutrition appears to help maintain nitrogen balance and the intracellular glutamine pool in skeletal muscle [16]. A recent trauma study reported a greater than 50% decrease in pneumonia compared to an isonitrogenous, isocaloric control population [17]. A decrease in bacteremia and sepsis was also noted. In critically ill patients, glutamine supplementation may attenuate villous atrophy and the increased intestinal mucosal permeability associated with parenteral nutrition. Intravenous glutamine supplementation in a randomized, blinded trial of 84 critically ill patients showed significant improvement in long-term mortality [18]. In another study bone marrow transplant patients were randomized in a blinded fashion to glutamine or an isonitrogenous formula, resulting in fewer infections, improved nitrogen balance, and significantly shorter mean hospital length of stay [19]. Glutamine supplementation has also been shown to aid in protecting the GI tract against chemotherapy-induced mucosal toxicity [20].

While a large volume of animal and human data support the concept that glutamine is beneficial in a variety of experimental models, the benefit of routine enteral glutamine supplementation in critically ill human patients remains somewhat controversial. Well-designed clinical trials are needed to assess whether the beneficial effects demonstrated in GI physiology, immune function and postoperative metabolism translate into a reduction in hospital stay and mortality rate.

Nucleotides

Nucleotides form yet another important component of immune modulation through their diverse array of function in cell metabolism. The average American diet contains 1–2 g/day of nucleotides. Nucleotides are made up of the purine and pyrimidine backbone with a ribose and one to three phosphates. As nucleotides are removed during processing for whey and casein concentrates in the production of commercial formulas, critically ill patients fed enteral formulas may in fact have inadequate supply of nucleotides. Several infant and animal models have shown that supplementation of nucleotides can decrease GI infections, increase natural killer cells, increase villous height and mucosal enzyme activity.

Nucleotides are available to the host via de novo synthesis or from salvage pathways of DNA and RNA degradation. Synthesis requires substrates of glutamine, aspartate, glycine, and formate. Activity and the contribution of the salvage pathways may vary among tissues and with phases of the cell cycle. Nucleotides serve an array of vital functions including signal transduction, regulation of enzyme activity, synthesis of macromolecular compounds such as glycogen and phospholipids, promotion of gut development and maintenance of mucosal integrity, tissue repair and cell turnover. Iwasa et al. [21] have reported various combinations of nucleotides in specific ratios to be cytoprotective, increase hepatic regrowth after partial hepatectomy, increase oxidative phosphorylation, and decrease total parenteral nutrition-induced gut permeability in a rat model.

Therefore, one may speculate that in critical illness, nucleotide requirements are elevated in the face of hypermetabolism and activated immune response. Numerous animal studies demonstrate impaired mucosal function in nucleotide-depleted diets that could be reversed by oral supply of these substrates [22]. In a model system for Crohn's disease involving indomethacin-induced enteritis in rats, supplementation of diets with 1% yeast RNA allowed a significant improvement in ulcer healing [23]. The benefits of nucleotide supplementation appear consistent across tissues and species in relation to gut barrier and immune function.

n-3 Fatty Acids

The importance of fatty acid metabolism in the inflammatory and immune response has been assessed in numerous studies [24]. The typical Western diet now contains significantly more n-6 than n-3 fatty acids. In addition it is now apparent that lipid membranes are strongly influenced by dietary lipid profiles. Dietary changes in lipids have been shown to alter T-cell proliferation, cell–cell adhesive properties, plasma membrane fluidity and cytokine response to various stimuli [25].

High levels of polyunsaturated fatty acids, especially linoleic acid, have a suppressive effect on neutrophils, lymphocytes, monocytes and macrophage function in both in vitro and in vivo studies. The more specific immunosuppressive influence includes inhibition of lymphocyte proliferation, decrease in neutrophil chemotaxis and migration, impairment of the reticuloendothelial system and decrease in the bactericidal capacity. Exchange of subtypes of fatty acids limits production of arachidonic acid metabolites such as thromboxane A_2, prostaglandin E_2 and I_2, as well as leukotriene B_4, all mediators of the systemic inflammatory response and hypermetabolism in sepsis. Therefore, the effect of n-3 fatty acids likely comes from a profound alteration in the immunoregulatory process achieved by elaboration of various cytokines, interleukins, and interferons [26]. Early studies in the Eskimo population of Greenland demonstrated that their diets enriched in n-3 fatty acids conveyed lower risk of coronary artery disease, likely due to diminished platelet aggregation and thrombosis, both of which are directly influenced by platelet-activating factor release stimulated by cytokines and other products of membrane phospholipid metabolism [27]. n-3 fatty acids have been associated with and reported to decrease cardiovascular disease, inflammatory diseases, autoimmune disease, type-I diabetes, and lower the incidence of colon and breast cancer. A number of animal studies have confirmed the benefit of n-3 fatty acids in terms of a reduction in post-burn metabolic rate, mortality from infection, bacterial translocation rate, and response to lipopolysaccharide. With regard to critically ill patients, the relevance of dietary n-3 fatty acids is clear in light of their attenuation of the inflammatory response, antithrombotic effects, prevention of overproduction of PGE-2 to stress stimuli, and depression of plasma triglyceride levels. In addition to the dietary influence in cell membrane changes, recent evidence now indicates that fatty acid ratio changes can have acute effects on platelet adhesiveness, neutrophil function, membrane stability and alteration in microvascular perfusion. An elegant study by Suchner et al. [28] defines the correlation of intravenous lipid infusion, prostaglandin-F/thromboxane B_2 ratios, pulmonary hemodynamics, and gas exchange. Acute respiratory distress syndrome (ARDS) patients enrolled in this trial demonstrated worsening oxygenation and increased pulmonary shunt shortly after administering a bolus of intravenous fat emulsion. Reduced production of vasoactive mediators by elimination of n-6 fatty acids likely limits splanchnic vasoconstriction thereby modulating gut ischemia during stress, minimizing bacterial translocation, and preserving GALT integrity. In general it is felt that, in the critical care setting, increasing n-3 fatty acid levels compete with cyclooxygenase metabolism to limit the n-6 production of PGE_2 and leukotrienes of the 4 series, all of which are proinflammatory and/or function to limit microvascular flow. Numerous animal studies and one very important clinical study in ARDS patients, using a formula enriched with n-3 fatty acids, reported fewer ventilator days and shorter duration of intensive care unit (ICU) stay [29].

Clinical Evidence

Since 1990 there have been 26 prospective randomized human trials investigating the effects of immunonutrition in hospitalized patients. Despite the variations in study design, the majority of the well-designed studies demonstrate a clear benefit in terms of reduced infection rates, decreased antibiotic use, and reduced ICU and hospital length of stay [30]. These studies may be best approached by categorizing each into subgroups including general ICU, GI surgery, trauma, burn, and sepsis/multiorgan system failure patients. Moore [30] examined a general ICU population of 296 patients, randomized to enteral feedings supplemented with arginine, dietary nucleotides, and fish oil (Impact®, Novartis) or a control formula, demonstrating a substantial reduction in length of hospital stay and a significant reduction in acquired infections. Five prospective randomized trials have been published limiting the study to include only trauma patients. Of these studies, four demonstrated advantages to early immune-enhancing enteral feedings in terms of incidence of systemic inflammatory response syndrome, resolution of hypermetabolism, infectious complications, length of hospital stay, incidence of intra-abdominal abscesses and multisystem organ failure.

Supplemented enteral formulas allowed comparable results in acutely burned patients as well. Similar analyses have been carried out in 'general surgery' patient populations, many of whom presented for resection of

Table 2. Immunonutrition: meta-analysis

Reference	Number of patients	Number of studies	Outcome
Heys et al. [8], 1999	1,009	11	Decreased infection rate Decreased hospital stay No change in mortality
Beale et al. [9], 1999	1,482	12	Decreased infection Decreased ventilator days Decreased hospital stay
Heyland et al. [33], 2001	2,419	22	Decreased infection Decreased hospital stay ?Mortality

GI cancer. The vast majority of these studies revealed a lower rate of postoperative infections and shorter length of hospital stay in patients given supplemented enteral formulas. Other benefits included earlier liberation from mechanical ventilation, shorter length of ICU stay, improved phagocytic ability of monocytes, and decreased IL-6 plasma concentrations. Three studies in particular were able to predict a cost savings per patient in treating fewer complications when using supplemented enteral formulations. It is likely that this result may be extrapolated to other studies when shorter length of hospital stay and decreased cost incurred by infectious complications are weighed against provision of an immune-enhancing enteral feeding [30].

There are now three meta-analyses encompassing most major prospective randomized clinical trials on supplemented enteral feeding [31–33] (table 2). Both studies published in 1999 demonstrated reduced infection rates and shorter duration of hospital stay in patients with critical illness who received enteral nutrition supplemented with key nutrients. In the meta-analysis by Beale et al. [32] of 1,482 patients in 12 trials, patients administered the supplemented enteral formula also spent significantly fewer days supported with mechanical ventilation. Heyland et al. [33] examined 2,402 patients in 22 randomized trials involving n-3 fatty acids, arginine, and nucleotide-supplemented enteral nutrient formulas. As in previous studies, immunonutrient formulas were associated with decreased infection rates and decreased length of stay. In a subset analysis, critically ill septic patients (as opposed to surgical patients) demonstrated a higher mortality rate when given supplemented formulas. Overall Impact® and Immunaid® produced lower mortality rates than in groups using other formulas. Therefore, the authors conclude that further study is necessary to identify subgroups of patients who will benefit from nutraceuticals.

Several recent reports using immune-modulating formulations preoperatively and/or pre- and postoperatively have shown significant benefit

Table 3. Consensus recommendation from the US Summit on
Immune-Enhancing Enteral Therapy

Probable benefit
    Major vascular with COPD
    Major head and neck resection
    Severe closed head injury (Glascow <9)
    Major burn (>30% TBSA)
    Ventilator dependent with high risk of subsequent infection
Expected benefit
    Major GI surgery
    Serious trauma (ISS >17, ATI >19)
No expected benefit
    Resuming per os intake within 5 days
    In ICU only for monitoring
    Incomplete/inadequate resuscitation

in decreasing postoperative infectious complications. Of particular interest is
the study by Gianotti et al. [34] giving an immune-modulating formula to well-
nourished patients preoperatively with significant improvement in outcome.
We are now able to examine a significant number of patients enrolled in
randomized studies on immune-enhancing nutrition. From these data we are
obligated to develop a new standard of care for the use of nutraceuticals in
critically ill patients. We may now be able to define which patients benefit
from this intervention as opposed to which patients incur higher mortality,
which formula should be given, when should it be used and for what duration.
Some of these issues were recently addressed at the US Summit on Immune-
Enhancing Enteral Therapy held in San Diego, Calif., May, 2000. The entire
proceedings were published in an attempt to clarify recommendations for use
[30] (table 3).

The Future of Immunonutrition

Recently a new interest has developed in certain probiotics and their
importance in critical illness. Probiotics consist of live microbes that when
ingested confer some benefit to the host organism as a result of microbial
influence on human physiology. Rapidly evolving concepts in this field suggest
that maintenance of the luminal microenvironment may prevent normally
nonpathogenic species from developing mucosal adherence and invasion.
These opportunistic microbes may then modulate the inflammatory and
immune response. Numerous bacterial and yeast species have been described
which have dramatically different effects on the GI system. In direct
association with critical care management is the use of *Lactobacillus* GG to
reduce antibiotic-associated diarrhea [35]. If success rates are similar in large

Table 4. Nutrients reported to have 'immune-modulating properties'

Arginine
Glutamine
Sulfur amino acids
Nucleotides
n-3 fatty acids
Fiber/probiotics
Glutathione/various antioxidants
Ornithine α-ketoglutarate
Probiotics
Taurine

randomized clinical trials, the use of probiotic therapy may become the routine.

Exciting new data in the realm of probiotics were recently unveiled by Popoff et al. [36] from the University of Alberta. Recent in vitro experiments demonstrate the role of epithelial cells in modulating the immune response at the mucosal level by sampling DNA of local organisms. These investigators used both a freeze-dried culture of live probiotic bacteria, as well as purified DNA from probiotic strains to pretreat human colonic cells in culture [36]. Cells subsequently exposed to pathogenic bacteria displayed significant reductions in activation of inflammatory pathway elements. This study is the first evidence that epithelial cells perform this level of receptor-based recognition, independent of immune surveillance cells. This new concept in epithelial biology opens the door to refinement of the ingredients of the probiotic 'cocktail' based on membrane receptor composition and the ability to maximize the anti-inflammatory effect.

In summary, we now have a wealth of animal and human data attempting to elucidate the appropriate mix of 'immune-modulating' nutrients (table 4), the adequate level of nutrient required to show benefit, the appropriate timing of delivery and, most importantly, the clinical scenarios yielding the best outcome with the use of immune-modulating formulas. The basic tenets outlined above should be observed prior to any attempt at nutritional immune modulation.

What is more controversial, yet apparent from multiple clinical trials, is that the concept of immunonutrition is now not only theoretical, but can yield clinical benefit. Subtle differences in patient selection, population studies, and nutrient mix can explain the outcome differences in the relevant studies. Additional research is needed in the arena of single nutrient supplementation to better define mechanisms in humans. Continued, rigorous, critical evaluations of the data are needed as more immunonutrients and 'nutraceuticals' are reported for modulation of immune function. Optimizing outcomes in critical care will be the reward for tenacious pursuit of further understanding of the potential beneficial pharmacologic effects of nutraceuticals.

References

1. Scrimshaw NS, Taylor CE, Gordon JE. *Interactions of Nutrition and Infection.* Geneva: World Health Organization, 1968, vol 57.
2. Wilmore DW. Homeostasis: Bodily changes in trauma and surgery. In: Sabiston DL, ed. *Textbook of Surgery: The Biological Basis of Modern Surgical Practice.* Philadelphia: Saunders, 1997.
3. Gottschlich MM, Jenkins M, Warden GD, Baumer T, Havens P, Snook JT, Alexander JW. Differential effects of three enteral dietary regimens on selected outcome variables in burn patients. *JPEN J Parenter Enteral Nutr* 1990; 14: 225–36.
4. De Bandt JP, Cynober LA. Amino acids with anabolic properties. *Curr Opin Nutr Metab Care* 1998; 1: 263–72.
5. Barbul A, Lazarou SA, Efron DT, et al. Arginine enhances wound healing and lymphocyte immune responses in humans. *Surgery* 1990; 108: 331–7.
6. Evoy D, Lieberman MD, Fahey TJ, et al. Immunonutrition: The role of arginine. *Nutrition* 1998; 14: 611–7.
7. Cynober L, LeBoucher J, Vasson MP. Arginine metabolism in mammals. *J Nutr Biochem* 1995; 6: 402–13.
8. Heys SD, Walker LG, Smith I, et al. Enteral nutrition supplementation with key nutrients in patients with critical illness and cancer. *Ann Surg* 1999; 229: 467–77.
9. Beale RJ, Bryg DJ, Bihari DJ. Immunonutrition in the critically ill. A systemic review of clinical outcome. *Crit Care Med* 1999; 27: 2799–805.
10. Wilmore DW, Shabert JK. Role of glutamine in immunologic responses. *Nutrition* 1998; 14: 618–26.
11. Ziegler TR, Bazargan N, Leader LM, Martindale RG. Glutamine and the gastrointestinal tract. *Curr Opin Clin Nutr Metab Care* 2000; 3: 355–62.
12. Griffiths RD. Glutamine: Establishing clinical indication. *Curr Opin Clin Nutr Metab Care* 1999; 2: 177–82.
13. Schloerb PR. Immune-enhancing diets: Products components, and their rationales. *JPEN J Parenter Enteral Nutr* 2001; 255: S3–S7.
14. Fukuchtl S, Bankhead R, Rolandelli RH. Parenteral nutrition in short bowel syndrome. In: Rombeau JL, Rolandelli RH, eds. *Parenteral Nutrition,* 3rd ed. Philadelphia: Saunders, 2001; 282–303.
15. Ikeda S, Zarzaur BL, Johnson CD, Fukatsu K, Kudsk KA. Total parenteral nutrition supplementation with glutamine improves survival after gut ischemia/reperfusion. *JPEN J Parenter Enteral Nutr* 2002; 26: 169–73.
16. Stehle P, Zander J, Mertes N, et al. Effects of parenteral glutamine peptide supplements on muscle glutamine loss and nitrogen balance after major surgery. *Lancet* 1989; i: 231–33.
17. Houdijk APJ, Rijnsburger ER, Jansen J, et al. Randomized trial of glutamine-enriched enteral nutrition on infectious morbidity in patients with multiple trauma. *Lancet* 1998; 352: 772–6.
18. Van Der Hulst RRW, Van Krell BK, Von Meyenfeldt MF, et al. Glutamine and the preservation of gut integrity. *Lancet* 1993; 341: 1363–5.
19. Ziegler TR, Young LS, Benfell K, et al. Clinical and metabolic efficacy of glutamine supplemented parenteral nutrition after bone marrow transplantation. A randomized, double-blind controlled study. *Ann Intern Med* 1992; 116: 821–8.
20. Houdijk AP, Rijnsburger ER, Jansen J, Wesdorp RI, Weiss JK, McCamish MA, Teerlink T, Meuwissen SG, Haarman HJ, Thijs LG, van Leeuwen PA. Randomized trial of glutamine-enriched enteral nutrition on infectious morbidity in patients with multiple trauma. *Lancet* 1998; 352: 772–6.
21. Iwasa Y, Iwasa M, Ohmori Y, Fukutomi T, Ogoshi S. The effect of the administration of nucleosides and nucleotides for parenteral use. *Nutrition* 2000; 16: 598–602.
22. Cosgrove M. Perinatal and infant nutrition. Nucleotides. *Nutrition* 1998; 14: 748–51.
23. Sukumar P, Loo A, Magur E, Nandi J, Oler A, Levine RA. Dietary supplementation of nucleotides and arginine promotes healing of small bowel ulcers in experimental ulcerative ileitis. *Dig Dis Sci* 1997; 42: 1530–6.
24. Furst P, Kuhn KS. Fish oil emulsions: What benefits can they bring? *Clin Nutr* 2000, 19. 7–14.
25. Grimble RF. Dietary lipids and the inflammatory response. *Proc Nutr Soc* 1998; 57: 535–42.

26. Suchner U, Kuhn KS, Furst P. The scientific basis of immunonutrition. *Proc Nutr Soc* 2000; 59: 553–63.
27. Dyerberg J, Bang HO. Lipid metabolism, atherogenesis, and haemostasis in Eskimos: the role of the prostaglandin-3 family. *Haemostasis* 1979; 8: 227–33.
28. Suchner U, Katz DP, Furst P, Beck K, Felbinger TW, Senftleben U, Thiel M, Goetz AE, Peter K. Effects of intravenous fat emulsions on lung function in patients with acute respiratory distress syndrome or sepsis. *Crit Care Med* 2001; 29: 1569–74.
29. Gadek JE, Demichcle SJ, Karlstad MD, Pacht ER, Donahoe M, Albertson TE, Van Hoozen C, Wennberg AK, Nelson JL, Noursalehi M. Effect of enteral feeding with eicosapentaenoic acid, gamma-linolenic acid, and antioxidants in patients with acute respiratory distress syndrome. Enteral Nutrition in ARDS Study Group. *Crit Care Med* 1999; 27: 1409–20.
30. Moore F. Effects of immune enhancing diets on infectious morbidity and multiple organ failure. *JPEN J Parenter Enteral Nutr* 2001; 25 (2 suppl): S36–S43.
31. Heys SD, Walker LG, Smith I, Eremin O. Enteral nutritional supplementation with key nutrients in patients with critical illness and cancer. *Ann Surg* 1999; 229: 467–77.
32. Beale RJ, Bryg DJ, Bihari DJ. Immunonutrition in the critically ill: A systemic review of clinical outcome. *Crit Care Med* 1999; 27: 2799–805.
33. Heyland DK, Novak F, Drover JW, Jain M, Su X, Suchner U. Should immunonutrition become routine in the critically ill patient? A systematic review of the evidence. *JAMA* 2001; 286: 944–53.
34. Gianotti L, Braga M, Nespoli L, Radaelli G, Beneduce A, Di Carlo V. A randomized controlled trial of preoperative oral supplementation with a specialized diet in patients with gastrointestinal cancer. *Gastroenterology* 2002; 122: 1763–70.
35. Heyman M. Effect of lactic acid bacteria on diarrheal diseases. *J Am Coll Nutr* 2000; 19: S137–S46.
36. Popoff I, Jijon H, Monia B, Tavernini M, Ma M, McKay R, Madsen K. Antisense oligonucleotides to poly(ADP-ribose) polymerase-2 ameliorate colitis in interleukin-10-deficient mice. *J Pharmacol Exp Ther* 2002; 303: 1145–54.

Discussion

Dr. Moldawer: I started my talk with the pharmaceutical side in which we were doing drug testing, and now we should perhaps talk more about these drugs in our food. So let me put a challenge to you that the pharmaceutical industry would never consider testing 3 or 4 different drugs simultaneously in septic patients, and in fact the Food and Drug Administration (FDA) is very leery about combination therapies without biological activities with single monotherapies. So I ask you an obvious question: have we failed in this approach to really do good science and do control trials with individual nutrients first?

Dr. Martindale: I think we have failed because there is very little or no data on single nutrients in that population. It would be very nice. I think with this group we could perhaps eventually get collaborative studies going to get enough patients. The problem is money, and I think that no one would fund this kind of study with single nutrients because they are going to site the data that are already out. It would be very nice to have the data, but it is going to be very difficult to show in humans.

Dr. Zazzo: In the same position I will ask you why your consensus statement did not mention the available data on trace elements?

Dr. Martindale: Our goal really was to look at these main nutrients or products that are already out there and there was such variability. You know the trace elements in those areas were just not addressed, it was not part of our specific question. This is a very good question, it definitely needs to be addressed but it was not in that consensus.

Dr. Cynober: I question the fact that ornithine α-ketoglutarate was totally ignored by you, and most of the American investigators, despite various clinical studies [1–3] that have been published in the *American Journal of Clinical Nutrition, Critical*

Care Medicine, and the *Journal of Nutrition*, which are all American journals and considered as not so bad. In addition I will especially focus on the results with ornithine α-ketoglutatate in burn patients because in my opinion 3 independent studies [4] show that this glutamine precursor improves wound healing. Taking this drug into consideration would probably have moved the ASPEN summit recommendation for burn patients from low to better level of recommendation.

Dr. Martindale: I can allude back to the fact that we used peer-reviewed literature, some of it with ornithine α-ketoglutarate, but we went back to the more clinical studies. What is available in the clinical studies that are using these formulas on the market, that was what we were looking at.

Dr. Cynober: But do you feel that wound healing is not a clinical end point in burn patients?

Dr. Martindale: No, no question but in this case we were looking very specifically. I agree, α-ketoglutarate is beneficial. I don't know where it all fits.

Dr. Rosenfeld: I have one doubt, we know the stores are decreased or the substrates are heavily mobilized. My doubt is that what you are providing improves full function, gives the cell new function or works better. Are we just restoring the normal functions or giving the starving cell the conditions to react to the situation?

Dr. Martindale: I think we are enhancing function and especially in case of arginine administration. I think the data support that T-cell function seems to be supported by arginine. So I think it is variable but in this case I believe we are helping, not just maintaining.

Dr. McClave: You tease out that group with pneumonia in the Ross study (unpublished data). What is the take-home message from that if we clearly identify somebody with pneumonia, is it the age, is it the sepsis, and we treat them differently? The second question is: if they aren't that well on admission and then we start immunonutrition and then they develop pneumonia, what do we do?

Dr. Martindale: If they have pneumonia I will not use immunonutrition, if they already have pneumonia and already are septic. That is my take-home message, and in elderly septic individuals I think we should be very careful. I think if nothing else as the whole controversy is brought up, the point is that we can't generalize, we have got to be specific. I think that nitric oxide has the ability to be a panacea or a toxic, depending on the situation.

Dr. McClave: What happens if you start them on immunonutrition and they develop pneumonia, would you stop it?

Dr. Martindale: Good question, I wouldn't stop it.

Dr. Déchelotte: I would like to comment on this point about pneumonia. If patients who have pneumonia are not to be included in a study with immunonutrition, I think it makes no sense with the major goals of immunonutrition. I think the right interpretation of these data should be that this type of immuno-enhancing diet, this type and given in this way, is not adequate for this kind of patient. I think it is a very important point to make that this word 'immunonutrition' is misleading because it covers a very wide field of many things, of many substrates, many combinations of substrates, differences in doses, differences in site and timing of delivery, and I think we should omit this word. Of course it is quite practical in common use, on an everyday basis, but it is very misleading, we should specify glutamine-enriched or arginine-enriched, it is actually more precise.

Dr. Martindale: I think that is a very good point and that is why I brought up the point about Optimental®, which was the formula used and has half the arginine of most of the other products. But I think you are right, should we just not use that product, and if supposedly arginine is the problem, it probably isn't because of the dose that is in there.

Dr. Steenhout: You just mentioned that this study was done with a product with half the dose of arginine. In your nice slide I realize that the product also contains structured lipids. So I don't know if that is involved in this bad effect or not. But what is your opinion about structured lipids in such a formula because it is coming slowly.

Dr. Martindale: The question on structured lipids is again very controversial. Most people would believe that the structured lipid is beneficial, but again we don't have enough data to confirm this.

Dr. Heyland: I am actually delighted to hear that. I don't think we are too far off in our view of immunonutrition, because what I heard you say, if I am correct, is that you do not give this to sepsis patients, it is alright for elective surgical patients, and perhaps we still have some disagreement in the average critically ill nonseptic patients. Again I wonder if this point of disagreement is not based on the interpretation of the different results from the studies. I tend to focus on the intention-to-treat analysis as you know, and I think that most focus on compliance analyses. You emphasized the point that we need to get an adequate dose of the nutrients or drugs, as may be, into the patients. What do you think about the hypothesis that giving an arginine supplement-containing formula to a relatively sick intensive care unit (ICU) patient, the effect that it would have on gastrointestinal motility and creating problems with tolerating feeds so that then the sickest patients are excluded from the analysis? In this sort of secondary analysis, you are really left with imbalanced groups which you favored, in the arginine-containing group you have excluded 6 patients because they did not tolerate enteral feeds. Would you tell me what you think about that analysis?

Dr. Martindale: I think first we don't have any data that a high arginine formula does decrease tolerance.

Dr. Heyland: In terms of nitric oxide, if you produce nitric oxide it will impair gastric emptying.

Dr. Martindale: But in many cases it increases blood flow.

Dr. Heyland: Yes, but the motility goes down. There are experimental data for that.

Dr. Martindale: With high levels, very high levels in it, in an already stimulated model but not in the normal patient.

Dr. Heyland: I am not talking about normal patients.

Dr. Martindale: You are talking about surgical and not immediate postoperative patients, so they are already induced.

Dr. Heyland: They are already induced. There is some form of information going on in the patients so you are probably producing nitric oxide.

Dr. Martindale: I think we get around that by the fact that we attempt gastric feeding and if unsuccessful we go to jejunal feeding, and as you know we can feed fairly sick patients very carefully in the jejunum if we watch them very closely. I am one of the bigger advocates of early feeding, but I also think that we have gone too far with our attempts to feed earlier. In fact that was the title of my talk at the ASPEN symposium, have we pushed too long and pushed too hard trying to use the gut? Maybe we should say alright there are some patients we can't feed and back off a little bit. So I think in that case we would enhance visceral blood flow, which may help us in the gastrointestinal tract. But you are all right, gastric emptying is a little bit of a problem but if we are intolerant then we use the gastrointestinal tract.

Dr. Heyland: Certainly in the future we are going to design better trials, from the gut we should be putting the tubes in the small bowels to deliver adequate nutrients or drugs.

Dr. Martindale: I personally like jejunal feeding for the sicker patients anyway.

Dr. Heyland: I think it biases the analysis and therefore the interpretation thereof if you are systematically excluding those patients who don't get fed enough because there is an interaction between the arginine, gastric emptying, tolerance, and outcome.

Dr. Martindale: I think your first statement I was omitting the septic patients, I wouldn't omit all the septic patients, I would omit the septic patients with severe pneumonia and the elderly, those patients I would say.

Dr. Heyland: I guess we still disagree with that.

Dr. Labadarios: You did say that we should look at these nutrients as drugs, but if we did that the chances are excellent that they would never really appear on the market because they have never been investigated the way a drug normally is investigated. So I think we have to be careful about what we consider to be a drug. Coming back to the question of pneumonia, do you think we are in an area here where in trying to treat a disease we are likely to be creating another disease, which is not necessarily a complication of the present disease? For instance, if you look at another field of nutrition. There is little doubt about the validity of vitamin A being an immuno-enhancing nutrient in high doses, but we have now realized that one of the side effects of these high doses of vitamin A supplements may be an increased risk for respiratory infections. It actually goes further because we have some data from Mozambique which show that it may not be advisable to treat children with cerebral malaria with high doses of vitamin A because if you follow the survivors for 2 years, as we have done, you find a tendency in these vitamin A-supplemented children to develop mental deficits. So quality-of-life aspects may arise from improved survival rates [5]. Do you think that we may be dealing with a situation like this? Have we got data to know what we are doing really?

Dr. Martindale: No, we don't have the data but I think that it would be a pretty big jump to say that the minor modifications we are making are going to produce a new problem. Now you are right in that select population, but I think we need to go back through and look at these under specific situations, and then look at the long term. We have the Griffiths data at 6 months talking about glutamine over a very short period making a difference at 6 months. We should go back now and look at the 6-month and the 1-year outcome of some of the immunonutrient studies.

Dr. Kudsk: This is the first time I have seen the Ross data. A question I would like to ask you, what is the pneumonia data, a post hoc analysis? If it is a post hoc analysis, it comes under all the other criticism of all studies that do post hoc analyses. It has to be tested, because if it was pre hoc then it should have been powered to show a difference in mortality in pneumonia and I suspect it wasn't.

Dr. Martindale: This was the intermediate analysis which went and looked at the data and said lets stop because we have a problem. I think the problem was the randomization, we would not have seen it if we had easily randomized pneumonia. These patients had pneumonia when they got the nutrient.

Dr. Ribeiro: Most of the studies were made with the first-generation immune-stimulant formulas. What about these newest formulas, named immune-modulating formulas, that have just emerged on the market?

Dr. Martindale: You are all right, this is the first-generation and 90% of the studies we have seen today were done with one product or two. I think there are minor changes in the new ones, in fact if anything they are coming down on some nutrients and going up on others, but they are not coming out very fast. The changes are not being made very fast. I think the newer ones, the second-generation, will have more trace minerals, will have a different absorption, will probably combine with probiotics or at least the prebiotics, not for all patients but some. When I think back to modulating formula there is a basic core in a modulating formula and it may be transition over time: in the first week treated, change from one and switch to a second, and change it over time, so very expensive.

Dr. Maiorova: You demonstrated the influence of several nutrients on immunological functions, but at the same time you showed several theoretic aspects.

Is it possible that using some amino acids, for example arginine, glutamine, influences the activity of drug-metabolizing enzymes, for example cytochromes and others, and does it influence the drug metabolism of patients in the ICUs or overall? What is your opinion?

Dr. Martindale: Certainly any nutrient, or as we would like to use it at a drug level, would clearly induce enzyme systems, we have not seen problems with toxicity in the liver with these products. Again that is why I think the FDA allows these things to be placed on the market with very low testing because they are classified as medical foods under the idea that they are generally recognized as safe, and so in most cases they are safe. I think where we can get into trouble is if we start displacing drugs from albumin binding and changing levels of drug. But in that case we haven't seen that problem, we haven't seen changes in drug metabolism.

Dr. Maiorova: Because I am interested in several drugs that have a very narrow therapeutic index, when their metabolism is altered we see some toxicity. I mean for example drugs used in cancer therapy.

Dr. Martindale: I have no data on the cancer therapy.

Dr. McClain: You could make a couple of postulates on the pneumonia patients, one would be that the alveolar macrophages were too jazzed up and released tons of tumor necrosis factor and every body got inflammatory respiratory distress syndrome and died, or you could say that they could not kill and so you just got over whelming sepsis. Has anybody looked at these patients carefully to try and separate that out?

Dr. Martindale: No. We can get the Ross data, which has been looked at now as part of the abstract which should be presented at the *Society for Critical Care Medicine,* but as far as individual patients are concerned, we can't really see any major difference, we haven't looked at individuals.

Dr. Nitenberg: I have been working in that field for many years and I am more and more confused about the conclusions. If we try to go back to the real world again and if we accept your conclusions, I don't say that I accept but suppose that we accept your conclusions, let's say that first for surgical patients, and I think that is the strongest evidence that we have presently, we can use immune-enhancing diets preoperatively and possibly postoperatively, but what type of immune-enhancing diet could I use in my hospital? If you look carefully at the results the only immune-enhancing diet that has been proven to be efficient in this case is Impact®. If you pick up Impact® you have no results. So the only thing I can say is in our hospital for surgical patients I can try to use Impact®, nothing more, and I don't know what is efficient in Impact®. Second point, in multiple trauma patients it is more confusing because to my knowledge there are the studies from Dr. Kudsk and Dr. Moore which have been made with Immun-Aid® if I remember well, which is another nutrition mix, but there are also the remarkable results from the Houdijk study which was made with something which is very closed to Alitraq® and which is only rich in glutamine and may be a little source of antioxidants I think. So in that case what do I have to recommend, I don't know. What is more amazing, you say that in septic patients, I do agree with that, but in very severe ICU patients we don't know. Unfortunately there is only one study by Galban that may prove that Impact® is efficient in septic patients and perhaps in pneumonia patients, and your conclusion does not, certainly not immune-enhancing diets in pneumonia patients. So finally what do I chose and why?

Dr. Martindale: I think in the Galban study, as you know only the mild and moderate septic patients would benefit from it, the severely septic patients would not. So I think that it is reasonable to say severe sepsis, as we have talked about it earlier, those are the patients for whom we really have to know what we are doing, nutritionally as well as metabolically. So I think that is part of the key, with severe sepsis you just have to be careful. The rest of it, you ask what should we give. I think the data are there and I think we have to say we can give Impact[®], we can give some similar products. I give what the data would support.

Dr. Berger: I probably have a silly question but it is my lack of knowledge of American products which is behind this. I have been amazed that many control studies in America have been done using Vivonex[®], which is an elemental diet. I haven't seen this myself, but I was told yesterday by 3 different American persons that in Vivonex[®] there is an amazingly large proportion of glutamine, or an enriched proportion, higher than any other standard enteral diet. How can we then compare, how can we interpret the trials where actually the control group was a glutamine group?

Dr. Martindale: I don't know that any of these studies up there today use Vivonex[®] as control.

Dr. Moore: Can I respond, because it is our study that used Vivonex[®].

Dr. Martindale: The first one.

Dr. Moore: If you go back into the history of Vivonex[®], it was actually created by a pharmaceutical company. Before they went and promoted it in the ICU they said we are going to test this like a drug, and that is the reason why all those studies were done with Vivonex[®]. They did not want to market it unless they had data. Over about 10 years we did 3 prospective randomized trials that showed whether you gave Vivonex[®] without anything or Vivonex[®] with total parenteral nutrition (TPN) or Vivonex[®] with delayed TPN you get a better outcome with Vivonex[®]. Therefore we went on to design the Immun-Aid[®] study and Dr. Kudsk was in the discussion. It was hard for us to take Vivonex[®] and spike it with something to make it isonitrogenous. So we said this is our standard of care with the plans that Dr. Kudsk was going to do the follow-up study and make an isonitrogenous diet and compare it. Then we did the Vivonex[®] versus Immun-Aid study and showed improved outcomes. Dr. Kudsk did the isonitrogenous isocaloric versus the Immun-Aid[®] and showed the same results. His patients were a little sicker.

Dr. Martindale: I would even go back a little further than that, Vivonex[®] was originally made for the space program as an elemental diet. The idea was that they didn't want the astronauts having a stool in space so give them a pure elemental diet, and in fact the Air Force troops that they studied went from 1 stool/day to 1 stool/week.

Dr. Moore: It is kind of funny.

Dr. Martindale: They didn't know the benefit of glutamine at the time of formula creation. The reason they put glutamine in there was because of the taste because literally the troops would not drink it without something to cover the taste. When they realized that glutamine was tasteless they put in more glutamine just because of the taste issue. Tang was developed to cover the taste.

Dr. Moore: Once they figured out that there was some pharmacological fact and that something was happening, ...,

Dr. Martindale: They sold it.

Dr. Moore: They ran with that for a long time, so I always said glutamine, I don't want to believe that. Maybe there is something with the glutamine.

Dr. Berger: Does it mean that the enteral Vivonex[®] studies against TPN are actually glutamine against nothing?

Dr. Martindale: They do. The original Vivonex[®] had less glutamine than the current Vivonex[®].

Dr. McClain: It just depends on which part of the animal you are looking at. For somebody studying liver disease like myself, when I want to make patients choline-deficient or if I want to make them deficient in methionine, I give them Vivonex[®]. So it is probably the worse thing to give somebody with liver disease or somebody in the ICU.

Dr. Déchelotte: I would like to come back to the pragmatic remark by Dr. Nitenberg. We have to make decisions together with our hospital administration. We have to make decisions on what product will be referenced or not in our hospital and for which patients. We made the decision 2 years ago that there wouldn't be any immune-enhancing diet. Last year we made the decision that Impact® would be taken only for heavy surgery in cancer patients, only, and we made the decision based on the available data in our hospital together with our colleagues that it should not be used for septic ICU patients. I think the new data from the Ross study (unpublished data) that you showed today, which I am very disappointed but also delighted to see, provide additional evidence from the previous meta-analyses that in severe ICU patients, septic or not, we should not routinely use Impact® which is at the present time the only nutrient diet that has been tested in this kind of patient. There are no studies with the other arginine-enriched compounds available in Europe. So we need to withhold from using these diets at the time.

Dr. Martindale: I think you made a good statement that you sit down with the colleagues and say are we using it and make the decision. I have to say I don't know that there is a huge difference between them if they are made with the same amount of nutrients, if they put similar arginine, similar n-3 fats from a similar source, I can't say there is going to be a huge difference between them. Now it may well be that going from 6 to 16 g/1,000 cal may make a difference. But remember that the mortality was in the group that had less arginine. Half the arginine of the Impact® is where the mortality was. So to say that we should not use Impact® for the same argument you are making, to say that we should not use a high arginine formula and there we can't really make that statement either.

Dr. Déchelotte: I agree that we should not use any arginine-enriched diet at the present time for very severe ICU patients because we don't have the rationale to make the difference in comparison to a standard product.

Dr. Martindale: But that product has very little more than a normal diet, than a normal standard formula, not much more. The standard formula has about 5.5 g and this one has about 7.5 as opposed to 14, so there is very little difference between that and the standard formula. So to say that 2 g for a 1,000 cal made all the difference, I can't make that jump.

Dr. Déchelotte: If I may go to another point again with glutamine and arginine. All these data that you showed are done with arginine-enriched diets and you are well aware of the Immun-Aid® papers with arginine plus glutamine which are positive and the Dutch paper on trauma patients. So I think there is a great difference. At the present time there are limited studies with enriched glutamine diets, but most of them are either equivalent to control or better than control. None of them show any increased morbidity or mortality in comparison to control, which is a big difference to arginine-enriched diets.

Dr. Martindale: And even to make it more confusing, in the US we now have got Impact® with glutamine, and so it is even more confusing.

Dr. Zazzo: Let us go back to the dosage recommendation in the consensus statement. The consensus said 1.2–1.5 liters/day. That is right?

Dr. Martindale: Over that by the 5-day period, try to get it to about 50% of caloric goal.

Dr. Zazzo: When we consider the few studies in elective surgery, before surgery, it is 1 liter/day during a week.

Dr. Martindale: 5 days to a week.

Dr. Zazzo: Yes, but 1 liter. How do you explain this discrepancy between elective surgery and the conclusions.

Dr. Martindale: I think there is a big difference. One is going to have the metabolic stress, the metabolic demands are down and the rate of metabolism has changed significantly. If you can preload prior to the insult, I think that is the key. I think this is sort of like carbo loading for a marathon run. We can change the membrane concentration of the n-3 fat.

Dr. Zazzo: This is only hypothesis, we have no data to recommend more or less?

Dr. Martindale: No, I can only go from the Braga and Gianotti data, and there are several others now, as you saw there are several papers now on the pre- or perioperative period. To me the most fascinating data are in the well-nourished population. Giving it for 1 week or 5 days preoperatively, 1 liter/day shows a positive outcome equivalent to giving it pre- and postoperatively. As you know the Heslin data used an immune-enhancing formula and they showed no benefit. Part of the problem there was most of those patients had albumin of >35g/l on entry for surgery and they showed no benefit. This is a very nice set up because if you can give it to the patient for 1 week preoperatively between admission and setting the patient up for surgery that can make a significant difference in a large number of patients. But again, how much to give, would 2 liters be better, would $500 \, cm^3$ be enough, we don't know.

Dr. Tepaske: There is a recently published Spanish study about multifibers compared to an isonitrogenous control which only showed some differences in infections in 1 versus 9 patients I believe. I am coming back to the septic patients and also looking from a nutritional and especially clinical point of view. First of all I am interested if I can feed or not feed the patients enterally, and I know if I can feed them enterally they are in the bad group, high morbidity, high mortality, I think there is no discussion about that. But then there is a second choice to make. If I can feed them nasogastrically with a tube, what do I have to choose? In my opinion there is the Bauer study and the Atkinson study showing that the best is immunonutrition. Do you agree with that?

Dr. Martindale: I feed septic patients with immunonutrients, so I go from there. The question is are they sick enough so that it is difficult to feed them enterally? I think you made that point very well. But I still use it in septic patients. Now I am a little more cautious if I am called for a consultation and the patient has got pneumonia, is on the ventilator, an elderly patient, but in general I would use immunonutrients in septic patients.

Dr. de Bandt: Haven't we overlooked the question of micronutrients in this situation? I don't know the specific requirements of pneumonia patients, but if we go back to basic biochemistry the toxicity of nitric oxide is not due to nitric oxide per se but to its reaction with superoxide anion, leading in the situation of an excess of superoxide anion to the toxic peroxynitrite anion. So if you prevent excessive superoxide anion production you enable a beneficial effect of nitric oxide which is the control of NF-κB and the activation of transcription systems such as expression of cytokines. So is there a problem in this field, have we not overlooked this question?

Dr. Martindale: You make a very good point. I am not sure that we have overlooked the question. I think that the reactions that are going on inside the cell are so compartmentalized that it is going to be very difficult to sort out whether it is going as a substrate for arginase versus nitric oxide synthetase, and I think that is compartmentalized and upregulated or downregulated depending on what is going on in the cell. I think that is why we see such a variation in outcome and we are overlooking it. But when we block nitric oxide synthetase we still see benefits in some cases, so it may not be nitric oxide production, but also we may get the benefit of vasodilatation.

Dr. De Bandt: If we take the example that Dr. Cynober gave this morning we have an increased mortality in a simple model of lipopolysaccharide toxicity when *L-nitro-*arginine methyl ester is administrated. When you block nitric oxide you have a dramatic increase in mortality. So it is not so simple.

Dr. Martindale: No it is clearly not simple.

References

1. Coudray-Lucas C, Le Bever H, Cynober L, et al. Ornithine alpha-ketoglutarate improves wound healing in severe burn patients: A prospective randomized double-blind trial versus isonitrogenous controls. *Crit Care Med* 2000; 28: 1772–6.
2. De Bandt JP, Coudray-Lucas C, Lioret N, et al. A randomized controlled trail of the influence of the mode of enteral ornithine alpha-ketoglutarate administraion in burn patients. *J Nutr* 1998; 128: 563–9.
3. Le Bricon T, Coudray-Lucas C, Lioret N, et al. Ornithine alpha-ketoglutarate metabolism after enteral administration in burn patients: Bolus compared with continuous infusion. *Am J Clin Nutr* 1997; 65: 512–8.
4. Cynober LA. The use of alpha-ketoglutarate salts in clinical nutrition and metabolic care. *Curr Opin Clin Nutr Metab Care* 1999; 2: 33–7.
5. Varandas L, Julien M, Gomes A, et al. A randomized, double-blind, placebo-controlled clinical trial of vitamin A in severe malaria in hospitalized Mozambican children. *Ann Trop Paediatr* 2001; 21: 211–22.

Cynober L, Moore FA (eds): Nutrition and Critical Care.
Nestlé Nutrition Workshop Series Clinical & Performance Program, vol 8, pp 265-277,
Nestec Ltd., Vevey/S. Karger AG, Basel, © 2003.

Lessons from Pharmacokinetics in the Design of New Nutrition Formulas for Critically Ill Patients

Luc Cynober

Biochemistry Laboratory, Hôtel-Dieu Hospital, AP-HP and Laboratory of Biological Nutrition
EA 2498, Pharmacy School, Paris 5 University, Paris, France

Severe injury causes alterations in protein metabolism [1], including net muscle protein breakdown, increased transfer of amino acids (AAs) from the peripheral to the splanchnic area, intense use of AAs for gluconeogenesis and consequently a marked increase in nitrogen loss, leading to a negative nitrogen balance [2]. When persistent and/or very severe, this process is responsible for protein wasting and in turn for morbidity and mortality.

Nutritional supply must therefore form an integral part of therapeutic strategy in critically ill intensive care unit (ICU) patients. But the qualitative intake of nitrogen has to match the requirements of such patients, which are specific and different from those of healthy subjects [1]. The specificity of their requirements arises from a number of factors, some of which are summarized in table 1.

However, because historically the technical aspects were mastered before knowledge of the physiopathological alterations became fully known [3], the specific AA needs of ICU patients unfortunately long went unrecognized, and recommended requirements were merely adapted from those set for healthy subjects. Most products tailored for enteral use supply nitrogen in the form of high nutritional value proteins, and most solutions for parenteral nutrition (PN) provide a mixture of free AAs that reproduce the composition of these high-quality reference proteins (egg and cow milk proteins), namely ≈ 45% essential AAs (EAAs) and a ratio of EAAs to total nitrogen of ≈ 3.1 mg/g.

It is clear that current formulas are unlikely to meet ICU patients' requirements fully [4]. The key questions that must be addressed are the following: (1) How do we determine the AA requirements of critically ill

265

Table 1. Specificity of AA requirements in ICU patients

Related to adaptation of metabolic pathways
Unrestrainable increase in liver gluconeogenesis
→ Increase in ALA, GLN, PRO, GLY, SER consumption by the liver
Increase in renal ammoniagenesis to counteract metabolic acidosis
→ Increase in GLN oxidation in the kidney
Increase in the synthesis of certain proteins
→ The AAs needed for the synthesis of proteins involved in host defense may differ from those provided by muscle proteolysis
Expression of certain pathways
→ Expression of inducible nitric oxide synthase leading to an increase in ARG requirements
Change in energy substrates
→ Activated immune cells switch from glucose to glutamine as primary fuel
Other
Defect in renal reabsorption of certain AAs
Organ failure
→ e.g. Decrease in phenylalanine catabolism in liver failure
Decrease in citrulline metabolism in kidney failure

patients? (2) Are there distinct disease-related qualitative requirements? (3) Should the requirements be fully individualized?

Isotope-based studies have yielded many important results [5]. However, these methods are difficult to implement for the non-EAAs (NEAAs), giving uncertain results that are possible for only one AA at a time, all other AA intakes remaining constant. Owing to overlapping and competition for cell transport and metabolism, it is likely that requirements for any given NEAA or EAA depends on the provision of a number of other AAs. For example, providing extra leucine (LEU) at pharmacological dosages (which is reasonable since this AA promotes protein synthesis at the translational step [6]) may modify valine (VAL) and isoleucine behavior (and therefore requirements) since these three AAs compete strongly for cell uptake and metabolism [7].

Another way to assess AA requirements is to use variations in AA concentrations in plasma [8], because AAs must pass into the bloodstream after oral, enteral or parenteral administration before any further cell metabolism or incorporation into proteins can take place. Although the plasma pool of AAs is quantitatively very small compared with its intracellular free pool, and almost insignificant compared with the AAs incorporated into the protein pool, the blood compartment may play a key role in controlling AA availability for protein synthesis [6] and for specific functions such as nitric oxide synthesis in the case of arginine (ARG) [9]. We have recently discussed the characteristics, regulation and metabolic significance of plasma AA levels [7].

Plasma AA concentrations at any particular time reflect an equilibrium between their rate of entry (Ra) into plasma and their rate of exit (Rd) from it. Ra sums AA intake and AAs released by tissues, and Rd sums AA oxidation, metabolism and incorporation into proteins and, to a minor extent, loss in urine, feces, etc. [7].

Thus hyperaminoacidemia in a patient in stable metabolic conditions results from an overload of one or several AAs. Conversely a hypoaminoacidemia reflects a shortage of one or several AAs because their rate of utilization exceeds the rate of de novo synthesis plus protein catabolism, with an insufficient intake of the given AA(s).

Merely looking at AA levels in the post-absorptive state, although it simplifies the problem (i.e. in this case Ra = AAs arising from protein catabolism + de novo synthesis), cannot predict the effects of feeding, and so is of limited usefulness and may even lead to erroneous conclusions [3]. To estimate whether intake matches requirements it is necessary to measure the plasma AA level both at the basal state (i.e. post-absorptively) and at various times during AA administration.

We [10, 11] and others [12–14] have found that during continuous enteral [11], oral [13] or parenteral [10, 12, 14] administration of AAs there is a first sharp increase in AA levels and then a plateau lasting several hours. The level of the plateau, which reflects the balance between Ra and Rd, appears to be related to the rate of perfusion of each AA for any given subject [8].

This finding prompted us [15] to construct a one-compartment model with first-order elimination kinetics [16], to study the relationship between the increase in plasma AA level (pAAl) and the rate of perfusion for a given AA (AAx):

$$(AAxt3 - AAxt0) = f \text{ (rate of perfusion)}$$

Where AAxt3 is the pAAl of a given AA after 3-hour perfusion and AAxt0 the pAAl of the same AA at the post-absorptive state. There is a consensus [16, 17] that nutrition must be interrupted 3 h before the start of the test infusion, this wash-out period representing a compromise between too-short and too-long fasting.

We tested this model in healthy subjects receiving a new AA solution (AFD 10%, B. Braun) for PN [10]. The plasma concentrations of the infused AAs were closely ($r^2 = 0.92$) correlated to their infusion rate (fig. 1). In addition, as expected, the steady state was reached within 3 h on AA infusion (except for glycine and lysine: 6 h). Renal reabsorption was over 99% for most of the AAs.

Our hypothesis and its related model were also tested in an interventional study in ICU patients [18] to determine whether a qualitative manipulation of AA intake could improve the nutritional status of patients. Surgical patients received total PN for two consecutive 5-day periods. The patients were randomized into 2 groups. The control group received the same standard AA solution for the full 10 days. The experimental group received the standard solution during the first 5 days, but was switched to a more individualized solution during the last 5 days. The composition of the second solution was determined from the dynamic test described above, i.e. choosing a solution

267

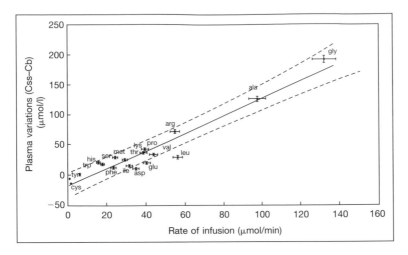

Fig. 1. Relation between the rate of infusion of amino acids and their plasma variations at steady-state $(t_{3h}-t_0)$ in healthy volunteers. — = Linear regression; ---- = 95% confidence interval. Reproduced from Bérard et al. [10] with permission.

available on the market that provided less of the AAs found to be oversupplied and more of those found to be undersupplied. AAs were defined as oversupplied or undersupplied when outside the 95% confidence interval (above or below the curve, respectively). Thus the selected solution provided (per gram of nitrogen) less of the AAs given in excess and more of those that were short.

During the second 5-day period (the test was performed again on day 8), imbalances persisted in the control group but were almost abolished in the experimental group. In addition, the mean of 5-day nitrogen balance was significantly higher during the second period in the experimental group than in the control group: 4.5 ± 0.8 vs. 0.2 ± 0.7 g nitrogen/day (p < 0.01). These findings suggest that the relationship between rate of infusion and plasma AA variations may offer a rational basis for choosing the most appropriate AA mixture for catabolic patients.

In our study on ICU patients [18], the relationship between (Aaxt3 – AAxt0) and rate of perfusion was less close (r^2 = 0.45–0.88 with no relationship in 1 patient) than in our study on healthy subjects [10], and varied from one patient to another. This emphasizes the fact that the behavior of perfused AAs is patient-specific, and argues for setting intake rates on a patient-by-patient basis, or at least according to pathology (see below).

Notably, in 5 of 12 patients, the alanine (ALA) increase was appreciably lower than predicted from its rate of perfusion, which was very high. This evidently reflects a very high utilization of this AA in gluconeogenesis. The search for a relationship between this observation and overproduction of hormones (e.g. glucagon) and mediators (e.g. tumor necrosis factor-α (TNFα), interleukin-6) in the concerned patients would be useful and deserves future study. Also of major interest was the observation on day 3 that all but one of the patients analyzed displayed abnormally high variations in levels of lysine (LYS), which was apparently infused in too high amounts for our population of catabolic patients. This was accompanied by a surprisingly high enrichment of plasma ARG; although on the contrary data from the literature [19] would have led us to expect that standard solutions would undersupply this AA. This may be because LYS and ARG share a common transport system, called CAT [9]. Therefore, oversupplying LYS may be responsible for a decrease in ARG uptake and further metabolism with an accumulation of both AAs in plasma. Decreasing LYS intake in the experimental group also normalized ARG levels [18].

A study of particular interest is that of Lerebours et al. [20]. Gastroenterological patients (mainly with Crohn's disease) received the same AA solution in two cross-over periods over 16 or 24 h. Plotting the plasma variations of each AA against the infusion rate showed a clear-cut relationship between the two parameters (NB: in this study AAt_0 was obtained after 7.5 h withdrawal of the perfusion and sample at steady state after 15.5 h of perfusion). Increasing the perfusion rate 1.5-fold (i.e. the same amount over 16 h instead of over 24 h) resulted in 2.5-, 4.5-, 2.0-, and 2.2-fold increases in proline (PRO), ALA, VAL and LEU, respectively. Increases for most of the other AAs were proportional to the increases in infusion rate. This suggests that PRO, ALA, VAL and LEU intakes are excessive compared with intake of other AAs in these patients. However, urinary elimination of AAs did not differ between the two rates of perfusion, indicating that the imbalance remained in the homeostatic range. Evidently then, a standard AA solution undersupplies ALA in ICU patients [18] but oversupplies it in gastrointestinal patients [20].

Thus a number of factors may affect the relationship between rate of perfusion and pAAl enrichment. These factors may include the type of pathology (depleted vs. hypermetabolic) [21], and the level of concomitant energy administration [8, 21]. Notably, the rate of plasma clearance after total parenteral nutrition (TPN) cessation also depends on the underlying pathology [17, 18].

Such a direct relationship between the rate of infusion and the patients' needs cannot be established for all AAs when they are provided by the oral or enteral route [13]. This is because, using this route of administration, the first absorption stage in the splanchnic area totally modifies the pattern of AAs appearing in the general circulation.

For example, a large proportion of glutamate (GLU) is extracted and metabolized in the gut [22], and a large proportion of glutanine (GLN) is metabolized by both the intestine and the liver [23]. Therefore, even though GLU + GLN represent ≈ 20% of total AAs in ingested proteins, they form only a small minimal proportion of the AAs appearing in the general circulation.

Conversely, branched-chain AAs (BCAAs) also represent $\approx 20\%$ of AAs in ingested proteins, but make up 40% of total AAs appearing in the general circulation, because BCAAs are only poorly metabolized in enterocytes and not at all in hepatocytes [24].

However, the kinetics of AAs appearing in the general circulation are particularly interesting because it is clear that there is a relationship between plasma enrichment of AAs and protein synthesis (especially in muscle) in the postprandial state [1, 6]. Recent studies [25, 26], strongly suggest that sarcopenia in elderly subjects may result from an abnormally high postprandial sequestration of AAs in the splanchnic area (twice that in young subjects). Providing 80% of the daily ration of proteins in a single meal affords similar protein synthesis in elderly and young adults [27]. This suggests that splanchnic sequestration of AAs is a saturable process. This may explain why a very high intake of GLN ($>30\,g$/day) by the enteral route is required to obtain a beneficial effect in critically ill patients, whereas lower intakes have no effect [28, 29].

Monitoring variations in plasma AAs during continuous enteral nutrition may also help to evaluate the efficacy of the form of nitrogen intake. For example, we demonstrated that when nitrogen was provided in the form of a peptide-based diet, LEU plasma levels and LEU enrichment ($LEUt_3$–$LEUt_0$), were associated with a higher insulin secretion [11].

Finally, the new and interesting concept of slow/fast proteins [30] is also relevant here: ingestion of fast proteins (e.g. lactalbumin) leads to a faster and higher increase in plasma LEU than that of slow proteins (e.g. casein), but this is a transient effect and the areas under the curves of pAAl after some hours, the amount of proteins oxidized and the protein turnover are equivalent, regardless of the type of protein. Since these proteins affect protein synthesis and protein catabolism differently, this concept may nevertheless have important applications in feeding ICU patients according to their underlying type of catabolism (decreased protein synthesis or increased protein catabolism).

In conclusion, kinetic measurements of plasma AAs following parenteral or enteral administration of AAs throw light on patients' qualitative requirements. These determinations can be used to define more closely adapted solutions for critical care patients and could be useful for individualized patient monitoring. In addition, these findings justify pharmacy facilities, the cost-effectiveness of which versus marketed ready-to-use bags is currently a subject of discussion.

References

1. Obled C, Papet I, Breuille D. Metabolic bases of amino acid requirements in acute diseases. *Curr Opin Clin Nutr Metab Care* 2002; 5: 189–97.
2. Biolo G, Toigo G, Ciocchi B, Situlin R, Iscra F, Gullo A. Metabolic response to injury and sepsis: Changes in protein metabolism. *Nutrition* 1997; 13 (suppl): S52–S7.

3. Fürst P, Stehle P. Are we giving unbalanced amino acid solutions? In: Wilmore DW, Carpentier YA, eds. *Metabolic support of the critically ill patient.* Berlin: Springer, 1993; 119–36.

4. Fürst P. Criteria underlying the formulation of amino acid regimens: Established and new approaches. In: Kleinberger G, Deutsch E, eds. *New aspects of clinical nutrition.* Basel: Karger, 1983; 361–76.

5. Young VR, El-Khoury AE. The notion of the nutritional essentiality of amino acids, revisited, with a note on the indispensable amino acid requirements in adults. In: Cynober L, ed. *Amino acid metabolism and therapy in health and nutritional diseases.* Boca Raton: CRC Press, 1995; 191–232.

6. Kimball SR, Jefferson LS. Regulation of protein synthesis by branched-chain amino acids. *Curr Opin Clin Nutr Metab Care* 2001; 4: 39–43.

7. Cynober L. Plasma amino acid levels with a note on membrane transport: Characteristics, regulation and metabolic significance. *Nutrition* 2002; 18: 761–6.

8. Waterhouse C, Clarke EF, Heinig RE, Lewis AM, Jeanpretre N. Free amino acid levels in the blood of patients undergoing parenteral alimentation. *Am J Clin Nutr* 1979; 32: 2423–9.

9. Morris SM. Regulation of arginine availability and its impact on NO synthesis. In: Ignarro LJ, ed. *Nitric oxide: Biology and pathobiology.* San Diego: Academic Press, 2000; 187–97.

10. Bérard MP, Hankard R, Cynober L. Amino acid metabolism during total parenteral nutrition in healthy volunteers: Evaluation of a new amino acid solution. *Clin Nutr* 2001; 20: 407–14.

11. Ziegler F, Nitenberg G, Coudray-Lucas C, Lasser Ph, Giboudeau J, Cynober L. Pharmacokinetic assessment of an oligopeptide-based enteral formula in abdominal surgery patients. *Am J Clin Nutr* 1998; 67: 124–8.

12. Iapichino G, Radrizzani D, Colombo A, Ronzoni G, Pasetti G, Bonetti G, Corbetta C. Plasma amino acid concentration changes during total parenteral nutrition in critically ill patients. *Clin Nutr* 1992; 11: 358–64.

13. Ashley DV, Barclay DV, Chauffard FA, Moennoz D, Leathwood PD. Plasma amino acid responses in humans to evening meals of differing nutritional composition. *Am J Clin Nutr* 1982; 36: 143–53.

14. Carpentier YA, Richelle M, Rubin M, Rossle C, Dahlan W, Bosson D, et al. Stabilisation of plasma substrate concentrations: A model for conducting metabolic studies. *Clin Nutr* 1990; 9: 313–8.

15. Abumrad NN, Darmaun D, Cynober L. Approaches to studying amino acid metabolism: From quantitative assays to flux assessment using stable isotopes. In: Cynober L, ed. *Amino acid metabolism in health and nutritional disease.* Boca Raton: CRC Press, 1995; 15–30.

16. Mosebach KO, Stoeckel H, Caspari R, Muller R, Schulte J, Lippoldt R, et al. Pharmacokinetic evaluation of a new maintenance solution for severely injured patients. *JPEN J Parenter Enteral Nutr* 1980; 4: 346–50.

17. Radrizzani D, Iapichino G, Bonetti G, Bozzetti F, Ammatuna M, Colombo A. Plasma amino acid concentration changes after total parenteral nutrition (TPN) interruption in critically ill and surgical neoplastic patients. *Clin Nutr* 1987; 6: 201–3.

18. Bérard MP, Pelletier A, Ollivier JM, Gentil B, Cynober L. Qualitative manipulation of amino acid supply during total parenteral nutrition in surgical patients. *JPEN J Parenter Enteral Nutr* 2002; 26: 136–43.

19. Yu YM, Ryan CM, Castillo L, Lu XM, Beaumier L, Tompkins RG, et al. Arginine and ornithine kinetics in severely burned patients: Increased rate of arginine disposal. *Am J Physiol* 2001; 280: E509–E17.

20. Lerebours E, Colin R, Hecketsweiler B, Matray F. Plasma amino acids in total parenteral nutrition comparison of continuous and cyclic parenteral nutrition. *Clin Nutr* 1987; 6: 143–9.

21. Iapichino G, Radrizzani D, Bonetti G, Doldi SB, Della-Torre P, Ferrero P. Dispensable and indispensable amino acid requirements in depleted patients receiving total parenteral nutrition. *Clin Nutr* 1987; 6: 5–12.

22. Matthews DE, Marano MA, Campbell RG. Splanchnic bed utilization of glutamine and glutamic acid in humans. *Am J Physiol* 1993; 264: E848–E54.

23. Darmaun D. Métabolisme de la glutamine in vivo chez l'homme: Implications pour la nutrition artificielle. *Nutr Clin Métabol* 1990; 4: 203–14.

24. Abumrad NN, Williams P, Frexes-Steed M, Geer R, Flakoll P, Cerosimo E, et al. Interorgan metabolism of amino acids *in vivo. Diabetes Metab Rev* 1989; 5: 213–26.

25. Boirie Y, Gachon P, Beaufrère B. Splanchnic and whole-body leucine kinetics in young and elderly men. *Am J Clin Nutr* 1997; 65: 489–95.

26. Walrand S, Chambon-Savanovitch C, Felgines C, Chassagne J, Raul F, Normand B, et al. Aging: A barrier to renutrition? Nutritional and immunologic evidence in rats. *Am J Clin Nutr* 2000; 72: 816–24.
27. Arnal M, Mosoni L, Houlier M, Morin L, Verdier E, Ritz P, et al. Protein pulse feeding improves protein retention in elderly women. *Am J Clin Nutr* 1999; 69: 1202–8.
28. Cynober L. Les pharmaconutriments azotés: du tube à essai à la pratique clinique. *Nutr Clin Métabol* 2001; 15: 131–43.
29. Alpers DH. Is glutamine a unique fuel for small intestinal cells? *Curr Opin Gastroenterol* 2000; 16: 155–9.
30. Boirie Y, Dangin M, Gachon P, Vasson MP, Maubois JL, Beaufrere B. Slow and fast dietary proteins differently modulate postprandial protein accretion. *Proc Natl Acad Sci USA* 1997; 94: 14930–5.

Discussion

Dr. Baracos: In the study by Bérard et al., did the amino acid infusion contain all 20 amino acids used in protein synthesis and any other amino compounds of interest, or was it a subset?

Dr. Cynober: Which one, on healthy subjects [1] or patients in the intensive care unit (ICU) [2]?

Dr. Baracos: Both, particularly in the ICU patients. I would say that it is perfect or has been nicely done.

Dr. Cynober: The product used in the ICU patient study was really a standard product, at that time it was most popular in France. The name is Vinténe®, containing 20 g of amino acids and all standard amino acids but no cysteine, no glutamine, and very low amounts of tyrosine. It was really a standard solution mimicking the composition of the most efficient proteins such as egg or milk protein.

Dr. Baracos: I would like to see that done with all the amino compounds of potential interest. I find this approach enormously helpful. I guess the difficulty that I have with the present discussion on mono amino acid therapy is that if you are giving glutamine or arginine or leucine, or whatever it is you may chose to supplement, what you might expect to be the outcome of that supplementation is only as good as your concept of what is likely to be the first limiting amino acid. If you are supplementing something which actually is in fact the second limiting amino acid or if there are two concurrent, or 3 or 4, I don't know how many concurrent amino acids which are limiting to an important degree, you supplement one of those, you can expect to see exactly nothing. I think the approach that you described could be quite useful, especially in those situations where you believe the amino acid requirements to be highly deviated from the normal condition but you do not have a clue as to where to start. So we very much look forward to seeing more work of this kind in different patient populations.

Dr. Breuillé: I have a small comment about Dr. Baracos proposal. I think it is true that there is a risk of losing some effect when you have secondary limiting amino acids, but it probably is worth a try. My other comment is that, with this kinetic study, it is in fact necessary to see the amino acids that are going to accumulate or not. We know that some amino acids accumulate easily or not at all. For instance amino acids like threonine or valine accumulate very easily in the blood, and others like tyrosine or cysteine do not. So my question is, is there a risk of missing some amino acids?

Dr. Cynober: I didn't answer Dr. Baracos, it was more a comment. I don't claim that these solutions, especially for the parenteral route, are totally inadequate for patients, especially those in the ICU with major stress. Of course then we can discuss a number of issues, for instance the reliability of the compartment that we are exploring, but it

In exactly the same problem of what is the best precursor pool when you are working with stable isotope, etc. Of course if we improve the alanine intake there is a risk that other amino acids become more limiting but it is not certain, we have to verify that. Remember that in the data I presented when we provided more alanine we corrected the imbalance and there was no new imbalance or almost no new imbalance appearing in patients, and the nitrogen balance was improved in that group. Now the second part of your comment/question, when you say that threonine accumulates, or tyrosine accumulates, to which study are you referring?

Dr. Breuillé: We know that some amino acids are very well controlled in their concentration in the blood, for instance for cysteine it is very difficult to see a large increase in this amino acid. It is true that it is even more pronounced if you look at the supplementation by the enteral route, and so it is very difficult to extrapolate the enteral administration.

Dr. Cynober: All amino acid increases are very well controlled for the simple reason that high amounts of most amino acids may induce brain disorders and the organism makes very big efforts to control the concentration of amino acids in fixed concentrations. It is my opinion, and if you look at the range of variation of amino acids in physiology and pathology, it is almost the same for most amino acids.

Dr. Zazzo: Some clarity about the critically ill patients in St. Antoine Hospital. We know that the amino acid profiles are different in liver disease, acute liver disease especially, and renal failure. I think these patients were not in renal failure, had no organ failure, but probably you must accept this kind of patient on the rationale of this prospective study.

Dr. Cynober: In that study patients with renal and hepatic failure were not included, and during the study those patients where excluded from the protocol. I mentioned that organ failure modifies the requirement of amino acids. Another thing related to this aspect is the problem of lysine. From a survey of the literature, I am certain that lysine is given in excess in ICU patients. But note that if we are afraid of the possibility of arginine giving rise to nitric oxide, perhaps it is a good thing to provide some patients large amounts of lysine. Furthermore, we have heard that it would be alright for ICU patients to have 50% essential amino acids. I don't share this view because essential amino acids are not used in large amounts in such situations and they recycle very well. I think that the true problem of availability is the amount of nonessential amino acids in this situation.

Dr. Nitenberg: I have two short questions. Maybe I missed something in the methodology of the Bérard studies [1, 2]. I don't know how to use the plasma concentrations of amino acids. Finally you show that you have a decrease in alanine, for example, in very severe patients, but did you measure what the uptake of alanine was in this situation, and what about excretion, because if uptake is improved it is very different from the situation in which there is a high excretion of amino acids. In one of your slides, at day 8, you show that suddenly the nitrogen balance was negative in the control group compared to the positive balance on day 3. Did the situation of these patients change to explain that? Finally, if you suggest that there is a shortage in alanine, do you suggest that the dipeptide alanyl-glutamine is perfectly suited for critically ill patients?

Dr. Cynober: It makes sense to come to such a conclusion. First, you said a decrease in alanine. There was no decrease in alanine, there was an increase which was lower than expected from the rate of perfusion. That is quite different because of course due to the activation of transporter controlled by the hormones, by cytokines and other mediators, there is a relationship between the use of this amino acid and further use in the tissues. As an example, if by using a pharmacological method or, in a model of perfused rat liver for example, you block alanine utilization in gluconeogenesis with the stimulation of glucagon, you will immediately see an increase in free alanine in the liver.

273

Then there is a control, which is called trans inhibition control, which causes the increase in intracellular alanine to exert a feedback on the cellular transport of alanine, and the uptake of alanine will immediately be decreased. In other words there is the same type of concept as developed by Newsholme et al. [3] some years ago about the control of the pathway. I think it is important to understand the mathematical manipulation well in that circumstance. Concerning your other question, it is not a negative nitrogen balance, it is a null balance, i.e. not different from zero, and I am not certain that this balance was significantly different from the two balances during the first period. Perhaps you were very impressed by the fact that from day 0 to day 5 it was up and down for the control group after that. It is true nitrogen, it is not derived from urea, and so I am confident with this parameter.

Dr. Déchelotte: I would like to make 3 different points. I am quite convinced that the pharmacokinetic approach may be helpful to design formulas, but I think when we make some pharmacokinetic calculations at best we would need to have several distinct and different infusion rates in order to check whether there are some linear pharmacokinetics or not. Probably our metabolic clearance of several amino acids is not linear. That could explain why in healthy subjects there is a very nice relationship between the infusion rate and concentration just because the metabolic clearance rate is supposed to be constant all the time for the people, and it is quite different in your patients in both studies, as you underlined, because some metabolic clearance of some distinct amino acids, such as valine, may be reduced in the case of valine or increased in the case of alanine. So I think before drawing definite conclusions about the ideal profile of the amino acid composition we need more information on the dose relationship, the infusion rate relationship to the whole pharmacokinetic approach.

Dr. Cynober: This is why the session is entitled 'towards the future'. I agree with you. Of course if you have increasing levels of perfusion you have additional information but by knowing the rate of perfusion you can calculate the rate of utilization of the whole body and you can calculate the central clearance, but note that it is exactly what Lerebours et al. [4] did, it was the same amount of amino acids at a different rate. We achieved exactly the same condition and we had the same linear regression. Also there is a classic paper, an American paper by Clowes et al. [5], which was published in *Surgery* almost 20 years ago. They made arteriovenous differences and made similar calculations, and made the same conclusions about the reliability between the rate of perfusion and tissue utilization of amino acids.

Dr. Déchelotte: Going on with the same point. The difference also in the Lerebours et al. study [4] was that during the night patients were fed cyclically or continuously, so they also received higher amounts of glucose and lipids during the night together with amino acids over 12 or 14 h instead of 24 h. Probably then there was some influence of energy intake on the metabolic clearance of amino acids. The second point is about this difference in kinetics between casein and whey proteins which was so elegantly shown by Boirie et al. [6]. Of course there was a difference in the acute effect on protein synthesis or protein degradation but, as you know, there was also a difference in the net leucine balance at the end and casein had a better global leucine balance than lactoserum because it has less influence on protein synthesis but a better beneficial effect on inhibition of protein degradation. This kinetic difference is mainly related to the gastric emptying profile of these proteins. I assume we should be cautious in extrapolating these data from healthy subjects to the situation of ICU patients where we know that there is a great incidence of gastroparesis. The difference in the profile of gastric emptying, degradation, absorption and influence on protein metabolism could be quite different for these two types of proteins.

Dr. Cynober: We have to rewrite this paper because I remember that the total balance was not different.

I feel that this type of approach may be very useful because we were discussing huge amounts of arginine, huge amounts of glutamine, and new products with huge amounts of both glutamine and arginine, nobody studied any competition. At the last ESPEN Congress in Glasgow several new products were displayed without any pharmacokinetics or clinical evaluation. On one hand we are discussing pharmacology and on the other we don't make the studies which are required for such products. Could you imagine that a new non-steroidal anti-inflammatory agent is released on the market without any pharmacokinetic or pharmacological study? I think we have to take note of all these elements, which is probably not feasible, but of course the protein nature of the different diets used, some are based on animal proteins which are very rich in lysine and poor in arginine. If you use soy proteins it is the reverse and the difference is huge, and therefore you can have major interference in the metabolism. Again we discussed the problem of giving immune-enhancing diets to elderly subjects. Why to elderly subject, because there are some data which indicate that this probably has something to do with the splanchnic sequestration of amino acids and the specific metabolism of arginine into citrulline in this tissue. We need data about that. Of course I agree with your interpretation of the Boirie et al. [6] study.

Dr. Déchelotte: My last point was about splanchnic uptake in older patients. The data by Arnal et al. [7] were gained in healthy old people, not in ICU patients. I agree with you that there are very little data in these old ICU patients. We studied the splanchnic uptake of leucine in operated patients with a cross-perfusion of stable isotopes. They were middle-aged, about 50-, 55-year-old cancer patients, and the splanchnic uptake of leucine and glutamine was quite similar in these patients to that observed in healthy subjects.

Dr. Berger: I am a bit confused about all those plasma levels and I need your help here. Of course we need pharmacokinetics, of course plasma is what we can get at, but our ICU patients are very unstable and their plasma levels, I know that from micronutrients, are just very difficult to assess regularly. Plasma levels reflect flow. You very nicely made the point that about 35–50% of enterally administered glutamine is likely metabolized into the gut. Not to have an increase in plasma level does not mean it does not work. What do you think about that, because of course we have to compare solutions which give the same amounts and if that was the point I fully agree, but not achieving the same plasma levels does not mean the solution is not working.

Dr. Cynober: Patients are unstable in the ICU but I studied burn patients for years and we can have a very reliable profile 2 or 3 days after burn injury. Again, and I agree with you, there are fluxes and there are concentrations. It is absolutely certain that the basal concentration or only the concentration under perfusion is of no interest. I am sure there are too many factors that can be involved in increase or decrease. That is why the difference in concentration and perfusion is mandatory. In that condition if you are able to saturate splanchnic sequestration of glutamine, you must see glutamine increasing the general circulation.

Dr. Moore: I used to be a disciple of Frank Cerra and read all his work. I really believed in it. We went through a phase, at least in the United States, of being very excited about altering the amino acid composition for these different solutions and thought that we were going to improve outcome. There were a number of trials done on branched chain amino acids suggesting that you could alter metabolic endpoints, improve protein synthesis, but we could never show an improved outcome. There was a small study from Spain [8] recently showing a decreased mortality. Similarly, in liver failure we can make people wake up in the ICU but not too many of them would walk out of the hospital as a result. With dialysis renal failure it is the same thing: we can decrease dialysis needs but at the end of the day there is the same number of dead patients. So my question to you is, is there a greater interest in Europe about this, and then the second question is, if you had to tell me what the ideal amino acid solution is for my ICU patients what does it need to be supplemented with?

Dr. Cynober: I am very happy with that because it will allow me to discuss a specific problem and to demonstrate how a potentially very interesting concept has been killed, the concept of branched chain amino acids. Because I have not discussed two things: one is galenic which does not concern branched chain amino acids, and the other is the cost of the products. As you mentioned there has been a lot of work on the possible pharmacological effect of branched chain amino acids, and most of the results were disappointing. I will take the example I know the best, which is burn injury. In total there are six experimental and clinical studies involving supplementation of branched chain amino acids by the parenteral route. Branched chain amino acids in burn injury improve protein metabolism, improve nitrogen balance, decrease 3-methylhistidine excretion and so on, but only in one condition, when the solution is enriched with leucine. If you look at most of the products available on the market, due to the cost of amino acids they are actually enriched in valine, in isoleucine. Because the 3 amino acids compete very tightly for cell uptake and metabolism, when you are providing this so-called enriched solution of branched chain amino acid, what you are actually giving in percentage is a leucine-poor solution, and this explains why most of the studies failed to provide results. Again simple pharmacokinetic studies show that and the recent study I mentioned by Kimball and Jefferson [8] on the control of protein synthesis regulation is exactly in agreement: only leucine has such properties. Again, of course there is nothing to expect by providing 80% of the diet in the form of branched chain amino acids included in the total amount of nitrogen given it is totally imbalanced. That is why in the introduction I mentioned the concept, especially for parenteral nutrition, as being established long before we had most of the helpful physiopathological knowledge that we have now. Finally we are of the opinion that most experts say that all solutions are equivalent, nobody has shown any difference in manipulating the standard composition of amino acids. It is not a special European interest, it is an ignored field of research and I think that now is a good time to readdress this type of question.

Dr. Martindale: We have all these fluxes of amino acids. You haven't addressed the fact that we have 5 systems to absorb some of these amino acids: system Y, system B, system B0, system CAT2, etc. You showed CAT2 competing with lysine. So not only do we have the confusion of the individual amino acids but the 4 or 5 transporters for which they compete, and those are changed by diseases. We don't really know what happens to these transporters in critical illness, we don't know in sepsis, we don't know in trauma.

Dr. Cynober: Yes, it is perfectly true. It is the type of study we are performing, realistic studies with a pragmatic approach, and we have global results. At the tissue level I would like to mention the work by Souba and Pacitti [9]. For example Pacitti et al. [10] studied the N system of transport for glutamine in various tissues and with various results. But I fully agree that we have a lack of knowledge in this specific area.

References

1. Bérard MP, Hankard R, Cynober L. Amino acid metabolism during total parenteral nutrition in healthy volunteers: Evaluation of a new amino acid solution. *Clin Nutr* 2001; 20: 407–14.
2. Bérard MP, Pelletier A, Ollivier et al. Qualitative manipulation of amino acid supply during total parenteral nutrition in surgical patients. *JPEN J Parenter Enteral Nutr* 2002; 26: 136–43.

3. Newsholme EA, Crabtree B, Ardawi MSM. The role of high rates of glycolysis and glutamine utilization in rapidly dividing cells. *Biosci Rep* 1985; 5: 393–400.
4. Lerebours E, Colin R, Hecketsweiler B, Matray F. Plasma amino acids in total parenteral nutrition: Comparison of continuous and cyclic parenteral nutrition. *Clin Nutr* 1987; 6: 143–9.
5. Clowes Jr. GHA, Mc Dermott WV, Williams LF, Loda M, Menzoian JO, Pearl R. Amino acid clearance and prognosis in surgical patients with cirrhosis. *Surgery* 1984; 96: 675–84.
6. Boirie Y, Dangin M, Gachon P, et al. Slow and fast dietary proteins differently modulate postprandial protein accretion. *Proc Natl Acad Sci USA* 1997; 94: 14930–5.
7. Arnal M, Mosoni L, Houlier M, et al. Protein pulse feeding improves protein retention in elderly women. *Am J Clin Nutr* 1999; 69: 1202–8.
8. Kimball SR, Jefferson LS. Regulation of protein synthesis by branched-chain amino acids. *Curr Opin Clin Nutr Metab Care* 2001; 4: 39–43.
9. Souba WW, Pacitti AJ. How amino acids get into cells: Mechanisms, models, menus, and mediators. *JPEN J Parenter Enteral Nutr* 1992; 16: 569–78.
10. Pacitti AJ, Austgen TR, Souba WW. Adaptive regulation of alanine transport in hepatic plasma membrane vesicles from the endotoxin-treated rat. *J Surg Res* 1991; 51: 46–53.

Cynober L, Moore FA (eds): Nutrition and Critical Care.
Nestlé Nutrition Workshop Series Clinical & Performance Program, Vol. 8, pp. 279–298,
Nestec Ltd.; Vevey/S. Karger AG, Basel © 2003.

Nutritional Support in ICU Patients: Position of Scientific Societies

Federico Bozzetti and Biagio Allaria

Istituto Nazionale per lo Studio e La Cura dei Tumori, Milano, Italia

The most prominent metabolic alterations which characterize the systemic inflammatory response syndrome and sepsis include hypermetabolism, hyperglycemia with insulin resistance, accelerated lipolysis and net protein catabolism [1–3]. The combined effect of these metabolic alterations associated with bed rest and lack of nutritional intake can lead to a progressive depletion of lean body mass.

Even if nutritional support in critically ill patients cannot fully prevent or reverse the metabolic alterations and, consequently, the disruption in body composition and the erosion of the body cell mass, it can nevertheless slow the rate of net protein catabolism by providing an exogenous load of energy and nitrogen [2, 4].

Recent publications demonstrate increased non-resting energy expenditure (i.e. activity) after the first week of critical illness [5]. Total energy expenditure in septic patients was in fact 25 ± 5 kcal/kg/day during the first week of critical illness and increased to 47 ± 6 kcal/kg/day during the second week. However, it remains to be determined if administering more than 25–30 kcal/kg/day is beneficial to these patients, and if providing more than 1 g amino acid/kg/day (a quantity sufficient to minimize loss of body protein during the initial 2 weeks of critical illness) carries further benefit [6].

We reviewed the official statements of some national and international scientific societies regarding the nutritional support of intensive care unit (ICU) patients: the Italian Society for Parenteral and Enteral Nutrition (SINPE) 1995 [7]; the French Speaking Society for Enteral and Parenteral Nutrition (SFNEP) 1996 [8] that only considered septic patients; the American College of Chest Physicians (ACCP) 1997 [9]; the French Speaking Society of Enteral and Parenteral Nutrition (F3NEP) 1998 [10]; the European Society of Intensive Care Medicine (ESICM) 1998 [11] that also published a position paper on Enteral Nutrition in Intensive Care Patients (ESICM, 1999) [12]; the American Society for Parenteral and Enteral Nutrition (ASPEN) together with the American Society of Clinical Nutrition (ASCN) (ASPEN-ASCN) 1997 [13]; the European Society for Parenteral and Enteral Nutrition (ESPEN) 2000 [14]; the American Gastroenterological Association (AGA) 2001 [15], and finally the American Society for Parenteral and Enteral Nutrition (ASPEN) 2002 [16].

It is worth noting that the guidelines of the ESPEN on this topic have not been properly published and all ESPEN statements refer to the book officially supported by the educational committee of the society [14].

Regarding the AGA, we refer to the medical position statement concerning parenteral nutrition only [15].

For each society statement, we considered the following issues: (1) selection of patients; (2) timing; (3) requirements of macronutrients; (4) composition of the nutritive admixture; (5) special nutrients, and (6) special conditions.

Selection of Patients

Even if data from patients recovering from major surgery cannot be fully extrapolated to other critically patients, morbidity and mortality increase significantly after 2 weeks of glucose infusion (250–300 g/day) when compared to nutritionally complete total parenteral nutrition (TPN) [17]. Initiating TPN after 2 weeks of glucose infusion does not improve outcome [17].

The Italian and the American societies have the most strictly defined criteria in the selection of patients requiring nutritional support.

SINPE 1995 [7] recommends nutritional support in all patients with hypercatabolism (>15 g urinary nitrogen/day) or 10–159 urinary nitrogen/day if they are unable to be adequately fed by mouth (<50% of the basal requirements) for 7 days. If patients are already malnourished and have a catabolism exceeding 10 g urinary nitrogen/day, they should receive nutritional support if 5 days of inadequate feeding is anticipated.

ASPEN 2002 [16] recommends 'that some form of nutritional support be started after 5–10 days of fasting in patients who are likely to remain unable to eat for an additional week or more'.

This statement confirms the previous recommendations of the ASPEN-ASCN 1997 [13] that suggested nutritional support for 'patients who are unlikely to consume adequate nutrient intake for prolonged period' (7–10 days).

The other societies have a less strict criterion of patient selection:

- ACCP 1997 [9]: 'clinical setting requiring at least 4 days of ICU confinement'.
- SFNEP 1998 [8]: malnourished patients (weight loss exceeding 10% of the body weight) and those unable to reassume 'normal' nutrition in a week after the acute episode.

- ESICM 1008 1009 [11, 12] recommends nutritional support in patients malnourished or well-nourished but candidates for fasting of more than 3 or 4 days and in severe trauma or burn patients.

With reference to enteral nutrition (EN) only, ESICM 1998–1999 [11, 12] suggests that enteral support is indicated in septic malnourished patients unable to eat, or in well-nourished candidates for prolonged fasting (>7 days).

EN may also be given as a supplement if one expects an insufficient oral intake for >7 days.

AGA 2001 [15] simply concludes that TPN does not affect mortality in trauma patients or length of time on mechanical ventilation. However, it points out that some but not all the randomized clinical trials (RCTs) comparing TPN to EN found less infections in patients receiving EN.

Timing

SINPE 1995 [7] and ACCP 1997 [9] recommend starting nutritional support as soon as possible after resuscitation. In fact, in critical states when splanchnic blood flow is compromised, EN can increase blood flow in the proximal part of the bowel (where EN is administered) and decrease blood flow in the distal part with consequent hypoxia, impairment in motility and damage to the intestinal mucosa.

FSNEP 1998 [10] also considers hemodynamic instability as incompatible with the start of nutritional support.

However, it is worth recalling the recent experience of Revelly et al. [18] who showed that enteral delivery of nutrients can be safely performed with good compliance and utilization of substrates also in patients with hemodynamic instability requiring inotropic drugs like catecholamines.

ESICM 1998–1999 [11, 12] suggests early nutritional support (within 24–48 h) in highly catabolic states (severe trauma, burns, etc.) and after 2–3 days in patients with moderate stress who are unable to eat.

In contrast, ASPEN 2002 [16] seems to propose a policy of wait and see: 'it appears reasonable to recommend that some form of specialized nutritional support be started after 5–10 days of fasting in patients who are likely to remain unable to eat for an additional week or more'.

With regards to EN, ESICM 1998–1999 [11, 12] suggests that 'EN should begin as soon as possible, not necessarily with the goal of providing total support, but with that of exerting the beneficial effects on the gut which can be obtained with even small amounts of enteral feeding. In many critically ill patients a 5- to 7-day delay before initiating EN has been considered reasonable, since no deleterious effects of short fasting have been demonstrated in these conditions However, if prior malnutrition or a simply catabolic condition are present, this delay should be shortened to 1–2 days.'

Requirements of Macronutrients

Energy
SFNEP 1996 [8] recommends for septic patients 34–44 kcal/kg/day, which should correspond to 1.3–1.5 times the estimated resting energy consumption.

ACCP 1997 [9] recommends 25 kcal/kg/day, SFNEP 1998 [10] 21–26 kcal/kg/day, SINPE 1995 [7] and ASPEN 2002 [16] recommend 25–30 kcal/kg/day, and ESPEN 2000 [14] warns to not exceed 30 kcal/kg/day.

ESICM 1998–1999 [11, 12] differentiates males who should receive 25–30 nonprotein kcal/kg/day from females who should be treated with 20–25 nonprotein kcal/kg/day. This society also specifies the reference body weight in malnourished and obese patients; this should be calculated as the mean between measured and ideal weight in severely malnourished patients, and as a value 20% higher than the ideal weight in obese patients.

SFNEP 1998 [10] suggests that energy intake should be very close to the resting metabolic expenditure. The estimate by the Harris-Benedict equation should be corrected by different factors depending on the nature of the injury: postoperative period 1–1.1; fractures 1.1–1.3; severe infection 1.3–1.6, and burns 1.5–2.1. However, different conditions may affect the metabolic expenditure: hyperthermia increases metabolic expenditure by 10%/1 °C, and infection also by 10%. In contrast, both hypothermia or sedation tend to reverse hypermetabolism to a value close to basal.

ESICM 1998–1999 [12] also specifies that the lower values should be followed in patients >60 years of age.

When body temperature is increased, 10% should be added to energy needs for every degree >37 °C, according to this society.

Glucose
SINPE 1995 [7] suggests that glucose should account for more than 80% of total energy requirements, whereas SFNEP 1996 [8], ACCP 1997 [9], SFNEP 1998 [10] and ESICM 1998–1999 [11, 12] suggest that glucose should cover 60–70% of the energy requirement.

Consequently SINPE 1995 [7] recommends a dosage not exceeding 5.7–7.2 g/kg/day, while ACCP 1997 [3] suggests 2–3 g/kg/day, SFNEP 1998 [10] 3.8–4.5 g/kg/day (15–18 kcal/kg/day) and ESPEN 2000 [14] a value ranging from 3 to 6 g/kg/day.

Fat
There seems to be an agreement that long-chain triglycerides (LCTs) should account for at least 3% of total energy intake [7] and n-3 PUFAs for at least 7% of total calories.

The requirement of fat is complementary to that of glucose and SINPE 1995 [7] and ESICM 1998–1999 [11, 12] recommend that fat should account for 20–30% and 90–40% of nonprotein calories, respectively, whereas according to ACCP 1997 [9] fat should represent 15–30% of total energy.

ESPEN's 2000 [14] indications are more concerned to avoid toxicity (no more than 1.4 g LCTs/kg/day or no more than 1.7 g medium-chain triglycerides (MCTs) as MCT/LCT emulsion/kg/day rather than to suggest the optimal dose of lipids.

SFNEP 1996 [10] recommends that lipid should not exceed 2 g/kg/day in septic patients.

FSNEP 1998 [12] recommends 0.7–0.9 g/kg/day (6–8 kcal/kg/day).

This society also states that there is no evidence of a significant clinical difference among LCTs and mixed emulsions of LCTs and MCTs and emulsions with a prevalent olive oil content (80%).

Amino Acids

ACCP 1997 [9] and ESICM 1998–1999 [11, 12] suggest amino acids be given at 1.2–1.5 g/kg/day. According to ACCP 1997 [9] recommendations for amino acids should account for 15–20% of total calorie intake, while ESICM 1998–1999 [11, 12] suggests that patients should never receive more than 1.8 g/kg/day unless they have exceptional losses (extensive burns, digestive losses, etc.).

This society also suggests that body weight used for this computation should be the mean between ideal and measured weight in severely malnourished patients, and 20% higher than the ideal weight in obese patients.

FSNEP 1998 [10] recommends 1.5–2.1 g/kg/day.

ESPEN 2000 [14] and SINPE 1995 [7] recommend higher quantities, 1.5–2.0 g/kg/day and also 2.5 g/kg/day in severe catabolism [7]. SFNEP 1996 [8] suggests that an amino acid intake of 2.5 g/kg/day is a maximum beyond which further supply is inefficient and even harmful, and an appropriate energy/nitrogen ratio should be in the order of 100–150 kcal/g nitrogen.

Micronutrients

There is no recommendation for an extra supply of micronutrients [10], except if patients are supported enterally with 1,500 ml of enteral formula or less or in the presence of severe conditions combining increased needs and large losses of trace elements.

Route of Administration

According to SINPE 1995 [7], ACCP 1997 [9], ESICM 1998–1999 [11, 12], and ESPEN 2000 [14], the enteral route and a continuous administration are preferred [10].

ASPEN-ASCN 1997 [13] and ASPEN 2002 [16] also prefer the enteral route but 'it is not clear whether EN provides a specific benefit or whether TPN itself or overfeeding by TPN is associated with an increased risk of infection'.

ESICM 1998–1999 [11, 12] recommends the use of standardized, industrially produced feeding as iso-osmotic (approximately 300 mosm/l) mixtures containing 1–1.5 kcal/ml, 45–60% of which should be in the form of carbohydrates, 20–35% as lipids, and 15–20% as proteins.

These mixtures should be gluten- and lactose-free.

The consensus of ACCP 1997 [9] also states the modalities of the EN: 'Intragastric feeding requires adequate gastric motility. In general, a gastric residual exceeding 150 ml will require a moderation of the infusion rate, consideration for supplemented intravenous nutrition, or the use of small bowel feedings. Small bowel feedings can usually be performed, even in the presence of gastric atony and colonic ileus … and the presence of bowel sounds and passage of flatus or stool are not necessary for the initiation of enteral feeding. … Diarrhea may occur with administration of enteral feedings. It is usually secretory and it is generally not an indication to discontinue enteral feedings. If it exceeds 1 liter/day, an evaluation is required. If a relevant medical or surgical cause is not found, including *Clostridium difficile* enterocolitis, antidiarrheal agents may be used.'

According to ESICM 1998–1999 [11, 12], EN is absolutely contraindicated in intestinal obstruction, anatomic disruption or severe intestinal ischemia.

EN should be administered with caution in patients with reduced intestinal perfusion due to a state of prolonged or severe shock. Such patients are unable to increase their splanchnic flow in response to enteral feeding, and thus are unable to sustain the process of digestion and nutrient absorption.

Many patients with severe pancreatitis or high output proximal intestinal fistulas are intolerant to EN.

Regarding some practical aspects, this society also recommends that bags containing 500 ml of feeding admixture should be used, due to easier storage, manipulation and convenience at the bedside. The tubing connecting the container to the patient's feeding catheter should be changed once a day to avoid contamination, even if clear evidence of an association between the latter and an increased risk of clinical infection are still lacking.

Immunomodulation and Special Nutrients

The consensus guidelines of the Italian, American, and European societies edited before 2000 mentioned immunonutrients, but did so only to state that their role was still to be defined.

ESPEN 2000 [14] defines glutamine as 'potentially useful'.

ASPEN 2002 [16] questions the benefits of branched-chain amino acids.

ASPEN 2002 [16] also considers intravenous glutamine as being efficacious in reducing the infection rate [19] and improving survival [20].

Regarding the immune-enhancing enteral formulas, ASPEN 2002 [10] states that they may reduce the incidence of infectious complications but do not alter mortality [21, 22], which in some subgroups may actually increase [23, 24]. This statement mainly relies on the meta-analysis of Heyland et al. [24] which showed that in studies of critically ill patients with a high-quality score, immune-enhancing formulas were associated with an increased mortality rate and a significant reduction in infectious complications, compared with RCTs with a low-quality score.

Monitoring Nutritional Support

SINPE 1995 [7], but mainly ACCP 1997 [9] and SFNEP 1998 [10] suggest modalities for preventing iatrogenic complications.

ACCP 1997 [9] recommends the following.

- Avoid overfeeding (i.e. RQ >1) and reduce calorie intake in patients with respiratory risks.
- Avoid protein overload by checking nitrogen balance every 5–7 days, decrease nitrogen if BUN exceeds 100 mg/dl. If there is no benefit with formulations for acute renal failure, dialysis should be considered.
- Avoid excessive levels of triglycerides (more than 500 mg/dl).
- SFNEP 1998 [10] advises to start at 25 ml/h during the first 24 h and to increase by 25 ml/h every 12–24 h depending on the digestive tolerance and the desired volume to be administered. Tolerance is checked every 6 h by measuring the gastric residue and temporaneously withdrawing the infusion should such volume be 200 ml or more.
- With reference to EN, ESICM 1998–1999 [11, 12] recommends obtaining an abdominal X-ray after placement of a nasogastric tube and to monitor tolerance to gastric feeding by, 'measuring the gastric residue once a day (normal <300 ml) in order to reduce the risk of bronchoaspiration, especially in patients without protection due to tracheal intubation. If gastric residues are >300 ml, the infusion rate should be decreased by 50% for 4–6 h, and then resumed progressively over 24–48 h, during which time gastric residues should be monitored twice daily. Prokinetic agents such as erythromycin should be used in this situation to improve gastric emptying'.
- Diarrhea persisting for more than 3 days after exclusion of other common causes in patients receiving antibiotics should lead to stool culture for *Clostridium difficile* toxin, as well as a decrease in the flow rate of EN administration. If necessary, transient use of TPN should be considered in this situation to ensure adequate nutritional support. Finally, the value of administering antidiarrheal agents or *Saccharomices boulardii* should be considered in individual cases.

285

Administration of EN and TPN

ESICM 1998–1999 [11, 12] provides more detailed indications on this issue.

- Gastric feeding is usually poorly tolerated, especially if volumes >1,000 ml/day are administered.
- Nasoenteric route is preferable for short-intermediate (2–4 weeks) EN.
- Small diameter (6–12 french) silicone or polyurethane tubes are preferable. Depending on the desired location (in stomach, duodenum or jejunum), the appropriate length of the tube (90,110, at least 120 cm) is chosen.
- Proper placement is easier if performed under fluoroscopic guidance or endoscopic assistance using tubes with inner stylets.
- Percutaneous route is advised if EN is extended for ≥4–6 weeks and 9- to 24-french tubes are available.
- SFNEP 1998 [10] does not recommend the use of cyclic TPN to avoid the potential risk of fluid overload if all the solution is infused over a limited period of time, and the possible toxic effects of lipids (increase of intrapulmonary shunts, possible immunosuppression) due to a fast or abundant administration.

Special Conditions

Some societies have differentiated special acute clinical conditions with particular reference to the energy and nitrogen requirements.

SFNEP 1998 [10] has considered that there is some specificity in the nutritional approach in patients with severe sepsis, trauma, burns, and organ failure.

Sepsis

In these patients maximal care must be made to not exceed the energy requirements especially if hemodynamic conditions are frail.

Even if nitrogen balance is negative, there is no particular interest in administering >2 g amino acids/kg/day.

Trauma

The energy requirements may increase to 1.1–1.3 times the basal metabolic expenditure and reach a value of 1.4–1.9 times if a septic state is associated.

Fat administration might have a deleterious effect on infectious complications should it be delivered in an excessive quantity. Increasing the glucose level to >9 mmol/l (180 mg/dl) plasma should be avoided in order not to worsen cerebral ischemia.

Organ Failure

In patients with acute respiratory failure the recommendation is to avoid an excessive calorie load which increases CO_2 production and the fast infusion of lipid [illegible] of the drop of the PO_2/FiO_2 ratio. Phosphorus deficiency should be prevented or corrected since it interferes with diaphragmatic function.

In patients with renal failure nitrogen intake should not decrease: in contrast, if patients undergo hemodialysis or hemofiltration, the administration of glucose and amino acid should increase because of their potential loss during the procedure.

Caution must be paid to vitamin C administration because of the risk of oxalose.

In patients with liver failure there should be no restriction in the supply of lipids and proteins if they are not encephalopathic. However, careful surveillance of glucose administration is required.

Burns

The energy requirements have to be tailored to the extent and depth of the burn. An approximate estimate is obtained by Curreri's formula (25 kcal/kg + 40 kcal/% burn surface). However, deep sedation and analgesia reduce the energy expenditure. The administration of glucose and amino acids may reach 7 and 2.1 g/kg/day, respectively. The administration of vitamins and trace elements is recommended to improve the healing process.

The ASPEN Board of Directors [16] has differentiated the chapter on 'Critical Care for Critical Illness' from that on 'Critical Care for Burns'.

Since nutrition is a transverse discipline, a discipline within a discipline, we can expect that future guidelines for ICU patients will differentiate the approach to subjects with prominent organ failure, such as patients with cardiac or respiratory or renal failure. This also is the policy of the new edition of SINPE's guidelines, which are currently being prepared.

The guidelines of ASPEN 2002 [16] also include those of the American Burn Association Clinical Guidelines [25]. They recommend measuring, if possible, the energy requirement using indirect calorimetry and to increase the measured energy expenditure by 20–30% if physical therapy is performed or wound care is required.

There is also evidence of an increased protein need (20–33% of total calories from protein and a calorie:nitrogen ratio of 110:1 in severely burned children). EN should be used in preference to TPN and should be started as soon as possible. TPN should be reserved for patients who require nutritional support and EN is contraindicated or is unlikely to meet nutritional requirements within 4 or 5 days.

Areas of Consensus and Discrepancy

An overall evaluation of the statements of these societies shows a general agreement on the majority of issues we have considered. There is no doubt that nutritional support, especially via the enteral route, is recommended by all societies. This is not because of a better nutritional effect of EN comparing to TPN but because of greater protection against infections probably due to better preservation of the immune system within the gut. In addition EN is less expensive. TPN as the only nutritional support is reserved for patients who cannot be fed enterally. The selection of patients varies in the recommendations of some societies that modulate the option for nutritional support according to the degree of hypermetabolism or to the prevision of some days of inadequate nutrient intake.

This probably reflects two different positions, a traditional one referring to nutritional support as a tool to maintain an adequate nutritional status of the patients, and a more innovative one which considers nutritional support as a pharmacological tool to control the metabolic response to trauma, regardless of the nutritional status of the patient.

Also the proper time to start nutritional support shows little difference between the societies' recommendations. The authors supporting an early (immediate) start of nutritional support do not rely on the results of RCTs which do not exist, but on experimental data and clinical experience with burn patients or surgical patients receiving immunonutrition.

Perhaps the area of major discrepancy regards the composition of non-protein energy substrates to be administered. A high glucose to lipid ratio may be preferred because glucose is able to improve the nitrogen balance better than fat and represents the preferred fuel for tissue repair and bone marrow, and does not have the immunosuppressive properties of lipids.

In contrast, authors in favor of lipids claim that they are well utilized in injured people who often present a respiratory quotient of <1 and fear the deleterious effects of an excessive CO_2 production on weaning patients from ventilator.

The outstanding study of Van den Berghe et al. [25] is too recent to be considered in the guidelines of these societies. These authors showed that an intensive insulin therapy significantly reduced the mortality of ICU patients, principally through a reduction in the incidence of multiple-organ failure with a proven septic focus in subjects receiving intensive care for more than 5 days.

It is noteworthy that these results were obtained with a glucose:lipid ratio of 60–80:40–20, respectively, and a calorie regimen of 18–19 kcal/kg/day, the clinical benefit was magnified in the weeks–months after admission to the ICU and the mean glucose level was 8.4 and 5.9 mmol/l (153 and 108 mg/dl) in conventional treatment and intensive treatment groups, respectively.

From a speculative point of view, it is noteworthy that neutrophil-impaired phagocytosis has been reported both in laboratory [26] and in postoperative patients [27] when the blood glucose level was 13.3 mmol/l (240 mg/dl) or >12.2 mmol/l (270 mg/dl), respectively. Therefore it would appear that the benefit of intensive treatment was not due to a lack of noxious effects of blood glucose levels (which were lower than those commonly recognized as capable of badly affecting the host's defenses), but rather to the positive metabolic effects of insulin and were achieved with administration of 3–4 g glucose/kg/day.

Discussion

There are some points that deserve consideration. First, there is a great discrepancy between the abundance of data in the literature and the scientific value of their evidence. Only two publications, both from the USA [13, 16], attempted to grade their statements on the basis of the strength of the supporting data, as follows.

- A = Supported by RCTs or meta-analyses of RCTs.
- B = Supported by well-designed nonrandomized prospective, retrospective or case cohort-controlled studies.
- C = Supported by uncontrolled published experiences, case reports, or expert opinion or editorial consensus.

The preference of the scientific community is to rely primarily on RCTs as the basis for establishing practice guidelines, because therapies that are accepted and widely used may subsequently be found lacking when prospective RCTs are performed [28].

However, we fully agree with the opinion of the ASPEN Board of Directors [16] when it states that 'a major distinction between therapeutic trials of the efficacy of a drug or a procedure and feeding of nutrients known to be essential to maintenance of human health and survival must be made. Withholding a drug or invasive procedure will not produce disease in otherwise healthy humans, whereas essential nutrients must be provided to both healthy and ill people. Patients with advanced malnutrition or who are at risk for becoming severely malnourished must be fed to prevent death by starvation.'

In ICU patients, many of the guideline statements of the different societies were developed on the basis of expert opinion and editorial consensus because of the ethical dilemma of conducting RCTs with patients at risk of starvation who could not be randomized to a control arm without nutritional support.

A further major difficulty in clinical trials on nutritional support in critical illness is the extreme heterogeneity and complexity of critically ill patients. We agree with the conclusions of the Workshop of the American Thoracic Society Critical Care Assembly on Outcomes Research [29] when it states that, '… to formulate a research question an investigator must be able to define a disease, treatment, patient population, or provider to study and operationalizing these variables for critical care outcome research is complex. … Critical care is a challenge to the outcomes researcher precisely because the key variables of disease, patient population, therapy, and provider are difficult to study.'

Adopting a pragmatic solution that is to define critical care geographically as that taking place in the ICU, by the intensivists working in an ICU, on patients admitted to an ICU, does not solve the problem. In fact '... flexible nurse staffing, mobile technology, intermediate care units, and the growth of subacute care for chronically ill patients make the assumption that critical care begins and ends at the ICU door problematic. In addition, some patients, such as those recovering from operative procedures, may receive care in an ICU but not be critically ill ...'.

Nutritional therapy, like ventilatory or renal support, is not a disease-specific treatment and the assessment of benefit should be based on correction of nutritional abnormalities.

The outcome of these subjects is primarily affected by organ function impairment and the higher the number of organs and apparatus compromised, the worse the prognosis. As a matter of fact, the common scoring systems of severity of illness as APACHE II and III and SAPS II are composed by multiple items (14 and 12, respectively), thus confirming that nutritional status is only one (and certainly not the most prominent) of the components of the risk of complication/mortality.

Moreover, these scoring systems have recently been criticized because variability in collecting and managing the data could affect an objective determination of risk factors included in the severity of these illness scoring systems.

Finally, the effects of nutritional support are usually measured in many days or weeks whereas the mortality of ICU patients often occurs few days after admission. ICU patients may die just after their admission to the ICU, even if well-nourished or well-supported by artificial nutrition.

Therefore, difficulty in assessing the role of the nutritional status and, consequently of the nutritional support, explains why in the most recent publication [16] the four practice guidelines included in the recommendations for nutritional support in critical illness are classified as B or C and there is no A class.

This finding corresponds with the coding of the ASPEN Practice Guidelines in Nutrition Support as reported by Wolfe and Mathiesen [30]. They found that only 16% of the guidelines were judged to rely on good research-based evidence (class A), 29% on fair research-based evidence, and 55% on expert opinion only.

Conclusion

There is a gap between the abundance of data in the literature on nutritional support in ICU patients and the scientific value of their evidence.

This may be due to the extreme complexity of the critically ill patients and to the fact that nutritional support in general is not a disease-specific treatment. Nutritional support aims to treat the metabolic component of the critical illness but this does not necessarily translate into a better outcome for the patient. This chapter reviews the position of some national and international societies with special reference to the role of nutritional support in ICU patients.

There was some agreement on the following points:

- Nutritional support, especially via the enteral route, is recommended by all societies for malnourished patients, patients who are candidates for prolonged fasting or patients who are hypercatabolic or suffering from major injury.
- Nutritional support should start in an early or relatively early phase, as soon as the hemodynamic conditions have stabilized.
- Most societies recommend an energy intake proportional to the energy requirement and, empirically, of about 25 ± 5 kcal/kg/day.
- The nitrogen intake should range between 1.2 and 2.0 g amino acids/kg/day; on rare occasions 2.5 g amino acids/kg/day should be administered.
- The role of immunonutrition is not scientifically validated.
- There is some discrepancy about the calorie composition of the admixture, since some societies recommended a high glucose:lipid ratio regimen, while others preferred a more balanced regimen.

On the whole, few recommendations relied on good research-based evidence and the majority on studies of lower quality or on expert opinion.

References

1. Plank LD, Hill GL. Sequential metabolic changes following introduction of systemic inflammatory response in patients with severe sepsis or major blunt trauma. *World J Surg* 2000; 24: 630–8.
2. Shaw JHF, Wolfe RR. An integrated analysis of glucose, fat, and protein metabolism in severely traumatized patients. Studies in the basal state and the response to total parenteral nutrition. *Ann Surg* 1987; 209: 63–72.
3. Wolfe RR, Martini WZ. Changes in intermediary metabolism in severe surgical illness. *World J Surg* 2000; 24: 639–47.
4. Streat SJ, Beddoe AH, Hill GL. Aggressive nutritional support does not prevent protein loss despite fat gain in septic intensive care patients. *J Trauma* 1987; 27: 262–6.
5. Uehara M, Plank LD, Hill GL. Components of energy expenditure in patients with severe sepsis and major trauma: A basis for clinical care. *Crit Care Med* 1999; 27: 1295–302.
6. Ishibashi N, Plank LD, Sando K, Hill GL. Optimal protein requirements during the first 2 weeks after the onset of critical illness. *Crit Care Med* 1998; 26: 1529–35.
7. Bozzetti F, Braga M, Dionigi P. Linee guida per l'impiego della nutrizione parenterale ed enterale nei pazienti adulti ospedalizzati. *Riv Ital Nutr Parenter Enteral Suppl* 1995; 2: 39–42.
8. Bozzetti F, (for the SINPE). Perioperative artificial nutrition in elective adult surgery. *Clin Nutr* 1996; 15: 223–9.

9. Cerra FB, Rios Benitez M, Blackburn GL, Irwin RS, Jeejeebhoy K, Katza DP, Pingleton SK, Pomposelli J, Rombeau JL, Shronts E, Wolfe RR, Zaloga GP. Applied nutrition in ICU patients: A consensus statement of the American College of Chest Physicians. *Chest* 1997; 111: 769–78.

10. Conférence de Consensus Nutrition de l'agressé. *Nutr Clin Métab* 1998; 12 (suppl).

11. Jolliet P, Pichard C, Biolo G, Chiolèro R, Grimble G, Leverve X, Nitenberg G, Novak I, Planas M, Preiser JC, Roth E, Schols AM, Wernerman J, Working Group on Nutrition and Metabolism, ESICM. Enteral nutrition in intensive care patients: A practical approach. *Intens Care Med* 1998; 24: 848–59.

12. Jolliet P, Pichard C, Biolo G, Chiolèro R, Grimble G, Leverve X, Nitenberg G, Novak I, Planas M, Preiser JC, Roth E, Schols AM, Wernerman J. Enteral nutrition in intensive care patients: A practical approach. *Clin Nutr* 1999; 18: 47–56.

13. Klein S, Kinney J, Jeejeebhoy K, Alpers D, Hellerstein M, Murray M, Twomey P. Nutrition support in clinical practice: Review of published data and recommendations for future research directions. *JPEN J Parenter Enteral Nutr* 1997; 21: 133–56.

14. Sobotka L. *Basics in clinical nutrition*, 2nd ed. Prague: Galén, 2000.

15. American Gastroenterological Association Medical Position Statement. Parenteral nutrition. *Gastroenterology* 2001; 121: 966–9.

16. August D, Teitelbaum D, Albina J, Bothe AL, Guenter P, Heitkemper M, Ireton-Jones C, Mirtallo JM, Seidner D, Winkler M. Guidelines for the use of parenteral and enteral nutrition in adult and pediatric patients. *JPEN J Parenter Enteral Nutr* 2002; 26: 1.

17. Sandström R, Drott C, Hyltander A, Arfvidsson B, Schersten T, Wickstrom I, et al. The effect of postoperative intravenous feeding (TPN) on outcome following major surgery evaluated in a randomized study. *Ann Surg* 1993; 217: 185–95.

18. Revelly JP, Tappy L, Benper MM, Gersbach P, Cayeux C, Chioléro R. Early metabolic and splanchnic responses to enteral nutrition in postoperative cardiac surgery patients with circulatory compromise. *Intens Care Med* 2001; 27: 540–7.

19. Houdijk APJ, Rijnsburger ER, Jansen J, Wesdorp RI, Weiss JK, McCamish MA, et al. Randomised trial of glutamine-enriched enteral nutrition on infectious morbidity in patients with multiple trauma. *Lancet* 1998; 352: 772–6.

20. Griffiths RD, Jones C, Palmer TEA. Six-month outcome of critically ill patients given glutamine-supplemented parenteral nutrition. *Nutrition* 1997; 13: 295–302.

21. Beale RJ, Bryg DJ, Bihari DJ. Immunonutrition in the critically ill: A systematic review of clinical outcome. *Crit Care Med* 1999; 27: 2799–805.

22. Heys SD, Walker LG, Smith I, et al. Enteral nutritional supplementation with key nutrients in patients with critical illness and cancer. A meta-analysis of randomized controlled clinical trials. *Ann Surg* 1999; 229: 467–77.

23. Bower RH, Cerra FB, Bershadsky B, et al. Early enteral administration of a formula (Impact®) supplemented with arginine, nucleotides, and fish oil in intensive care unit patients: Results of a multicenter, prospective, randomized, clinical trial. *Crit Care Med* 1995; 23: 436–49.

24. Heyland DK, Novak F, Drover JW, et al. Should immunonutrition become routine in critically ill patients? A systematic review of the evidence. *JAMA* 2001; 286: 944–53.

25. Van Den Berghe G, Wouters P, Weekers F, Verwaest C, Bruyninckx F, Schetz M, Vlasserlaers D, Ferdinande P, Lauwers P, Bouillon R. Intensive insulin therapy in critically ill patients. *N Engl J Med* 2001; 345: 1359–67.

26. Tan Js, Anderson JL, Watanakunakorn C, et al. Neutrophil dysfunction in diabetes mellitus. *J Lab Clin Med* 1975; 85: 26–33.

27. Pomposelli JJ, Baxter JK III, Babineau TJ, Pomfret EA, Driscoll DF, Forse AR, Bistrian BR. Early postoperative glucose control predicts nosocomial infection rate in diabetic patients. *JPEN J Parenter Enteral Nutr* 1998; 22: 77–81.

28. Pocock SJ, Elbourne DR. Randomized trials or observational tribulations? *N Engl J Med* 2000; 342: 1907–9.

29. Rubenfeld GD, Angus DC, Pinsky MR, Curtis JR, Connors AF Jr, Bernard GR, and the Members of the Outcomes Research Workshop. Outcomes research in critical care: Results of the American Thoracic Society Critical Care Assembly Workshop on Outcomes Research. *Am J Respir Crit Care Med* 1999; 160: 358–67.

30. Wolfe BM, Mathiesen KA. Clinical practice guidelines in nutrition support: Can they be based on randomized clinical trials? *JPEN J Parenter Enteral Nutr* 1997; 21: 1–6.

Dr. Zazzo: Before we start the discussions, for more information I want to repeat that Dr. Bozzetti has no responsibility except for the last two slides.

Dr. Bozzetti: I think there are some French doctors here who are also responsible for the statement of the French-Speaking Francophone Society.

Dr. Déchelotte: All of us have some responsibility in this situation because we either performed studies in the last years or participated in round tables or conferences. I think it is quite disappointing that over the last 5 years experts in many countries have spent so much time working almost in parallel and we are not even able to draw the same conclusions from the same literature. I think it is quite a pity that so much scientific energy has been misused. I suggest that we take this into account when we plan new consensus round tables, to try to work more together and to obtain some good evidence for everybody, because it should not be so different from one part of the Alps to the other.

Dr. Bozzetti: I think that some discrepancies are untrue but only depend on the fact that we are considering different kinds of patients. For instance if we look at the result of immunonutrition in surgical patients and in critically ill patients, the results are quite different. So perhaps the first thing is that it is better to define which patients we are considering.

Dr. Déchelotte: And the second point is more optimistic. The literature, the good literature, I mean well-performed, high-scale, prospective studies, has probably increased in the last 5–10 years. So we can expect that our next discussion of guidelines will be more roughly based on good literature.

Dr. Labadarios: On the point of the cost-ineffectiveness of all these efforts, it might be an idea that one recommendation of this workshop should be for the International Council of Nutritional Support Organizations, in which all the relevant societies are represented, to be given a mandate to issue unified guidelines which would be a little bit more helpful than the ones we have at present.

Dr. Berger: We all agree that nutrition is perhaps the field where the biggest beliefs have been added. We all agree that we should improve world science and our studies. But aren't you fed up with this evidence-based trend, absence of evidence is not evidence of absence, and maybe we should start rethinking a few things.

Dr. Bozzetti: I completely agree with you. I would like also to stress that one major limitation of the study, and this in complete agreement with what you said, is that you can study in the proper way, that means a randomized way, patients undergoing a short period of starvation, comparing different types of nutritional support, but when you consider a long period of artificial nutrition as a life-saving treatment, you can't have a control group and, I agree with you, this lack of evidence does not mean that there is no evidence.

Dr. Carlson: I don't think it is reasonable to expect massive international agreement between different groups, especially when there is an absence of very clear evidence-based studies and what you end up with is philosophy. It has often been said that you can expect to get agreement between clocks more frequently than between philosophers. The second point is that I am not at all despondent that there are differences in opinions between different expert groups and the lack of clear categorical evidence, because in fact if you look at most of other areas of medical practice and really ask where is the evidence to support this or that course of action, there often isn't very good categorical evidence from randomized control trials for many things, particularly surgical issues. Lastly, perhaps we are expecting too much of nutritional support if we are expecting to see big differences in outcome in critically ill patients when there are so many other variables. Most people I think don't die of nutrition-related complications these days, or at least easily identifiable nutrition-related complications. On a pragmatic level if you look at differences in outcome between different surgeons, they are several fold greater than any potential benefit that you might expect to see with different strategies for nutritional support. So I think that is the problem we face.

Dr. Allison: If we are allowing philosophical thoughts and I guess it is a bit late in the day for science, penicillin was introduced without any data to support its use. When Alexander Fleming applied to the Medical Research Council for a grant to develop his work, he was turned down on the grounds that it was unlikely to be of any practical use.

Dr. Herndon: I would like to respond to your personal reflection. Point number 3, I think it is very difficult to look at short-term outcomes and perhaps that is the reason for the lack of consensus as alluded to in the previous discussions. But I think as people interested in metabolic support we may have harped too much on short-term outcomes and not looked at long-term outcomes about patient populations, strength, longitudinal growth in children, and that type-1 evidence-based data can be obtained by looking at interventions that we perform in the intensive care units (ICUs) that may affect the long-term outcomes, particularly if we carry through with our therapies and follow our patients as we should. I think the area here is really our own, and not following patients to the outcome and defining the outcomes that we should. Perhaps we should ask the international or national societies to help design studies that look at outcomes that can be achieved.

Dr. Berger: Those guidelines, many of us have given much time to them, and I think they are better than nothing. We all lack education and training in all our countries for nutritional support. These are just meant to be as you said, and I fully agree with you, the minimal standard we are supposed to go for. So having them repeated, having them improved over time is perhaps a limited way to just try to overcome the lack of training and perhaps we can do it better through implementing training in all our countries on this topic. That will produce better studies, better things, and I go also in your direction, I fully agree with you on long-term outcomes.

Dr. Zazzo: In the same way I agree with your proposition. We don't know the gap between the literature and academic recommendations and practice in clinical units, and I think this has to be evaluated first of all. How can we give credibility to the concept of nutrition in postoperative patients or in the ICU and improve diffusion of this recommendation and expert reports? I think this is probably the future and the name of the session is 'from now to the future'. It is probably a challenge for the future, an educational challenge. I think this is a very important point.

Dr. Ribeiro: We try to make guidelines in Brazil, the Brazilian Society, and our worry is about guidelines. They all decide who makes good or bad medicine based on rules, and I think medicine is based in experience and evidence is just a little part of medicine. This is my first concern that the guidelines can decide who makes good or bad medicine. My second concern is that this is also the case in the Health Medicine Organization, to decide what you are going to do and what you are not going to do. I don't know if you have these worries in Europe or in United States, but it is some worry we have in Brazil right now with guidelines.

Dr. Endres: I would not be afraid of this I think because it is only our guidelines or recommendations, and all this is based on consensus conferences, and we all know that the reason for organizing consensus conferences is the lack of data.

Dr. Nitenberg: Perhaps we have to stay modest about the impact of guidelines. I remind you about an exploration of that field recently. There was recently an article, I think in the *American Journal of Medicine*, on why doctors are so reluctant to apply guidelines. I remember well that there was a consensus conference on the utilization of albumin in ICUs a few years ago. There was an inquiry in ICUs and the first question was: Do you know that there was a consensus conference on the utilization of albumin? About 50% of the doctors said yes. Do you know the conclusions of this conference? 20% of the doctors said yes. Do you apply the conclusions? Less than 4% of the doctors said yes. So I think we spend an incredible time making consensus conferences and guidelines, but in fact we have to think about other measures to implement what we call guidelines and good recommendations for the utilization of nutritional support or any type of support in our patients.

Dr. Heyland: Just to follow up on some of the previous comments about the value of evidence-based medicine and practice guidelines. I want to make people aware that a study has been completed in Canada in which evidence-based guidelines were developed, in a randomized design, randomized hospitals, for different implementation strategies. So rather than passively disseminating a piece of paper we employed academic detailing, feedback as strategies to actively disseminate the guidelines. Then we demonstrated significant differences in the practice of nutritional support that was associated with a reduction in hospital mortality with the implementation of those guidelines. So I think there is a potential for guidelines to have an impact in optimizing the best practice with nutritional support. I think there is tremendous potential for the misapplication of nutritional support. We have the potential to do harm with our nutritional support and so there is a need to try and raise the level of practice, optimize care and you can influence patient outcomes. So I see the way for it is to generate more evidence that contributes to the scientific body of what best practice is, and then look further at aggressive strategies to implement those guidelines across the various societies.

Concluding Remarks

This morning we decided that I would make some summary statements and let Dr. Cynober talk about the manuscripts. I was trying to figure out how to approach this. I thought I should first give you a background of where I come from. About 18 years ago when I was a surgery resident, I made the observation that feeding patients into the gut improves their outcome. I was in an environment that was very heavily weighted toward research and I was promoted to work on that. In the mid 1980s, like most surgeons, I became very interested in nutritional support, and we actually ran two nutritional support teams in two hospitals. I became quite interested in total parenteral nutrition (TPN), and then somewhere around the 1990s I became more interested in just what the role of the gut was in MOF. When interest in nutrition slowly waned, I shifted my research in that direction. So I don't really consider myself to be at the cutting edge of nutritional support. When I was approached by Nestlé to co-chair a symposium on nutrition in the intensive care unit (ICU), I thought it would be a wonderful opportunity to be able to invite the leaders of the nutrition to come and lecture me and test my knowledge against what should be the gold standard. So I thought a very quick review of what I have got from the conference would be a nice summary.

The first session was the metabolic response to stress. The physiologic consequence of the stress response is fairly well characterized. It is hard to relate to individual patients. What trajectory a patient is going to go on isn't very clear. I thought the concept of nutritional stress was valid. I am not quite sure how to characterize it but that is probably something I haven't thought of. Genomics and proteonomics are going to enable us to better characterize this physiologic response, and I think it is going to give us the ability to pharmacologically manipulate that response to improve outcome, and in fact in burn patients it appears to work. How that relates to my patients, I am not sure. I think for somebody who is not septic, who is persistently hypermetabolic that perhaps anabolic agents would work, and this whole concept of intensive insulin therapy needs to be better implemented. While we think it is glucose control perhaps it really has some metabolic response to protein metabolism that we just don't understand.

The second session was on specific nutrients that might be used in critically ill patients. Clearly critically ill patients require high proteins, but the optimal amino acid composition of these solutions is not known. I already gave Dr. Cynober a little bit of hard time about this. It seems to be something we were quite interested in the past. What I came away with was perhaps glutamine, possibly alanine, could have some favorable impact. It appears that most of you are all fairly nervous about arginine, a lot more nervous than I am. Clearly similar to the amino acids, lipids were really designed to prevent essential fatty acid deficiencies and not to be used in high doses in septic patients. There appears to be a lot of concern about the use of lipids in high doses in septic patients and I concur with that. While we seem to know a lot about the n-3 fatty acid story, the real proof that it helps patients is lacking. Several people talked about the Gadek study, and while I reviewed that study I can't believe that anybody would give the control diet to septic patients. It is probably the worst thing to give. Vitamins, antioxidants, what a great idea, it certainly fits with my understanding of acute inflammation. As I told Dr. Berger I take a handful antioxidants every morning, I have yet to prescribe them to my patients. I am anxiously awaiting the results of Dr. Berger's trials. Most ICU practitioners do not even think about trace elements. In the era of when we were interested in TPN, people talked about it but I think we all need to go home and review these data and make sure we are adequately addressing this issue in our patients. About the route and goal of administration, I really appreciated the observation that we should not be in there, pushing really hard at the beginning. I certainly thought that positive nitrogen and positive caloric balance really should not be an early goal, but it should be a goal sometime later. In regards to the enteral versus parenteral nutrition debate some mechanisms to explain this have now emerged. The gut is a very important immunological organ and we need to promote its function. Now if we accept this to be true, which it appears everybody does, then the major impediment is just how do we achieve this. There is a great variety of gut dysfunctions that occur in ICU patients which are not very well characterized, and the monitoring tools are very crude. With dedicated effort you can achieve surprisingly high tolerance. There appears to be a lot of variability in opinions on how aggressive we should be in getting jejunal access. I think that we should get away from enteral nutrition and talk about enteral therapy. Get in there early and doing something to the gut to make it work, and then think about providing adequate nutrition.

Now the next session was about specific nutritional diseases, and I certainly don't know too much about neonates but I did find the correlation with adults to be surprisingly similar. The concept of minimal enteral therapy in the sphere of necrotizing enterocolitis, the high protein needs that must be acutely replaced. This is consistent with elderly patients coming to the ICU with no muscle or fat stores. They are not going to do well if we don't get in there. Similar to the adult population, the first studies on the potential use of glutamine were very favorable. The concept of a mandatory enteral circuit shows that the gut is an important antigen processor. Similar to adults, the role of lipids has not been very well studied. In regards to obesity, this major health care issue which clearly adversely affects the impact of long-term outcome, but the impact on ICU outcome is not as clear. A hypocaloric, high nitrogen strategy is a valid concept, and this is an area where a lot of prospective studies could be done. In pancreatitis, enteral nutrition challenges the traditional wisdom. The small studies are very impressive, at least to me, but this clearly is not the standard of care across the United States. I think the use of clinical markers to identify severe pancreatitis will be the way to identify these patients, I am still not so clear about the role of CT scan. Jejunal feeding is optimal, and this was a major obstacle to people during the discussion, but as long as there is no gastroenterologist to place the tube, the stomach will still be fed. With multiple organ failure and sepsis, we are talking about a very heterogeneous group of patients and therefore it is difficult for studies to show any difference in outcome. There were the comments that these people have a very bad outcome and the things that are probably going to save them are resuscitation, optimal antibiotics and a draining pus, and to think that enteral nutrition or parenteral nutrition is going to really change their outcome is probably a bit naïve. I agree with the idea that, once the patients survive this and we are trying to get them back into society, they need to have muscle mass and this should be an important part of their rehabilitation. We certainly don't want to hurt these patients by aggressively pushing enteral nutrition on them. I think enteral nutrition is feasible but again it should be taken carefully. The role of lipids is again an area of confusion. Now for the immune-enhancing diets, we have had a huge amount of discussion about this. I don't want to get into it other than to say that if you just look at the way the studies were done you can't expect that going into a heterogeneous ICU and enrolling a lot of patients that you are going to see a difference in outcome. The only way this is going to work is that homogeneous groups of patients are studied. They have to be patients for whom risk can be quantitated, trauma and burns, and postoperative major surgical patients. How this is to be translated into other patient populations, I don't know. One should be very cautious about saying that because it works on a trauma patient it should be used in a pneumonia patient. Until those studies are done I would not advise it. The other thing that becomes clear in those studies is that we are using the gastric route because it is clinically practical, but from a prospective study it is not very good because you don't know what you are giving the patients. So if you really want to do the study, put the tube in the right place. I think we can all get over the fact that there is one product that has been widely tested and pushed by a pharmaceutical company. There is one product that works but I would not get all excited about how we want to use that product in all the patients that we might encounter.

I think this has been a great meeting, I hope that it could be repeated in 5 years; it would be nice to see if we have made any advances. Thank you for your attention and participation.

Frederick A. Moore

I have some additional comments. I feel really that we had a very good combination of good science, practice, recommendations, and I am convinced that it is important to have such multidisciplinary meetings to try to have a continuum from high-tech molecular biology to the care of the patients at the bedside. I personally believe that in a few years physicians will ask for a genetic map, and this will work very quickly with an automatic R-PCR machine. From the results and the apparent risk to the patients the physician will be able to select or not select specific diets, and this will probably be very helpful in the discussion of overexpression of nitric oxide and arginine utilization, for example. Perhaps at this moment we will realize that the simple C-reactive protein measurement provides exactly the same information, and we will have to discuss the cost-effectiveness of different approaches. I really enjoyed all the talk and the discussions, the concept of the 40 min of discussion is excellent. I am also especially grateful to have had the pleasure of meeting 'Dr. Ross internal file' because we had the privilege to get some data and I understand that this paper will now be published. It is very important to have direct access to this up to now phantasmagoric study because, from these results, we can achieve quite different conclusions the about arginine story.

Thank you very much, I feel that we have had 3 exceptional days.

Luc Cynober

Subject Index